**Fetal Physiological Measurements**

# Fetal Physiological Measurements

Proceedings of the Second International
Conference on Fetal and Neonatal
Physiological Measurements

**Edited by**

**Peter Rolfe,** BSc, MA, PhD, CEng, MIEE
Head of Bio-Engineering Unit, Department
of Paediatrics, University of Oxford, John
Radcliffe Hospital, Oxford, UK

**Butterworths**
London Boston Durban Singapore Sydney Toronto Wellington

First published, 1986



**British Library Cataloguing in Publication Data**

International Conference on Fetal and Neonatal
Physiological Measurements (*1984 : Oxford*)
Fetal and neonatal physiological measurements.
1. Fetus—Physiology—Measurement
2. Infants (Newborn)—Physiology—Measurement
I. Title II. Rolfe, Peter
612'.647 RG610
ISBN 0-407-00378-9
ISBN 0-407-00450-5 v.1
ISBN 0-407-00451-3 v.2

**Library of Congress Cataloging-in-Publication Data**

International Conference on Fetal and Neonatal
Physiological Measurements (2nd)
Fetal physiological measurements.

Includes bibliographies and index.
1. Fetal heart rate monitoring—Congresses.
2. Fetus—Physiology—Congresses. 3. Blood gases—
Analysis—Congresses. I. Rolfe, Peter. II. Title.
[DNLM: 1. Fetal Monitoring—congresses. 2. Fetus—
physiology—congresses. W3 IN1748 2nd / WQ 209
I594f]
RG628.3.H42I58 1986 618.92'01 86-20753
ISBN 0-407-00450-5

Produced by computer-controlled phototypesetting by Unwin Brothers Ltd., The Gresham Press, Old Woking, Surrey.
A member of the Martins Printing Group.



Printed and bound in England by Robert Hartnoll Ltd, Bodmin, Cornwall

# Contents

Part 1

# Fetal General

Chapter 1

# A new look at fetal phonocardiography using a transducer of improved sensitivity and bandwidth

**D G Talbert, D P Southall**

## Introduction

Several factors cause fetal heart sounds to differ from those after birth, the most important being firstly, that the two ventricles are of similar size near term and, secondly, they pump between similar pressures. Whereas postnatal heart sounds are dominated by left side events, both sides of the heart can contribute equally to the sounds detected in the fetus. As the fetal lungs are fluid filled, sound travels in all directions through the fetal body into amniotic fluid. There is no acoustic screening by an air-filled lung, but as sounds are detected about ten heart diameters away, the transducer cannot be placed over a particular area to emphasize a particular heart sound. Part of the fetal blood volume lies outside the body in the placenta, and blood may flow into or out of the fetus in response to changes of pressure in the fetus relative to that in the uterine cavity. Uterine contractions thus have the capacity to produce changes in the heart sounds. Similarly, fetal breathing movements alter blood flow and apart from their known effect on beat-to-beat fetal heart rate, may alter the characteristics of the individual component sounds.

Goodlin (1), reviewing the history of fetal monitoring, notes that in 1833 late deceleration patterns were considered an indication of fetal distress, in the 1870s bradycardia was known to be associated with head compression, and De Lee was observing fetal breathing in 1913. The fetal systolic murmur was reported by Schroeder in 1878, that due to compression of the cord in 1833, and placental flow sounds were described by Braxton-Hicks, again in the late nineteenth century. All these discoveries were made by listening to the fetal heart sounds.

The wealth of information potentially available from fetal heart sounds has not been exploited so far, because of the weak, narrowly filtered signal that has been produced by machines designed primarily for heart rate determination. When the total acoustic phono signal (TAPHO - a term suggested to differentiate the process from narrow band phonocardiography) can be obtained, detailed changes of valve closure times become visible in a similar manner to that postnatally. The TAPHO signal thus provides a simple, non-invasive tool to study not only changes in heart rate and systolic timing but changes in fetal blood flow, distribution, or pressure, that are reflected in the forcefulness or timing of valve closures, heart recoil, or blood turbulence.

## TAPHO signal interpretation

The signal obtained is a series of shock excited pressure wave trains which are generated when the various valves snap shut. It was once thought that the sounds were caused by the impacting of the valves themselves, but it has since been realized (2) that they originate from vibrations set up in the heart by the pull on the valve attachments as the valves close. Both the frequency (period) and the variation of magnitude of these waves carry information.

Consider first a single valve. Just before it closes, blood is flowing through it with a velocity which depends on the pressure difference across it. When it snaps shut, it attempts to arrest this flow abruptly by generating a reverse pressure on the column of blood approaching it. It would require an infinite pressure to do this instantaneously, so the valve and its attachments are stretched 'downstream' until the flow is arrested. At this time, the valve is overstreteched and it returns to its natural position carrying some of the blood with it. The momentum of this blood may then cause a second overshoot, and a decaying oscillation occurs. The associated pressure waves appear at the mother's skin surface. In any one case and for a fixed relative position of fetus and transducer the magnitude of the signal varies with the mass of blood being stopped and its velocity at that time.

The period of the oscillations varies with the elasticity of the valve and its supports and with the mass of blood coupled to it. The mitral and tricuspid valves are larger and more elastic than the aortic and pulmonary valves and usually give pressure waves of longer period than the latter.

Now consider the signal from a pair of valves, the second closing while the first is still 'ringing', such as mitral/tricuspid, aortic/pulmonary pairs. The first valve of the pair to close will produce the same signal as before, but when the second valve closes, the TAPHO signals represents the sum of the two pressure waves. Depending on the delay between closures, the waves may add, substract or combine in some indeterminate manner. In general, there will be a discontinuity in the resultant tracing at the moment of second valve closures. The delay between closures of each pair of valves has fixed components depending on structure and changing components which, in turn, are dependent on atrial and outlet pressures. If, for simplicity, we assume that the mitral and tricuspid valves close passively, they will close when intraventricular pressure just exceeds atrial pressure. A rise in atrial pressure will delay closure of the corresponding valve until the new higher pressure has been achieved. Thus, changes in relative atrial pressures will appear in the TAPHO signal as changes in delay of the discontinuity from the start of the mitral/tricuspid complex and broadening or narrowing of the complex. A similar effect occurs on the outlet side, though here an increase in aortic pressure causes the aortic valve to closer earlier. The ventricles contract iso-volumically until their pressure exceeds the aortic pulmonary pressures. The sudden onset of flow causes the heart to recoil in a similar manner to the fireman holding a hose when the water starts to come through. This signal, together with that caused by the sudden enlargement of the aortic and pulmonary vessels, form a characteristic low frequency complex occurring soon after the mitral/tricuspid complex (marked Ej, see Figure 2).

## Construction of a TAPHO transducer

The philosopy of design has been previously described (3). The transducer is relatively simple to construct, details are given below and in Figure 1.

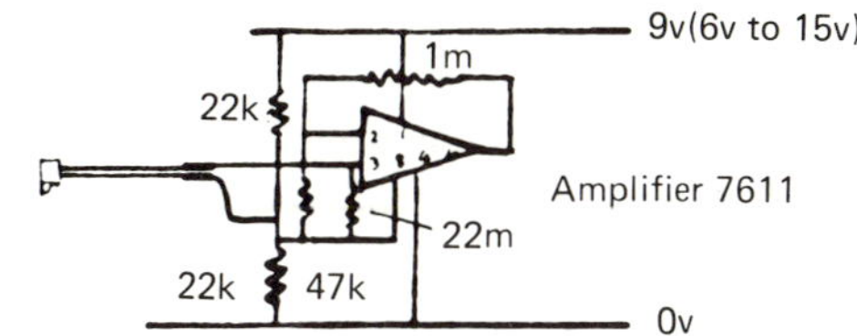


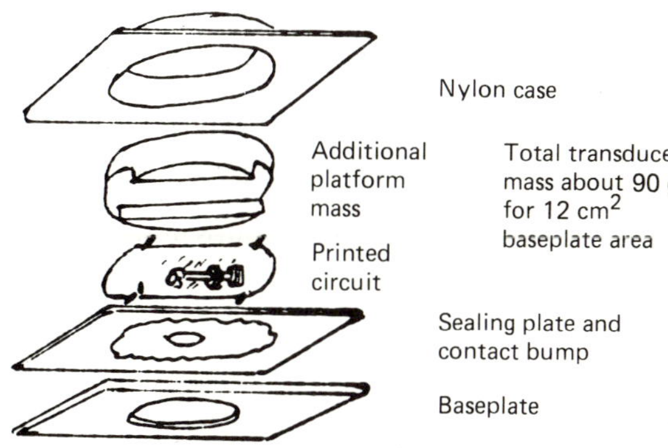


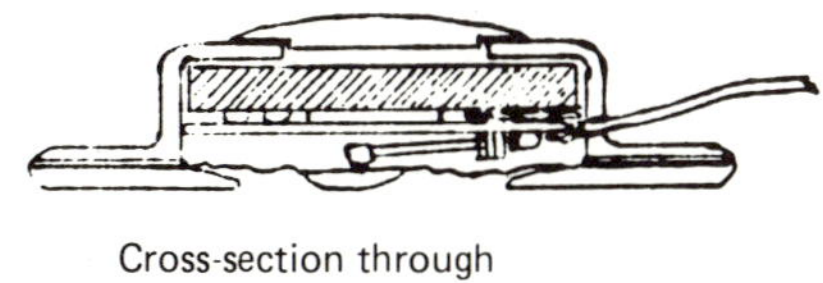


*Figure 1.* Construction of a TAPHO transducer

Two piezo-electric elements can be obtained from a replacement stereo record player pick-up head having a sensitivity greater than 100 mV. We have used BSR SX6H and ACOS 104 types successfully. Remove the stylus and carefully drill through the rivets or break open the plastic welds holding the upper and lower halves of the shell together and separate them. Two elements will be found inside usually attached at the stylus end by a soft plastic link and at the plug end by a common electrical connection. Cut through the plastic symmetrically to preserve a projection on both elements. Clip off the plug terminals preserving as much connecting foil as possible. Position the silicone rubber supports near the fixed end of the element. The optimum position of these components will vary with element parameters, contact bump area, platform mass etc, and must be found later by experiment. Bend the contact foils and solder directly to the underside of the amplifier printed circuit to minimize the lead length which will be exposed to electrical interference; the lower side and all unused printed circuit should be taken to the bias point, to screen the upper, active side and minimize DC leakage current.

The electrical signal obtained is at a high impedance, typically less than 1000 pf, and must be buffered and amplified. The element is mounted directly on the printed circuit by gluing the silicone rubber supports with Bostik No 1, which can readily be dissolved away should a different active length be desired.

The element detects movements of the mother's skin under the contact bump relative to the reference platform formed by the printed circuit and the lead weight to which it is attached. Ideally, this platform should not be significantly displaced by the forces generated by the sounds in the mother's skin under the base plate supporting the device. We have found the ratio of 1 $cm^2$ of base plate area for each gram weight satisfactory as a compromise between low frequency sensitivity and convenience of attachment. The printed circuit is attached to it by four stiff wires soldered between them.

The other major components are the nylon case, a sealing plate, and a base plate. The sealing plate has a hole, 2 cm diameter, cut in it which is covered by thin rubber from a toy balloon to form a limp sealing membrane below the active end of the sensing element. The base plate also has a 2 cm hole to form an annulus, mechanically isolating the contact bump from the surrounding skin under the base plate, which is acoustically immobilized by the platform mass.

An adult heart sound from the front of the chest should give a signal strength more than 100 mV peak-to-peak from the amplifier. The circuit will work satisfactorily from 5 V to 15 V taking less than 0.5 mA.

We have found that belts are an unsatisfactory means of attachment as they introduce noise if the patient moves. The transducer is quite light and we have found it better to stick it on. The optimum position is found and a barrier layer of Micropore tape is laid down on the skin, leaving a gap where the contact bump is to be. The transducer is then stuck to this with double sided sticky pads.

## Some observations of the fetus using TAPHO signals

Measuring the time between successive beats of the TAPHO signal produces accurate measurements of fetal heart rate and of beat-to-beat variability. Unlike fetal ECG or Doppler ultrasound, it is also possible to record extra information during each beat; for example valve timings, ejection timings, etc. As mentioned above, the narrow band filtering used by previous fetal phonocardiographic systems has meant that, although the user may have been able to hear subtle changes in heart sounds, a written printout was always disappointing. Provided the TAPHO transducer can be placed within about 7 cm of the fetal heart, many phenomena can now clearly be seen in the last trimester of pregnancy. Since there is no interference between TAPHO and ultrasonic systems, the relationship of the sounds to fetal breathing and fetal heart valve closures can be identified.

For example, during fetal breathing, a systolic murmur often occurs (Figure 2a, systolic interval $S_2$ ). This information is lost after filtering (Figure 2b). The force of the mitral/tricuspid valve closures has also been found to vary depending on the phase of the breathing cycle (Figures 3a and 3b on a longer time scale). Variations in the return of blood to the heart during fetal breathing are to be expected and probably result from large pressure differentials generated by the diaphragm. The resultant changes in atrial filling pressure and hence end-diastolic ventricular volume might be expected to explain some of the changes seen in the TAPHO signal.

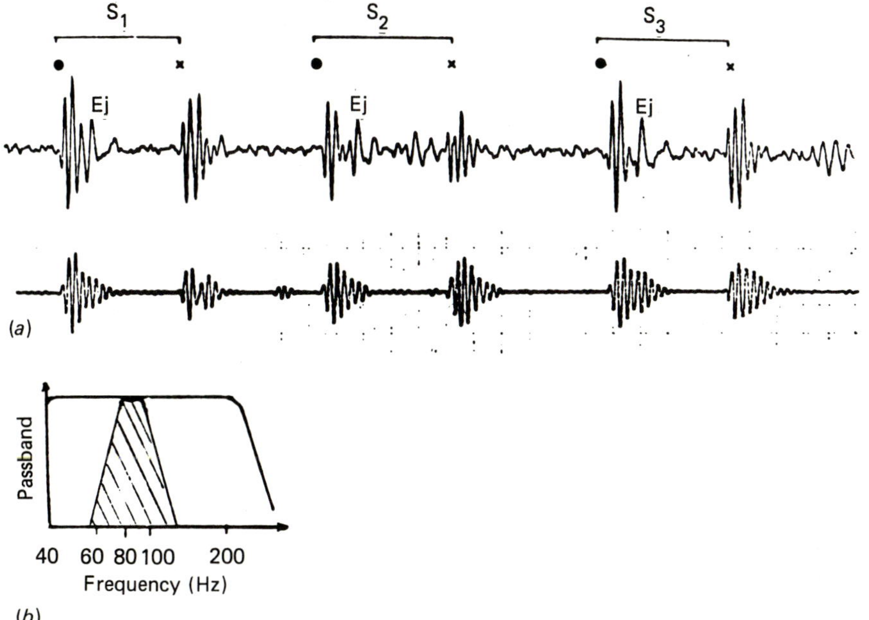


*Figure 2.* Significance of the components in the TAPHO signals. (a) The vibrations set up by three successive fetal heart beats. The start of each systole (S) occurs just before the start of the mitral/tricuspid closure complex. The start of flow into the aortic or pulmonary artery is marked by the heart recoil complex. The end of systole occurs just before the aortic/pulmonary valve closure complex. (b) This is the same signal conventionally filtered as shown shaded in the spectral plot. • = Mitral/tricuspid closure complex; x = aortic/pulmonary closure complex; Ej = ejection recoil complex; S = systolic period (approx)

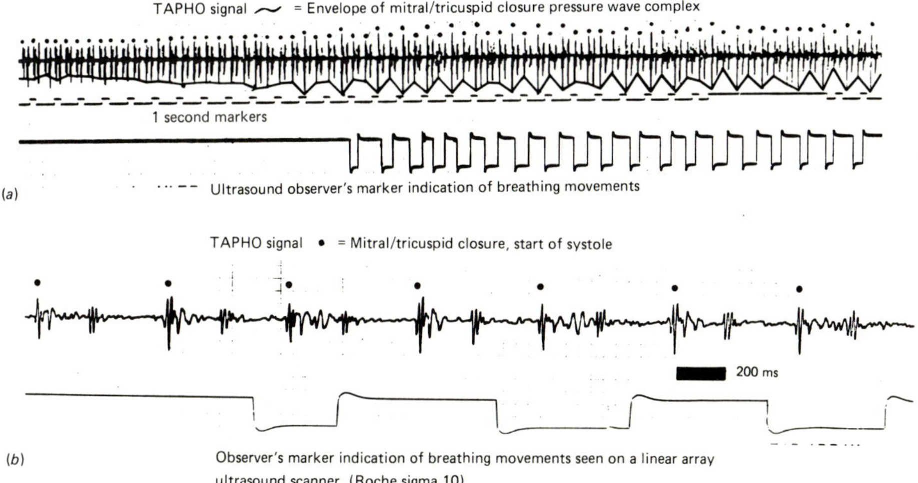


*Figure 3.* The effect of fetal breathing movements on TAPHO signal. (a) Variations of mitral/tricuspid closure complex amplitude. (b) Detail of (a) at higher speed to show systolic murmer during one phase of the breathing cycle

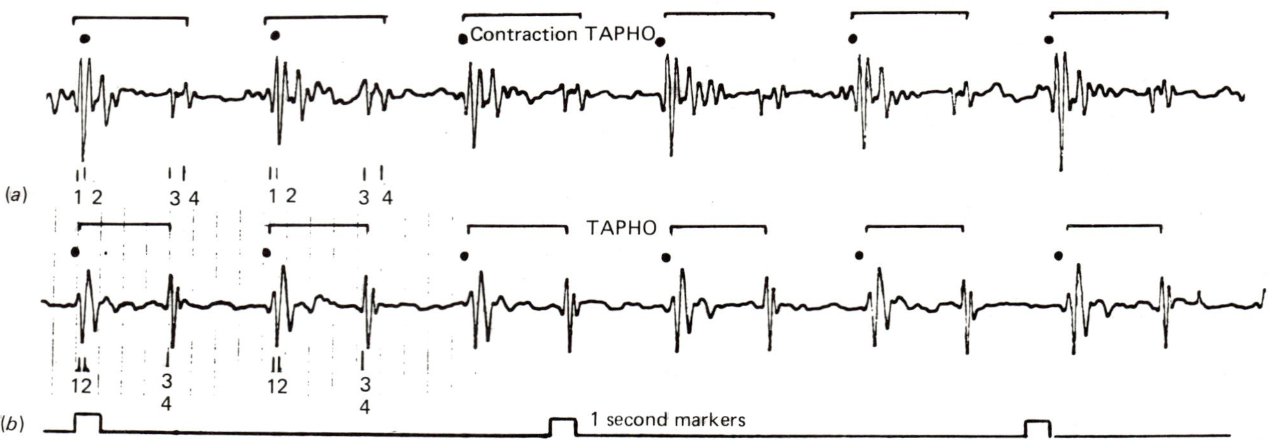


*Figure 4*. Split first and second heart sounds during Braxton-Hicks contractions (a) compared to signals between contractions (b). • = Mitral/tricuspid complex; — = systole

Changes in the relative timing of the component parts of the heart sounds are also of value. It will be remembered that an increase in atrial pressures will delay closure of the corresponding inlet valves. On the other hand, increases in aortic or pulmonary pressures will cause the corresponding outlet valves to close earlier. Thus, if pressures in one side of the heart diverge from those in the other, differences in valve closure times may be sufficient to produce splitting of the heart sounds. An example is shown in Figure 4 where the signal obtained during a Braxton-Hicks contraction (a) is compared with that occurring between contractions (b). Between contractions (b), valve pair closures are almost synchronous. During a contraction (a), the aortic and pulmonary complexes, and to a lesser extent the mitral and tricuspid complexes, have separated, indicating pressure differentials between the right and left sides of the heart. Such differences might be due to either a constriction of the ductus arteriosus or to a disturbance of the ratio of flows between the two sides of the heart. At present it is not known which valves are delayed or which are early, or both, but such changes indicate a possible means of non-invasively monitoring cardiovascular changes in the fetus.

## Conclusion

It would seem that much of the knowledge from the phonocardiographic techniques which are common place in postnatal studies could now be applied to the fetus, once differences due to similar right- and left-sided signal strengths have been elucidated. This ancient technique can now reveal things previously heard but not seen.

## References

1. Goodlin R C. History of fetal monitoring. *American Journal of Obtetrics and Gynecology,* 133, 323-352 (1979).
2. Luisada A A and Portaluppi F. *The Heart Sounds.* New York, Praeger Scientific (1982).
3. Talbert D G, Dewhurst J and Southall D P. New transducer for detecting fetal heart sounds: use of compliance matching for maximum sound transfer. *Lancet,* 1, 425-427 (1984).

Chapter 2

# The spectrum of the fetal phonocardiogram as an indicator of fetal maturity

**Joachim H Nagel**

## Introduction

Relatively few techniques offer a non-invasive means of investigating the fetus. Thus the expansion of diagnostic opportunities is a great challenge for biomedical engineering. Instead of searching for new, complicated measuring techniques, we have been trying to meet this challenge by developing suitable procedures aimed at improving the analysis of the data provided by present routine examinations. One highly promising result of our work has been the discovery that the power spectrum of the fetal phonocardiogram (PCG) can be used as a reliable indicator of fetal maturity.

## Physical basis of the PCG

In phonocardiography the mechanical energy of the heart sounds is picked up by a microphone. At present the only reason for analysing the PCG is to evaluate the heart rate and determine various electromechanical time intervals. In this way the function of the fetal cardiovascular system may be monitored. If we consider the generation of the heart sounds from a more physical standpoint, it seems obvious that more information about the heart must be contained in the PCG than merely the time course of the contractions. Because the heart is a rather complex oscillation system, the PCG is a compound signal whose spectral power distribution is determined by numerous factors such as the various valves, the heart muscle and the intracardiac blood volume. Even without a knowledge of all the interactions involved, we may suppose that variations in any one of these parameters will lead to a shift of the PCG spectrum.

In order to obtain an idea as to the effects that may result, we may consider the vibration of the heart valves. In a very simple model the valves may be compared to a stressed membrane, the two-dimensional equivalent of a vibrating string. The resonance frequencies of a square membrane are given by the equation:

$$\nu_{h,k} = \frac{1}{2l} \sqrt{(1+h)^2 + (1+k)^2} \cdot \sqrt{\frac{S}{\rho}} \qquad \mathbf{1}$$

where l = edge length, $\rho$ = density, S = tension h,k= series of the integer numbers 0,1,2,3 . . .

The fundamental frequency is:

$$\nu_{\infty} = \frac{\sqrt{2}}{2l} \cdot \sqrt{\frac{S}{\rho}} \qquad 2$$

Figure 1 shows the fundamental frequency in relation to the edge length for different tensions. Variations in the frequency caused by changing parameters can be

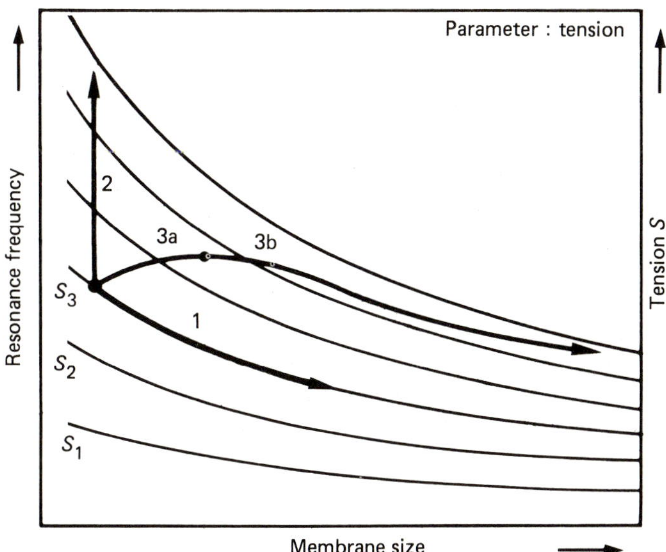


*Figure 1.* Fundamental frequency of a stressed membrane dependent on size and tension

investigated. For a given tension, an increase in the dimensions of the membrane results in a decrease in frequency (trace 1). Increasing tension at a constant membrane size augments the resonance frequency (trace 2). Changes in both parameters complicate the course of the frequency curve. When the influence of increasing tension predominates, the frequency increases (3a), whereas predominance of an increase in the membrane dimensions results in a decrease in the vibration frequency (3b). In each individual case there is an unequivocal relationship between frequency, tension and membrane size.

## Spectral changes of the PCG with fetal maturity

Applying these findings to the fetal heart valves, and assuming that during pregnancy both heart valves are growing and the contractile strength of the cardiac muscle is increasing (i.e. membrane tension is being augmented), we would expect to find spectral changes in the PCG as a function of the stage of fetal maturity. It is, of course, not realistic to describe the fetal heart in such a simple way - there are too

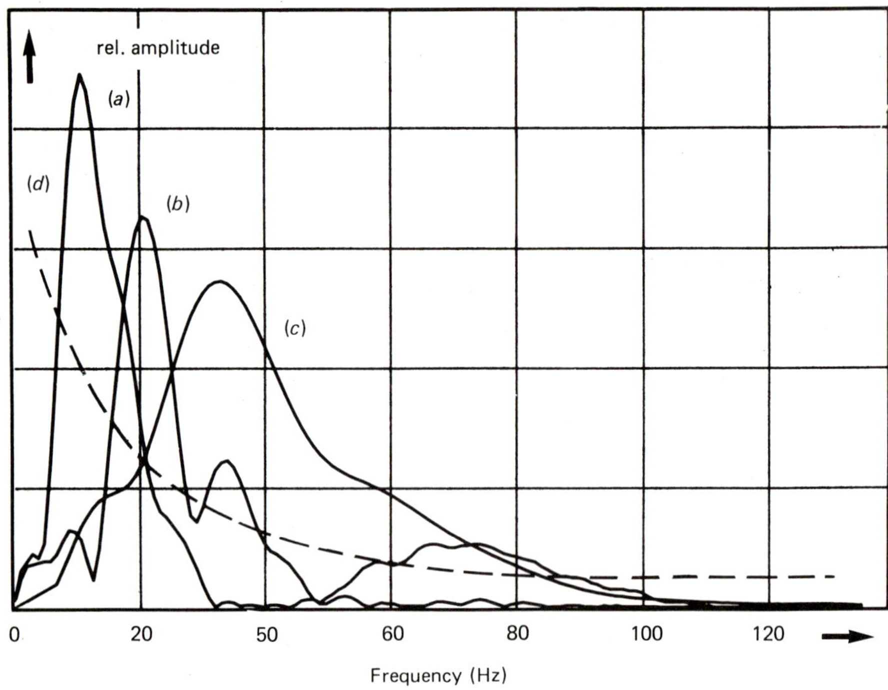


*Figure 2.* Frequency spectrum of the abdominal PCG. (*a*) maternal signal; (*b*) first heart sound of the fetus; (*c*) second heart sound of the fetus; (*d*) background noise

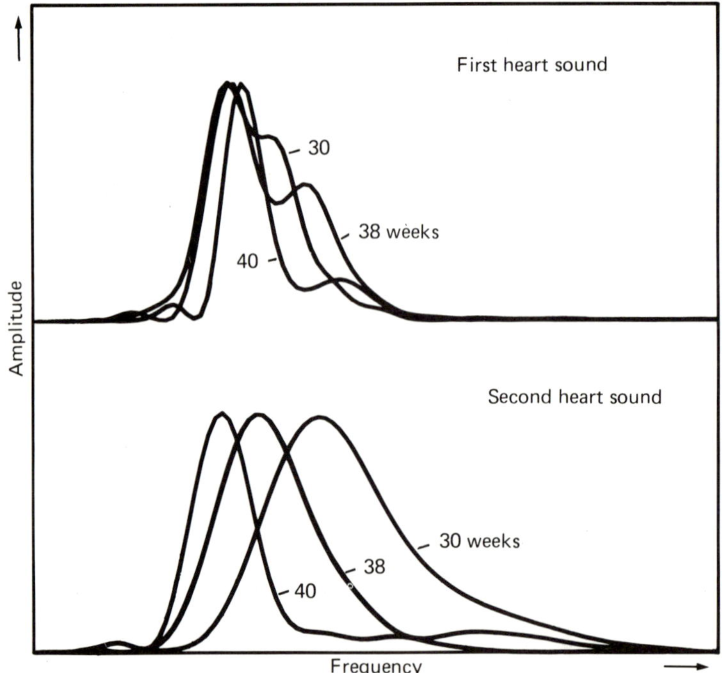


*Figure 3.* PCG spectra from different gestational ages

many differences between this simplified model and the complex structure and function of the heart. Nevertheless, the tendency for spectrum changes to occur as a function of fetal growth should be apparent. In order to verify this assumption and to investigate the course of the PCG spectrum during pregnancy, extensive experimental studies have been necessary. Our initial findings showed that the conventional phonotransducers did not have suitable transmission characteristics. In order to pick up the PCG over its full bandwidth we first had to develop an improved microphone.

Spectral analysis was effected by discrete Fourier transformation of the abdominal signals which were recorded unfiltered. Prior to the transformation the PCG was broken down to obtain the separate spectra of the maternal background sounds, the first and second fetal heart sounds, and noise. Figure 2 shows a typical example of such a power spectrum. From the membrane model a clear shift of the fetal spectra would be expected at different stages of maturity. Differences can indeed be seen (Figure 3). Unfortunately, however, the location of the maxima does not always reveal an unequivocal systematic shift.

A reconsideration of the model makes clear the reason for this discrepancy. The previous assumption is valid only for one characteristic frequency of one single valve, whereas the PCG results from the superimposition of many components of the heart's complex oscillation system, each with a different vibration frequency and amplitude. The maximum power density is determined by the distribution of the characteristic frequencies and need not necessarily express the changes in the individual vibration modes. But, in every case, an increasing frequency of the individual oscillators shifts the mean value of the PCG spectrum towards higher frequencies. Thus, both physical

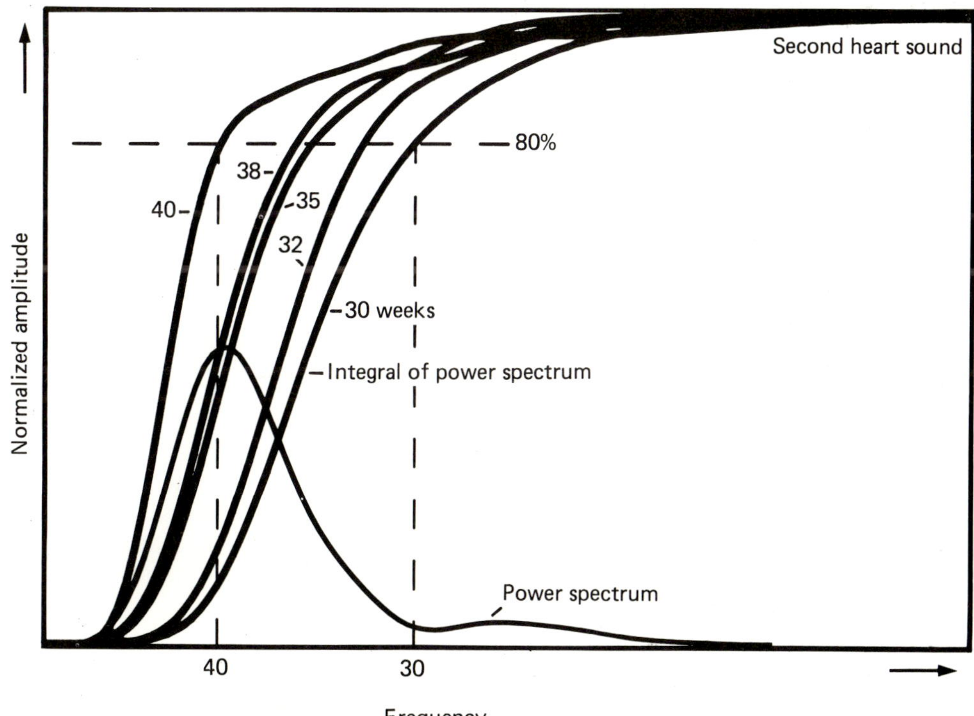


*Figure 4.* Normalized integrals of PCG spectra from different gestational ages

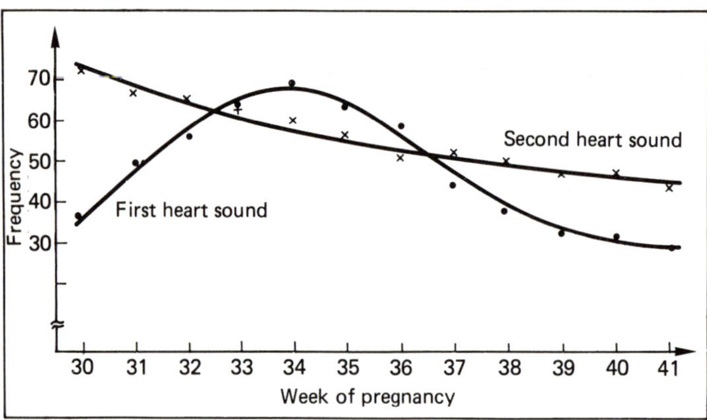


*Figure 5.* 80% power marks of the fetal PCG

considerations and experimental analysis show that spectral shifts can be detected best from the power spectrum integral. As a measure of spectral distribution we use that frequency, up to which 80% of the total signal power is contained. Figure 4 shows the integrated power spectra of different PCGs. The systematic shift of the 80% mark as a function of the gestational age is apparent. The mean values for the first and the second heart sound are shown in Figure 5. There is an unequivocal relationship between the spectrum of the PCG and the week of gestation. Of course, to obtain this picture, which may serve as a calibration curve, we considered only the spectra of fetuses that were known to be developing normally. The first heart sound reveals a steady shift towards higher frequencies up to about week 34 of gestation. Thereafter the shift reverses its direction. The spectrum of the second heart sound steadily shifts to lower frequencies. The reason for the decrease in the frequencies is known to be the growth of the heart, while the ascending slope of the spectrum of the first heart sound is, according to our model, caused by a predominance of the increase in aortic valve tension that results from the increasing contractile strength of the heart muscle.

## Conclusions

On the basis of these experimental results we believe that analysis of the spectrum - a passive measuring technique - may be a real alternative to such well-known active measurements as ultrasonic imaging in the determination of fetal maturity. Besides the information on physical dimensions, it also contains data on the function and the strength of the heart muscle. We must, of course, also consider possible disturbing influences such as changing cardiovascular conditions (e.g. the heart rate). So far we have found no such effects. It should be mentioned that the PCGs have always been picked up at the basal heart rate with no labour activity, and not during acclerations nor decelerations. At the present time we are investigating the reliability of this method, and its applicability to routine examinations.

Chapter 3

# A fibreoptic pressure transducer for intrauterine monitoring

**Leif Svenningsen, Øystein Jensen, M S Dodgson**

## Introduction

Monitoring of the fetal heart rate and of uterine contractions is essential in the active management of labour. Each uterine contraction represents a stress for the fetus, resulting in changes in the fetal heart rate (2, 10). The importance of the relationship between the fetal heart rate patterns and uterine activity is well established (1, 7). External detection of uterine activity using tocodynamometers gives a good indication of the duration and frequency of the contractions (2, 3), but measurement of the amniotic fluid pressure is essential if the intensity of the contractions is to be estimated. This is especially important when oxytocin is used to stimulate or augment contractions, and when maternal sensation has been reduced by epidural analgesia.

Until now, intrauterine pressure measurements have been made using either a fluid-filled open-ended catheter coupled to an external pressure transducer, or a microelectronic intra-amniotic catheter-tip pressure transducer (3, 9-11, 13, 14). The extraovular balloon techniques developed by Csapo (3) have been less well accepted. Solid state (microelectronic) catheter-tip pressure transducers are fragile, expensive and suffer from lack of stability in physiological fluids (6, 9, 11, 13). A new generation of commercially available miniature catheter-tip pressure transducers (4, 5, 6) using previously developed fibreoptic techniques (8, 12) has recently become available. We present a new application of the miniature fibreoptic catheter-tip pressure transducer in the measurement of intrauterine pressures. We have compared the fibreoptic catheter-tip pressure transducer with a conventional fluid-filled open-ended catheter system by means of simultaneous measurement of intra-amniotic pressures.

## Methods

### Patients

The pressure-measuring systems were compared in seven patients who were admitted for induction of labour because of postmaturity (four patients), pre-eclampsia (two patients), and previous caesarian section (one patient). Their ages ranged from 17 to 31 years; five were primiparous and two multiparous. All of the patients gave their consent before being included in the study. Ultrasound examination had confirmed the presence of a singleton fetus, head presenting, and had established the position of the placenta.

Labour was inducсd with an oxytocin infusion followcd by amniotomy. Thc fibreoptic transducer and the fluid-filled open-ended catheter were introduced into the uterus using full aseptic techniques once labour was clinically established (cervical diameter 2-5 cm). An introducer was used in both cases, placed between the posterior lip of the cervix and the fetal head. A scalp electrode to monitor fetal heart rate was applied at the same time. One patient was delivered by caesarian section because of prolonged labour; the others had normal vaginal deliveries. All the neonates had Apgar scores of eight or more at one minute and five minutes. There was no evidence of intrapartum or postpartum infection in any of the patients, apart from a slight wound infection after the caesarian section. At the end of each recording session, both transducers were calibrated against an air-filled reference aneroid manometer.

## Intra-amniotic pressure measuring techniques

### *Open-ended catheter*

The fluid-filled open-ended catheter recordings were made using a Fetal Monitoring Intrauterine Pressure Kit (Hewlett Packard 14099C) connected to a conventional external pressure transducer. The pressure transducer was placed at the level of the xiphoid process and the zero point set to atmospheric pressure before insertion of the catheter. The catheter was flushed with sterile water every half hour, or whenever the recording indicated that the catheter might be blocked.

### *Fibreoptic transducer*

The transducer consists of a bifurcated fibreoptic bundle with a pressure-sensitive stainless steel membrane at the common end. Light is transmitted and received through the fibre bundle by means of an appropriate electronic interface unit. An optic fibre emits light in the form of a cone (Figure 1, $A_1$) whose dimensions are determined by the physical properties of the fibre. Similarly, there is a cone of acceptance from which a fibre can receive light ($A_2$). About 300 fibres are divided randomly between an emitting and a receiving bundle. Infrared light from a GaAs

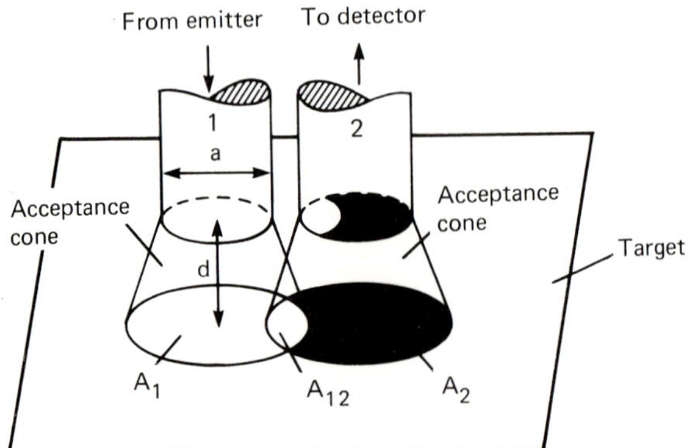


*Figure 1*. The principle on which the fibreoptic pressure transducer is based. $A_1$ is the cone of light from the transmitting fibre; $A_2$ is the cone of acceptance of the receiving fibre; $A_{12}$ is where the cones overlap; d is the distance between the reflecting surface and the fibreoptic fibres

light-emitting diode is conducted down the emitting bundle, reflected off the polished pressure-sensitive membrane, to be led back through the receiving bundle to a silicon PIN photodiode. The amount of light received by the photodetector depends on the degree of overlapping of the two cones ($A_{12}$), which in turn depends on the distance (d) between the pressure-sensitive reflecting surface and the fibreoptic bundles. The electronic interface unit is able to detect movement in the reflecting membrane with an accuracy of 1 nanometre. An air channel through the catheter connects the space behind the membrane to the atmosphere.

The pressure-sensitive membrane is 1.6 mm in diameter and 10 $\mu$m thick, and is contained within a protective stainless steel dome 3 mm in diameter containing two 2 x 4 mm side holes (Figure 2).

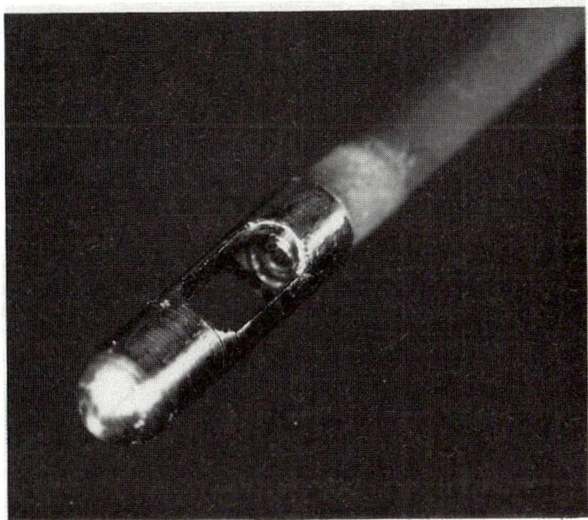

*Figure 2.* The membrane of the fibreoptic pressure transducer which can be seen within the protective dome

The membrane responds to pressure waves in the audio range, although, in practice, the bandwidth of the recording is limited to 50 Hz by the electronic interface unit. The interface unit contains circuits for zero setting and calibration, and a display showing the instantaneous pressure in millimetres of mercury. The fibreoptic bundles are contained within a catheter 2.5 mm in diameter and 1.8 m in length. The transducer has an operating range of -50 to 300 mmHg (-7 to 40 kPa), but can be subjected to ±1500 mmHg (±200 kPa) without damage. Non-linearity and hysteresis are ±1%. The complete transducer/interface unit has a zero drift with changing temperature ±0.6 mmHg (±0.05 kPa) per degree Celsius. Thermal responsitivity drift (mV/kPa per °C) is less than 1 part per 1000 (4).

The transducer was cold-sterilized for one hour in 2% glutaraldehyde, and then rinsed with sterile water before being placed in the amniotic fluid with the aid of a Shiley 3.5 mm endotracheal tube used as an introducer. Before use, the transducer was calibrated against a 75 cm fluid column, and then brought up to body temperature (by holding it against the labia minora for about ten seconds) and the zero point reset at the working temperature.

## Analysis

The measurements made by the two transducers were recorded on a conventional two-channel chart recorder. The recordings covered periods of labour ranging from three to six hours. Thirty contractions from each patient were used for detailed analysis. The contractions analysed were the first ten, the last ten, and ten from the middle of the strip chart. The pressure change from baseline of each contraction to its peak was calculated from the strip chart, and the ratio of the pressures measured by the two transducers was calculated. The mean of the pressure ratios and the standard deviation within each group of ten contractions were calculated, as well as the coefficient of variation defined as: (standard deviation/ mean) x 100. The use of the coefficient of variation of the ratio of the contraction amplitudes eliminates effects due to calibration errors between the transducers. The difference in the amplitude ratios measured for the individual contractions can thus be subjected to statistical analysis. The computation of ratios also makes it easier to see variations in pressure measurement accuracy, independent of physiological variations in the system being measured. This form of analysis for comparing two pressure transducers has been established by Neuman *et al* (9).

## Results and discussion

Figure 3 shows a typical tracing of the two simultaneously measured intra-amniotic pressures. It also demonstrates the disturbance caused by turning the patient into the supine position for a vaginal examination.

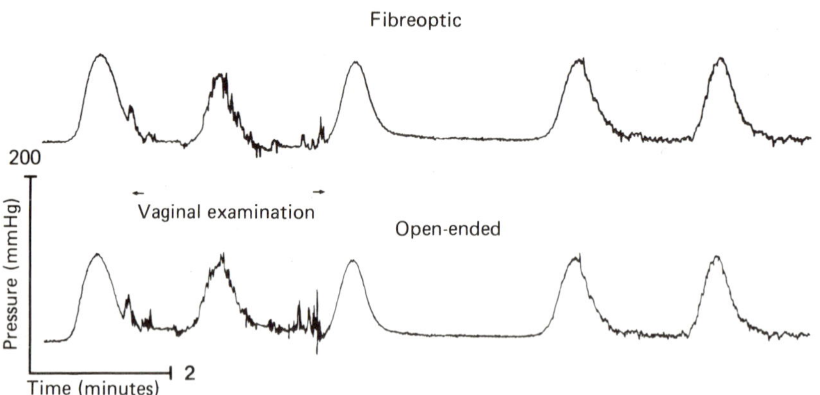


*Figure 3.* A typical pressure recording, showing the good correspondence between the two systems. The irregularities seen in the record were caused by the author

We have compared the two transducers by analysing 210 contractions, summarized in Table 1. There was substantial variation in the ratios of the pressure amplitudes measured by the fibreoptic and external transducers. However, the coefficient of variation within each subgroup is low enough to indicate a good correlation between the two methods in a clinical situation. This was in spite of the fact that no attempt was made to select the smooth bell-shaped curves which are usually considered to be 'good contractions'. Neuman (9) has shown, in a similar study, that the coefficient of variation can be reduced by half when contractions which are not bell-shaped are excluded. Our analysis is based on the first ten, middle ten, and last ten contractions recorded for each patient, irrespective of the shape of the pressure wave, thus representing clinically different situations. Furthermore, the fluid-filled open-ended catheter changed its position in patient number 2 and, by the end of the recording,

**TABLE 1. Summary of 210 contractions. Each series marked by A, B, C, represents 10 contractions. In ratio column, P1 is contraction pressure amplitude measured by fibreoptic transducer, P2 is contraction pressure amplitude measured by open-ended catheter. The coefficient of variation is defined by (standard deviation/mean) ×100%.**

| *Patient no.* | | *Fibreoptic transducer mean pressure (±s.d.)* | *Ratio (±s.d.) P1:P2* | *Coefficient of variation P1:P2* |
|---|---|---|---|---|
| | A | 55.1±10.0 | 1.34±0.17 | 18.2 |
| 1 | B | 61.7±9.8 | 1.36±0.06 | 15.9 |
| | C | 104.5±45.1 | 1.51±0.19 | 43.2 |
| | A | 51.5±8.3 | 1.73±0.26 | 15.2 |
| 2 | B | 42.0±9.6 | 1.66±0.92 | 55.7 |
| | C | 43.4±8.1 | 1.71±0.53 | 30.9 |
| | A | 45.1±3.5 | 1.18±0.04 | 3.2 |
| 3 | B | 42.6±6.1 | 1.12±0.05 | 14.3 |
| | C | 44.9±6.0 | 1.12±0.02 | 13.4 |
| | A | 41.9±3.2 | 0.62±0.07 | 7.8 |
| 4 | B | 38.7±3.0 | 0.58±0.02 | 7.7 |
| | C | 36.8±6.8 | 0.59±0.02 | 18.6 |
| | A | 27.7±6.5 | 1.00±0.11 | 23.6 |
| 5 | B | 29.1±4.0 | 0.91±0.08 | 13.8 |
| | C | 26.8±5.0 | 0.72±0.06 | 18.7 |
| | A | 27.0±6.5 | 0.70±0.11 | 16.7 |
| 6 | B | 31.1±3.1 | 0.74±0.07 | 10.0 |
| | C | 31.1±2.4 | 0.81±0.11 | 13.8 |
| | A | 23.6±4.7 | 0.60±0.15 | 24.6 |
| 7 | B | 26.4±8.0 | 0.71±0.23 | 32.6 |
| | C | 61.9±26.0 | 0.56±0.01 | 2.12 |

the catheter was probably lying between the fetal head and the uterine wall, and the recording had to be terminated. Patient number 1 started bearing down during the last ten contractions, which correlated with a large coefficient of variation in this subgroup. Patient number 3 showed a remarkably constant ratio between the pressures measured by the two systems, as well as a low coefficient of variation.

There are several reasons for the discrepancy in the absolute ratios between the pressures measured by the two systems. The catheters were inserted 'blindly', and it is reasonable to assume that they were at different points in the amniotic fluid since the exact positions of the catheter tips were not known. Neuman (10) has pointed out that if the tip of the open-ended catheter lies in contact with the endometrium, the transducer will measure the compression forces on the catheter wall as much as the intra-amniotic fluid pressure. The fluid-filled open-ended catheter can become obstructed by vernix or blood, thus damping the pressure wave relayed to the external transducer. The fibreoptic transducer has two large orifices in its protective dome. Vernix was sometimes seen within the dome, but there was no evidence that the transducer membrane was obstructed in any of the patients. The protective dome makes the fibreoptic transducer insensitive to direct forces, and even if the catheter tip should become impacted between the fetus and the uterine wall, it would not record an artefactually increased pressure.

The fibreoptic catheter is stiff when cold, becoming flexible at body temperature. In our earlier measurements, we tried to use it like the Gaeltec catheter-tip pressure transducer (13) and insert it without an introducer. However, it was difficult to pass the fibreoptic catheter between the fetal presenting part and the membranes. At present, there is no introducer available for the fibreoptic transducer, but we found that Shiley 3.5 mm endotracheal tubes made reasonable introducer sheaths. We have experienced no failures or complications with this technique in more than 30 insertions.

Because of their fragility, solid-state catheter-tip pressure transducers are usually removed before the cervix is fully dilated, but this is not necessary with the fibreoptic pressure transducer which is more robust because there is no mechanical linkage from the metal pressure sensitive membrane. The fibreoptic transducer has been deliberately left in the uterus throughout the second stage of labour as part of a study of the compressive forces on the fetal head during delivery (Svenningsen and Jensen, see p.77).

Intrauterine pressure measurement must not harm either the fetus or the mother. Fluid-filled open-ended catheters have been shown to be safe (15) because they are soft and flexible, giving way to any resistance. The fibreoptic catheter is as flexible as the open-ended catheter, and the transducer dome is smooth and round, so it should be as safe in use as the fluid-filled open-ended catheter technique. As far as electrical safety is concerned, the fibreoptic pressure transducer offers complete galvanic insulation of the patient, because it is made entirely from non-conductive materials.

Fetal and maternal safety is of paramount importance when intrauterine pressure is to be measured. The flexible fibreoptic pressure transducer fulfils this requirement. It is easy to use, as well as offering a superior mechanical strength. The membrane is protected from direct mechanical forces, and gives a reliable and accurate recording of the intra-amniotic fluid pressure.

## Acknowledgements

We are grateful to A/S Mikro-Elektronikk, Horten, Norway, for their kind co-operation during this project.

## References

1. Beard R W, Filshie G M, Knight C A and Roberts G M. The significance of the changes in the continuous fetal heart rate in the first stage of labour. *Journal of Obstetrics and Gynaecology of the British Commonwealth,* 78, 865 (1971).

2. Cereveka J, Scheffs J E and Vasicka A. Shape of uterine contractions (intra-amniotic pressure) and corresponding fetal heart rate. *Obstetrics and Gynecology,* 35, 695-703 (1970).

3. Csapo A. The diagnostic significance of the intrauterine pressure. *Obstetrics and Gynecology Survey,* 25, part I, 403-435, part II, 515-540 (1970).

4. *Fiber-tip data sheet,* Aksjeselskapet Mikro-Elektronikk, Horten, Norway (1983).

5. Hansen T E and Munkhaugen A. Fiber-optic sensors for medical and electrotechnical applications using bifurcated fibre bundles. Paper F14, Conference on Lasers and Electro-optics June 1981. Washington DC (1981).

6. Hansen T E. A fiber-optic micro-tip pressure for medical applications. *Sensors and Actuators,* (in press) (1984).

7. Hon E H G. *An Atlas of Fetal Heart Rate Patterns* . New Haven, Ct, Harty Press (1968).

8. Menadier C, Kissinger C and Adkins H. The fotonic sensor. *Instruments and Control Systems,* June (1967).
9. Neuman M R, Jordan J A, Roux J F and Knoke J D. Validity of intrauterine pressure measurements with transcervical intra-amniotic catheters and an intra-amniotic miniature pressure transducer during labor. *Gynecological Investigation,* 3, 165-175 (1972).
10. Neuman M R. Pressure measurements in obstetrics. In *Indwelling and Implantable Pressure Transducers,* edited by D G Fleming, W H Ko and W R Neuman, Cleveland, Ohio, CRC Press, 85-95 (1977).
11. Odendaal H J, Neves Dos Santos L M, Henry M J and Crawford J W. Experiments in the measurement of intrauterine pressure. *British Journal of Obstetrics and Gynaecology,* 83, 221-224 (1976).
12. Saito K and Matsumoto H. Development and evaluation of fiberoptic pressure catheter. *Digest of the 11th International Conference on Medical and Biological Engineering,* 690, Ottawa (1976).
13. Steer P J, Carter M C, Gordon A J and Beard R W. The use of catheter-tip pressure transducers for the measurement of intrauterine pressure in labour. *British Journal of Obstetrics and Gynaecology,* 85, 561-566 (1978).
14. Thomas D, Hansen S, Torbet E and May D. A comprehensive system for monitoring the fetal heart rate and uterine contractions. *Medical and Biological Engineering,* November (1973).
15. Trudinger B J and Pryse-Davies J. Fetal hazards of the intra-uterine pressure catheter. Five case reports. *British Journal of Obstetrics and Gynaecology,* 85, 567-572 (1978).

Chapter 4

# Objective recording of fetal movements in early pregnancy

**N-P Jörgensen, K Maršál, K Lindström**

## Introduction

The assessment of fetal motor activity in utero became feasible after the introduction of real-time ultrasound into obstetrics. The examination of fetal movements in early pregnancy provides important information on the physiological neuromuscular development of the fetus. In a clinical situation, e.g. in cases of threatened abortion, a change in the movement pattern might signal an increased fetal risk (8). Attempts have been made to record fetal movements in early pregnancy by objective methods (3,9). However, none of these methods has been used on a large scale and most published studies have evaluated fetal movements qualitatively by observing the screen of the ultrasound real-time scanner (7). The aim of the present study has been to develop and to evaluate an easily applicable ultrasound method for quantitative recording of fetal movements in early pregnancy.

## Method

### Technical equipment

The fetal movements were visualized with a real-time linear ultrasound scanner (Advanced Diagnostic Research, Tempe, Arizona, USA) with a 3.5 MHz transducer. The movements of the fetus were recorded by a time-distance recorder (TD-recorder; Teltec, Lund, Sweden) (6) connected to the scanner. The TD-recorder enables a semi-automatic measurement of the movements of the selected echo-giving structure along any line in the real-time ultrasound image. Two electronic markers are displayed on the screen of the scanner as horizontal lines. The first marker, nearest to the transducer serves as a reference point. The second marker is positioned proximally to the echo of interest. The leading edge of the first marker opens an electronic gate, which is then closed by the leading edge of the first echo following the second marker. During the time the gate is open, 4 MHz clock pulses are transmitted to a counter. The number of pulses is a digital measure of the length of the signal. After converting to an analogue signal, an output is produced which is proportional to the distance between the reference point and the selected echo. The measured distance is visualized on the scanner screen as an intensified part of the selected line. The analogue output signals are recorded on a polygraph (Recomed, Hellige, Freiburg im Breisgau, GFR).

**Recording procedure**

During the recording of the fetal movements the women were comfortably resting in a semi-recumbent position. Their bladders were moderately filled. The real-time image of the cross-section through the uterus was displayed and the fetal echoes identified. The real-time transducer was then kept in position by a special holder. The reference point (electronic marker 1) was situated at the level of the anterior uterine wall and the marker 2 was positioned within the echo-free part of the image representing the amniotic fluid (Figure 1).

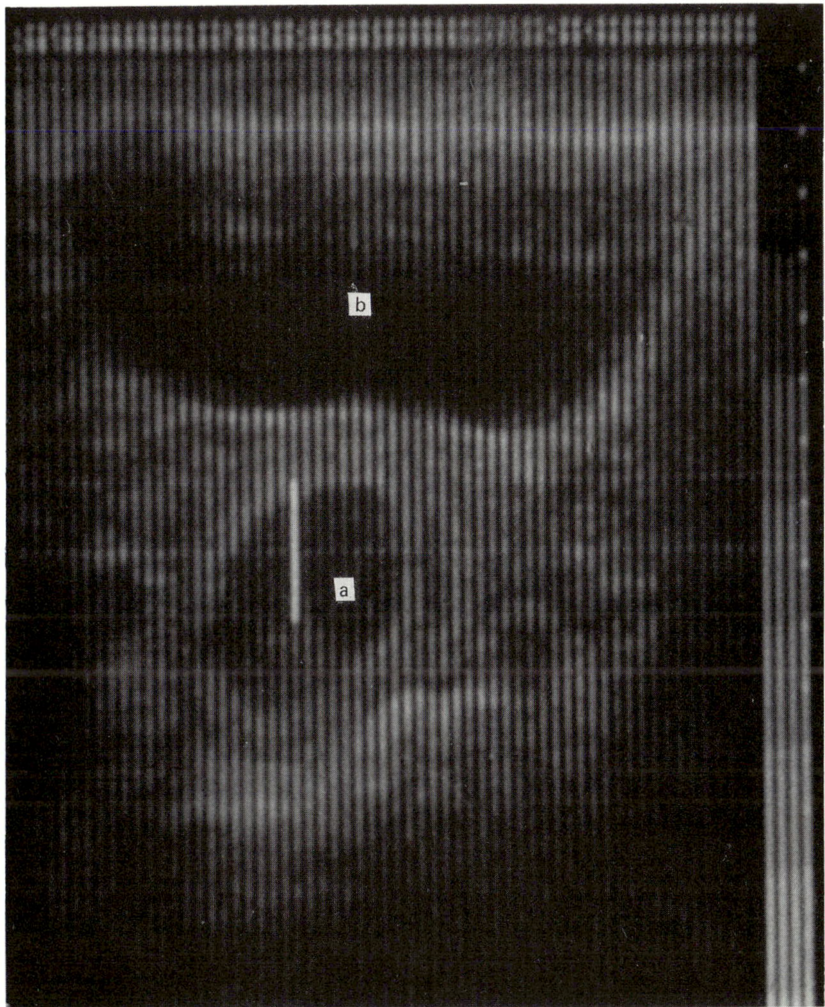


*Figure 1.* Real-time image of the transverse section through the uterus in the ninth week of pregnancy. The horizontal lines represent the positions of the two electronic markers. The bright vertical line represents the distance measured by the TD-recorder from the reference point to the fetal echoes. (a): amniotic cavity; (b): urinary bladder

The instantaneous changes in the distance between the reference point and the fetal echoes were recorded as a function of time, and they reflected fetal movements along the image line. After a 10 minute period allowed for settling down, the recording was started and it lasted for 30 minutes. The screen of the scanner was continuously observed and marks indicating fetal movements recognized in the real-time image were registered simultaneously with the output signals of the TD-recorder. If the fetus moved out of the scanning plane for more than 10 seconds, the transducer was readjusted. Such readjustment was only seldom necessary as the fetus usually returned to its original position within a few seconds.

## Quantification of the fetal movement signals

Figure 2 gives an example of the chart record of the fetal movement signals. In some recordings, baseline disturbances occurred due to passive displacement of the fetus caused by the maternal pulse and/or breathing. Such artifactual signals were always easily identified due to their repetitive character. The chart speed was set at 150 mm/minute. The trace deflections representing fetal movements were quantified manually. Fetal movement signals appearing within 2 seconds of each other were considered as a single movement. The frequency and the incidence of the fetal movements per recording time were calculated.

Recently, an interface has been designed for the automatic quantification of the fetal movement signal. The block diagram and the sequence function diagram of the interface are presented in Figures 3a and 3b. In the following, the letters in parentheses refer to the diagrams. The baseline of the input signal (A) is stabilized by the use of a differential slew rate filter (b). The filtered signal (B) is subtracted from the input signal (A) and the resulting baseline stabilized signal (C) is then passed through a variable squelch (d) which eliminates the recurrent artifactual signals from the mother. The signal (D) may contain artifactual negative signals which are eliminated

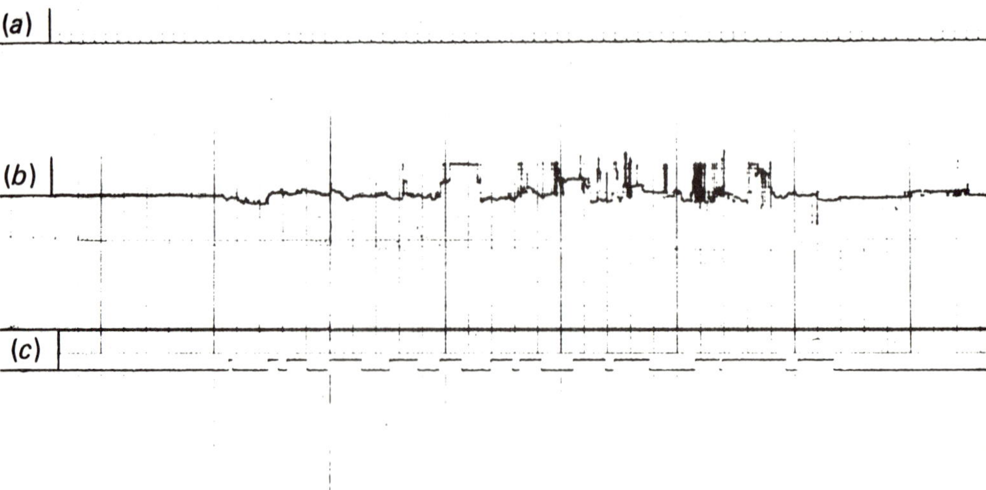


*Figure 2.* Chart record of the fetal movements in the 11th week of pregnancy. Trace (a): time in seconds; trace (b): fetal movement signals measured by the TD-recorder; trace (c): fetal movements marked by the observer

by a precision rectifier (e). The output signal from the rectifier (E) is then applied to an integrator (f). The integrator is automatically reset to zero when the output signal (f) reaches a level of 10 volts. The output signal of the interface represents the area under the fetal movement curve and is a quantitative arbitrary measure of the fetal motor activity during the given time period.

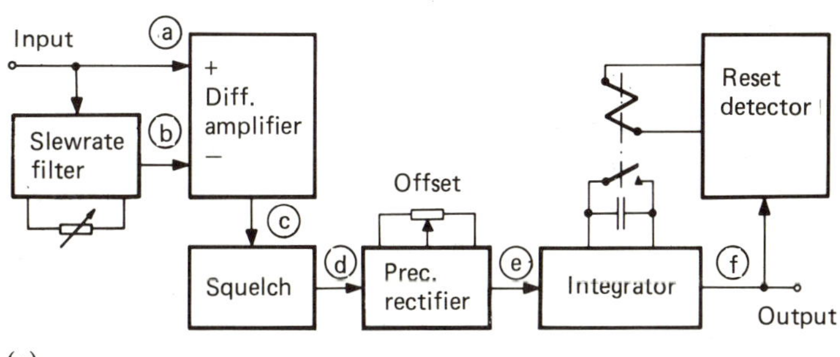


(*a*)

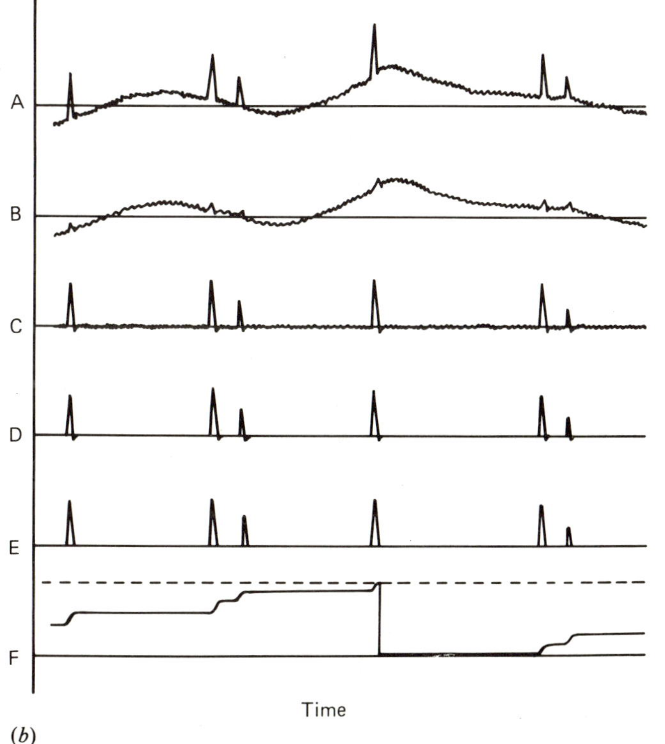


(*b*)

*Figure 3.* (*a*) Block schematic of the interface for the automatic quantification of the fetal movement signals (see text for details). (*b*) Function diagram of the interface for the automatic quantification of the fetal movement signals. (See text for details)

## Evaluation of the method for the recording of fetal movements in patients

### Patients

Twenty pregnant women with uncomplicated pregnancies participated in the study after giving their informed consent. The median age of the women was 28 years (range 20-40 years), 11 women were primiparae. The gestational age of the pregnancies was estimated by measuring the crown-rump length and varied from 11 to 13 weeks.

### Results

The number and the time incidence of the fetal movements recorded during a period of 30 minutes are given in Table 1. The table also gives the longest active and the longest inactive periods recorded. The number of movements recorded by the TD-recorder correlated significantly with the number of movements marked by the observer (r = 0.94; p less than 0.001); 100% of all movements observed and marked by the observer agreed in time with the movements recorded by the TD-recorder.

**TABLE 1. Fetal movement activity recorded for 30 minutes in 20 normal early pregnancies.**

| | *Median* | *Range* |
|---|---|---|
| Number of movements | 176 | 58–302 |
| Incidence of movements (% of time) | 19.5 | 6.4–35.1 |
| Longest active period | 2′10″ | 56″–6′28″ |
| Longest inactive period | 4′40″ | 2′10″–8′20″ |

Of the fetal movements detected by the TD-recorder, 86% (median; range 60-99%) were in agreement with the mark indications of the observer. The time incidence of the movements detected by the TD-recorder (median 19.5%; range 6.4-33.6) was not significantly different from the time incidence of the movements observed on the screen (median 16.2%; range 3.9-35.1) (Wilcoxon's test for paired observations).

## Discussion

Hofmann and Holländer (4) demonstrated fetal movements in the 12th week of pregnancy in their report on the use of the real-time scanner Vidoson. The real-time ultrasound technique visualizes even very small movements of the fetus provided that the movements occur in the plane of scanning. Reinold (8) was the first to examine and classify systematically the fetal motor behaviour in early pregnancy. The observed movements were quantified by counting the number of movements observed on the screen of the scanner during a period of 5 minutes. The modern, technically improved real-time scanners allow more detailed studies of fetal movements. The developmental pattern of fetal motor activity has been studied by several groups (1,2). Up to 16 different movement types were described in the first half of pregnancy (2). All these studies base their conclusions on the visual observation of the ultrasound scanner screen and may be considered subjective and difficult to reproduce. A detailed analysis of the fetal movement pattern is only possible in an off-line display of the videotape-recorded ultrasound image.

In the literature, two reports have been published on the objective examination of fetal movements in early pregnancy. Schillinger (9) recorded time-motion tracings of the fetal echoes as indicators of fetal movements. Henner et al (3) analysed video recordings of real-time images by following a chosen moving echo manually on the video screen with an electronic graticule. Obviously, the latter method was very laborious and did not find any further application.

The present method, providing a semi-automatic recording of the fetal motor activity has proven to be useful in practical application. However, the method has some obvious limitations. Due to the two-dimensional character of the real-time scanning, movements outside the scanning plane are not displayed. This, however, only seldom occurs in early pregnancy, when the movements usually involve the whole fetal body. The TD-recording is performed along only one of the image lines. This has not been found disadvantageous as the fetal body in the first trimester of pregnancy usually moves in the vertical direction. In the pilot study presented, the TD-recorder detected more movements than did the observer. This suggests a higher sensitivity of the TD-recorder. However, the possibility of false movement signals must be considered. Therefore, to minimize possible errors in the recording, the screen of the scanner is continuously supervised by the observer.

The preliminary results from a pilot study showed that the number of fetal movements recorded during a period of 30 minutes in normal early pregnancy was higher than that given for fetuses in the second half of pregnancy (5). The time incidence, however, was similar, suggesting that the duration of the movements is shorter in early pregnancy than in late pregnancy. The median length of the longest inactive period was 4 minutes and 40 seconds. This supports findings by Reinold (8) who described that, in normal early pregnancy, fetal movements always occur within 5 minutes of observation. He suggested this to be one of the criteria of fetal motor normality.

The output signals of the TD-recorder representing fetal movement have to be further quantitated. The use of a microcomputer with appropriate software would probably be the best method of quantitation, but the costs of such an approach would be considerable. Therefore, a method for the filtering and integration of the signals was developed. Normal limits have now to be established for this quantitative measure of the fetal movements. The method will then be applied to pharmacological studies on the acute effects of barbiturates and other medicaments on fetal motor behaviour.

## Acknowledgements

This study was supported by grants from the ‘Expressen’ Prenatal Research Foundation and the Swedish Society of Medical Sciences.

## References

1. Birnholz J C, Stephens J C and Faria M. Fetal movement patterns: a possible means of defining neurological developmental milestones in utero. *American Journal of Roentgenology*, 130, 537-540 (1978).

2. de Vries J I P, Visser G H A and Prechtl H F R. The emergence of fetal behaviour. I. Qualitative aspects. *Early Human Development*, 7, 301-322 (1982).

3. Henner H, Heller U, Wolf-Zimper O, *et al*. Quantification of fetal movement in normal and pathologic pregnancy. In: *Ultrasonics in Medicine,* edited by E Kazner, M de Vlieger, H R Müller and V R McCready, 316-319. Amsterdam, Excerpta Medica, (1975).
4. Hofmann D and Holländer H J. Die Anwendung des Ultraschallschnittbildgerätes Vidoson in der Gynäkologie und Geburtshilfe. *Elecktromedica,* 4, 105-107 (1968).
5. Lindström K and Maršál K. Fetal breathing and movement. In: *Non-Invasive Measurements:* 2, edited by P Rolfe, 61-101. London, Academic Press Inc, (1983).
6. Lindström K, Maršál K, Gennser G, Bengtsson L, Benthin M and Dahl P. Device for measurement of fetal breathing movements. I. The TD-recorder. A new system for recording the distance between two echo-generating structures as a function of time. *Ultrasound in Medicine and Biology,* 3, 143-151 (1977).
7. Marša K. Ultrasonic assessment of fetal activity. In: *Clinics in Obstetrics and Gynaecology,* Vol 10, no 3, edited by S Campbell, 541-563. London, W B Saunders Co (1983).
8. Reinold E. Ultrasonics in early pregnancy. *Contributions to Gynaecology and Obstetrics,* Vol 1, 102-127. Basel, S Karger (1976).
9. Schillinger H. Quantitative Untersuchungen zur embryonalen Motorik mit dem Ultraschall Time-motion Verfahren. *Archiv für Gynäkologie,* 222, 137-147 (1977).

Chapter 5

# Echocardiographic assessment of haemodynamics in small-for-gestational age fetuses

**Andrzej Piela, Jerzy Kuźniar, Andrzej Skret, Tadeusz Zaczek, Zbigniew Szmigiel**

## Introduction

A great deal of evidence has now been accumulated indicating that marked quantitative and qualitative changes appear in the fetal circulation during acute and chronic oxygen deprivation (3,11). It was shown that chronic diminished oxygen supply produces central redistribution of fetal cardiac output, and increase in total blood volume and left ventricular mass (6,9,15). However, these haemodynamic findings are based predominantly on invasive experiments in animals or extrapolated from data obtained on human newborn infants. The circulatory adjustment of the human fetus to such a condition has not been reported.

M-mode echocardiography has provided a unique opportunity to evaluate non-invasively the cardiac structure and function of the fetus *in utero* (4). This study was undertaken to evaluate the mechanisms of circulatory adaptation of the human fetus to low-grade prolonged asphyxial stress. The echocardiographic examination of haemodynamics was performed on a group of appropriate-for-gestational age (AGA) fetuses as well as those small-for-gestational age (SGA) due to chronic placental insufficiency.

## Materials

Thirty-seven fetal echocardiograms were selected retrospectively for the study.

The following criteria were used for selection:

1. the fetus was delivered no later than 2 weeks after echocardiographic examination (mean: 7 ± 4 days);
2. the recordings were of good quality and interventricular septum motion was normal;
3. obstetrical and neonatal assessment excluded congenital heart disease, hydrops fetalis and other congenital malformations.

The study population was divided into two groups according to postnatal findings. The first group (AGA) consisted of 21 fetuses and their gestational age ranged from 30 to 38 weeks of pregnancy (mean: 36 ± 2.1). Fetuses were defined as appropriate-for-gestational age (AGA) when fetal birthweight fell between the 10th and 90th percentiles. The mean birthweight of infants averaged 2952 ± 527 g (Table 1).

**TABLE 1. Time of gestation and birthweight (mean ± 1 s.d.) in adequate-for-gestational age group (AGA) and small-for-gestational age group (SGA).**

| | *AGA* (n=21) | *SGA* (n=16) |
|---|---|---|
| Time of gestation (weeks) | 36.0 ± 2.1 | 34.9 ± 3.1 |
| Birthweight (g) | 2952 ± 527 | 1675 ± 516 |

The second group (asymmetrical SGA) consisted of 16 fetuses, their gestational age ranged from 28 to 40 weeks of pregnancy (mean: 34 ± 3.1). Fetuses were defined as growth retarded when the birthweight fell below the 10th percentile and neonatal clinical examination revealed an asymmetrical type of intrauterine growth retardation. The SGA infants were delivered to mothers whose pregnancies were complicated by severe pre-eclampsia (10 cases), chronic renal disease with superimposed hypertension (four cases) or essential hypertension (two cases). The mean birthweight of infants averaged 1675 ± 516 g. Cardiotocograms performed on all patients in this group before M-mode examination were either reactive (nine cases) or non-reactive (seven cases). However, none of them showed decelerations on cardiotocographic recordings.

## Methods

Fetal left ventricular M-mode echocardiograms were performed using a Picker Echoview System 80C with 2.25 MHz transducer. The ultrasonoscope was coupled to a stripchart recorder. Recordings were obtained at a paper speed of 50 mm/s. The investigation of moving structures of the fetal heart was started at the umbilical region of the pregnant patients. After a picture of the moving structures was obtained on the screen an attempt was made to visualize the characteristic ventricular pattern of the fetal heart echo by changing the position and angulation of the transducer.

The sensitivity of the ultrasonoscope was adjusted to display simultaneous echoes of the endocardium of the interventricular septum and the endocardium of the left ventricular posterior wall. The representative fetal echocardiogram is presented in Figure 1. Fetal left ventricular identification was carried out on the typical systolic pattern of motion of the interventricular septum.

The left ventricular internal diastolic diameter (EDD) was measured as the distance between the endocardial surfaces of the left ventricular posterior wall and the interventricular septum in its maximal separation. The systolic diameter (ESD) was measured as the shortest possible distance during the cardiac cycle.

Interventricular septum thickness was measured at diastole including right and left endocardial echo thickness. Left ventricular posterior wall thickness was measured as the distance between the endocardial surface and the epicardial-pericardial line at diastole.

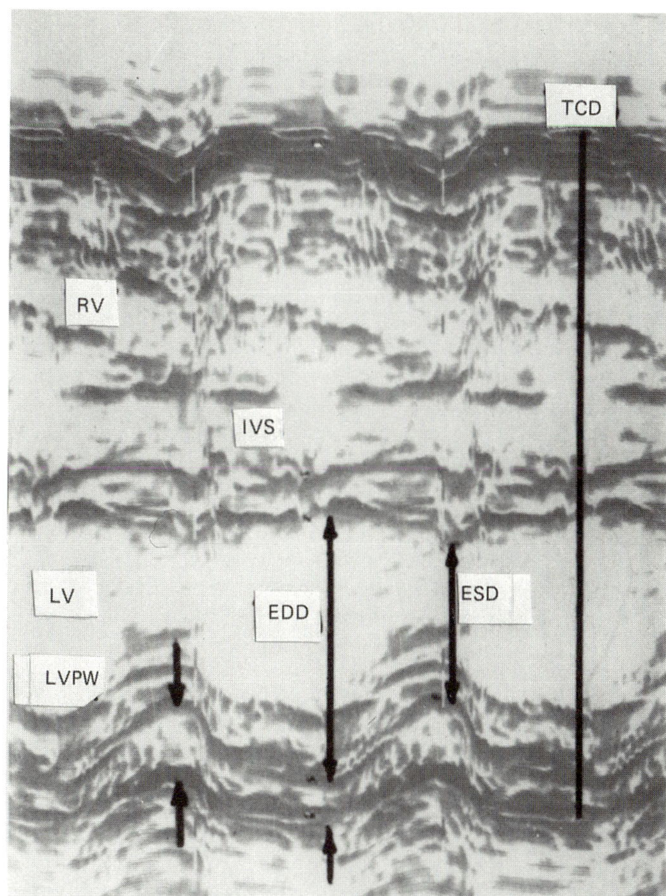


*Figure 1.* M-mode fetal echocardiogram demonstrating where dimensions were measured. RV, right ventricle; LV, left ventricle; IVS, interventricular septum; EDD, end-diastolic dimension; ESD, end-systolic dimension. Arrows indicate thickness of interventricular septum and left ventricle posterior wall. (Paper speed: 50 mm/s)

The following values were derived from these echocardiographic measurements:

1. the left ventricular volumes at systole (ESV) and diastole (EDV) were calculated from the cube of respective dimensions (10) ESV (ml) = $ESD^3$; EDV (ml) = $EDD^3$
2. the stroke volume (SV) was the difference between diastolic and systolic volume: SV (ml) = EDV - ESV
3. the left ventricular output (CO) was derived by multiplying the heart rate by stroke volume: CO (ml/min) = SV x HR. The heart rate was calculated from the echocardiographic record
4. left ventricular mass (LVM) was calculated according to the cube function geometry (12):

$$LVM\ (g) = ((EDD+IVS+LVPW)^3 - EDD^3) \times 1.05$$

(IVS = interventricular septum thickness, LVPW = left ventricle posterior wall thickness).

Corrections were made to account for differences in fetal body weight dividing diastolic volume, stroke volume, left ventricular output and left ventricular mass by birthweight, respectively.

Student's t-test was employed to assess statistically significant differences between AGA and SGA groups.

## Results

The left ventricular volume at end-diastole was found to be significantly higher in the SGA group compared with the AGA group (1.83 ± 0.58 ml/kg vs 1.34 ± 0.44 ml/kg, respectively; p less than 0.01) (Figure 2) With respect to the left ventricular end-systolic index no significant differences were found. The respective values for the SGA and AGA groups averaged 0.55 ± 0.26 ml/kg vs 0.41 ± 0.24 ml/kg (Table 2). The left ventricular stroke volume index was significantly higher in SGA (1.31 ± 0.40 ml/kg) as opposed to that of AGA group (0.93 ± 0.24 ml/kg; p less than 0.01).

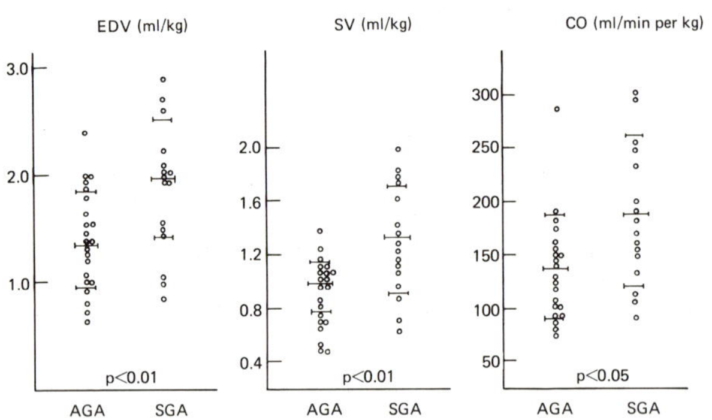


*Figure 2.* Distribution of end-diastolic volume index of the left ventricle (EDV) (left panel), stroke volume index (SV) (centre panel) and left ventricular output index (CO) (right panel) in adequate-for-gestational-age fetuses (AGA) and small-for-gestational-age fetuses (SGA). The middle horizontal bar indicates mean values, and top and bottom horizontal bars indicate 1 s.d.

**TABLE 2. Haemodynamic parameters (mean ±1 s.d.) of the left ventricle of fetuses in adequate-for-gestational-age group (AGA) and small-for-gestational-age group (SGA).**

| | *AGA* (n=35) | *SGA* (n=17) | *Significance* |
|---|---|---|---|
| Heart rate (beats/min) | 141.3±13 | 141.5±15 | NS |
| End-diastolic volume (ml/kg) | 1.34±0.44 | 1.83±0.58 | p<0.01 |
| End-systolic volume (ml/kg) | 0.41±0.24 | 0.55±0.26 | NS |
| Stroke volume (ml/kg) | 0.9±0.24 | 1.32±0.40 | p<0.01 |
| Left ventricular output (ml/min per kg) | 143±63.1 | 187±64.2 | p<0.05 |
| Left ventricular mass (g/kg) | 2.44±0.68 | 2.53±0.78 | NS |

NS=not significant.

The left ventricular output index of the SGA group averaged 187 ± 64.2 ml/min per kg while the respective value in the AGA group was 143 ± 63 ml/min per kg which was found to be statistically significant (p less than 0.05).

With respect to left ventricular mass index, we did not find any significant differences. The respective calculated values for the SGA and AGA groups averaged 2.53 ± 0.78 g/kg and 2.44 ± 0.68 g/kg.

There was no significant difference in heart rate between the groups.

## Comment

The measurement of cardiac output in the fetus has been hampered by difficulties in access to the subject and by the presence of large central shunts in the fetal circulation. Most previous studies of haemodynamic parameters have been made in fetal lambs either exteriorized or *in utero* with their umbilical placental flow maintained (2,5,8).

For obvious ethical and legal reasons, the use of invasive techniques for the study of the human fetus is not possible. Recently, M-mode echocardiography has been successfully applied to estimate the transverse diameter of the left ventricle of the fetal heart at diastole and systole (14). With the use of a geometric formula the end-systolic and end-diastolic volumes can be calculated and thus stroke volume and left ventricular output can be obtained (10,13).

With the use of this method we have found that the value of left ventricular output amounts to 143.2 ml/min per kg in the group of normal AGA fetuses aged 28-38 weeks of gestation. This value is in agreement with the results reported by Wladimiroff *et al* (14); however, it is slightly higher than that found by Winsberg (13).

Furthermore, our results are comparable with those obtained by authors using invasive methods for studying the cardiac output in fetuses of experimental animals. Assali *et al* (2) studied left ventricle output in lambs by means of electromagnetic flowmeters and obtained a value of 140 ml/min per kg.

Also, Goodwin *et al* (5) measured the output of the left ventricle in fetal lambs and obtained a value of 136 ml/min per kg with the use of indicator dilution techniques. Similar results (150 ml/min per kg) were quoted by Heymann *et al* (8) who used the microsphere method. In order to assess the haemodynamic alterations caused by chronic oxygen deprivation, we investigated a group of fetuses with asymmetrical growth retardation due to placental insufficiency. We believe that such a group represents a natural model for the study of adaptative mechanisms generated by chronic hypoxia.

Our data indicate that there are significant differences in haemodynamics of the SGA group fetuses as contrasted to those of AGA group. The former exhibited higher end-diastolic left ventricular volume index, stroke volume index and left ventricular output index.

The higher output of the left ventricle in the SGA group appears to be secondary to augmented stroke volume since the heart rate is not significantly different between the two groups. As the end-diastolic volume reflects, to some extent, a cardiac pre-load, it may be suggested that the volume load of the left ventricle is augmented in the SGA fetuses. If so, an increased end-diastolic volume in SGA fetuses may account for the higher stroke volume by initiating a Frank-Starling mechanism of cardiac reserve. These data may suggest that in the fetuses exposed to chronic hypoxia, the left ventricular output is regulated by an increase in the volume load of the heart.

Our findings are in accord with the results obtained from animal experiments performed by Goodwin *et al* (6) who indicated an increased left ventricular output in fetal lambs exposed to artificial conditions simulating hypoxia. These authors suggested that hypoxic stress produces a pulmonary vasoconstruction and impairment of ductus arteriosus blood flow, which would account for significant regurgitation of blood through the foramen ovale to the left side of the heart. This phenomenon of central redistribution of the cardiac output may lead to an increase in volume loading of the fetal left ventricle.

On the other hand, the increased end-diastolic volume, stroke volume and left ventricular output indices, which we have found in the group of growth retarded fetuses may be accounted for by a higher blood volume in these subjects. This assumption is supported by the findings of Yao *et al* (15) who reported evidence of higher values of haematocrit and haemoglobin levels in asymmetrically growth retarded infants as opposed to those appropriate-for-gestational age.

The low arterial level of oxygen partial pressure is essential for the rapid rates of myocyte division and cardiac growth in normal conditions. This is the reason why prolonged hypoxia was found to be a stimulus for increased ventricular mass, resulting from proliferation of myocytes and fibroblasts (9). Despite this evidence we did not find any significant differences in the left ventricular mass between the groups studied. This observation is in agreement with the previous pathological report of Gruenwald (15) which showed that fetal heart weight is less affected by growth retardation then total body mass.

In conclusion, the results of our non-invasive study with the use of M-mode echocardiography in the human fetus confirm positively the known results obtained so far from animal research. Thus it seems that this method may be useful in the clinical *in utero* assessment of the human fetus under various pathological conditions.

## References

1. Allan D L, Joseph M C, Boyd E G, Campbell S and Tynan M. M-mode echocardiography in the developing human fetus. *British Heart Journal,* 47, 573 (1982).

2. Assali N S, Bekey G A and Morrison L W. Fetal and neonatal circulation. In *Biology of Gestation,* 51-116. London, Academic Press (1968).

3. Behrman R E, Lees M H, Peterson E N, De Lannoy C W and Seeds A E. Distribution of circulation in the normal and asphyxiated fetal primate. *American Journal of Obstetrics and Gynecology,* 108, 956 (1970).

4. De Vore G R, Donnerstein R L, Kleinman C S, Platt L D and Hobbins J C. Fetal echocardiography. *American Journal of Obstetrics and Gynecology,* 144, 249 (1982).

5. Goodwin J W, Mahon W A and Paul W M. Fetal cardiac output as studied by dye dilution techniques. In *The Heart and Circulation in the Newborn and Infant,* 1-15. London, Cassels (1966).

6. Goodwin J W, Milligan J E, Thomas B W and Taylor J R. The effect of aortic chemoreceptors stimulation on cardiac output and umbilical blood flow in the fetal lamb. *American Journal of Obstetrics and Gynecology,* 116, 48 (1973).

7. Gruenwald P. Chronic fetal distress and placental insufficiency. *Biology of the Neonate,* 5, 215 (1963).

8. Heymann M A, Creasy R K and Rudolph A M. Quantitation of blood flow patterns in the fetal lamb *in utero.* In *Foetal and Neontal Physiology: Proceedings of the Sir Joseph Barcroft Centenary Symposium,* edited by S Comline, K W Cross, G S Dawes and P W Nathanielsz, 641. Cambridge, Cambridge University Press (1973).

9. Hollenberg M, Honbo N and Samorodin A J. Effect of hypoxia on cardiac growth in neonatal rats. *American Journal of Physiology,* 231, 1445 (1976).

10. Pombo J F, Troy B L and Russel R L. Left ventricular volumes and ejection fraction by echocardiography. *Circulation,,* 43, 480 (1971).

11. Saling E. Neue Gesichpunkte uber den ablauf fetaler Hypoxien. *Zentralblatt für Gynaekologie*, 88, 76 (1966).
12. Warburton D, Singer D, Bell E F, Corvin R and Oh W. Anatomic confirmation of echocardiographic measurements in neonatal hearts. *Pediatrics*, 64, 468 (1979).
13. Winsberg F. Echocardiography of the fetal and newborn heart. *Investigative Radiology*, 7, 152 (1972).
14. Wladimiroff J W, Vosters R and McGhie J S. Neonatal cardiac geometry and function during the last trimester of pregnancy and early neonatal period. *British Journal of Obstetrics and Gynaecology*, 89, 839 (1982).
15. Yao A C, Lind J, Tiisala R and Michelsson K. Placental transfusion in the premature infant with observation on clinical course and outcome. *Acta Paediatrica Scandinavica*, 58, 561 (1969).

Chapter 6

# Antenatal measurement of beat-to-beat fetal heart rate variation: accuracy of the Hewlett-Packard ultrasound autocorrelation technique

**A J Murrills, T H Wilmshurst, T Wheeler**

## Introduction

Antenatal measurement of fetal heart rate (FHR) variation from beat-to-beat has always posed problems, and the continuing difficulty in achieving adequate accuracy accounts in part for the lack of practical application of such measurements, in spite of claims for their clinical significance. For example, Kariniemi and Ämmälä (4) and Lauersen *et al* (6) report that recordings of beat-to-beat variation of only 5 minutes and 30 seconds duration respectively, can reliably predict fetal outcome. Such short recordings have an obvious clinical attraction when compared with the more usual 20-60 minute antenatal cardiotocogram (CTG).

The R-wave of the fetal ECG remains the ideal signal from which to make measurements of beat-to-beat variation but complex signal processing is required to obtain the maximum information from this waveform when it is recorded from the maternal abdomen (9,13). The ECG technique also has the serious drawback of a low success rate which, in the authors' experience, is only around 50% in late pregnancy (12,13). Some workers have achieved higher success rates (5,8), but most would agree that this problem limits the clinical usefulness of the method. It is still a valuable research tool, however, and its relative accuracy (11) means that it can be used as a standard against which other methods of measuring FHR variation can be compared.

Until recently the ultrasound method of recording FHR had suffered from poor accuracy due to the complexity of the signals, but a considerable improvement in record quality has now been achieved through autocorrelation processing of the Doppler signal envelope. This has helped to renew interest in beat-to-beat variation and we have therefore investigated the accuracy with which the new Hewlett-Packard 8040A cardiotocograph measures beat-to-beat variation from Doppler ultrasound signals.

Recordings were made with the new ultrasound equipment and its measurements compared with those obtained simultaneously by our own abdominal fetal ECG technique (9,13). A specially programmed microcomputer, connected to the cardiotocograph equipment, was used to collect and analyse all the data.

## Patients, equipment and methods

The investigation was carried out with antenatal patients, rather than those in labour, for two reasons: first, to avoid intrusion at a stressful and emotional time, and second because fetal breathing, which is a major cause of beat-to-beat heart rate variation (12), is uncommon during labour (1). However, these considerations had to be set against the lower success rate and poorer signal-to-noise ratio of the antenatal fetal ECG compared with the direct fetal ECG obtainable during labour.

All the patients in the study were resting in hospital with various complications of pregnancy. Forty-one combined ECG and ultrasound recordings of 30 minutes' duration were attempted in 36 patients between 34 and 42 weeks' gestation.

The equipment consisted, on the ultrasound side, of a Hewlett-Packard 8040A cardiotocograph with its digital output connected to an Apple II microcomputer via a DI-09 serial interface. Unlike earlier instruments, the HP 8040A does not produce trigger signals accurately related to the times of fetal heart beats and all measurements must be derived from either the digital or analogue representations of the FHR. (The 'flash' signal which accompanies each 'valid' heart beat is not intended as an accurate indicator of beat period and cannot be used as such.)

The Apple computer was programmed to interrogate the 8040A 16 times per second and to store the new heart rate value each time the 'flash' signal was detected. The FHR was measured by the 8040A to a resolution of 0.25 beats per minute (bpm) and stored to this same resolution. The computer also recorded the following information from the 8040A: (a) the presence or absence of the red signal- quality light (which is directly equivalent to pen 'off' or 'on' for the FHR chart recorder), and (b) the occurrences of the 'flash' signal. This allowed two data quality parameters to be computed: (i) the proportion of time for which the red light was not on, i.e. for which the FHR trace was actually marked on the chart paper and (ii) the proportion of time occupied by 'flashed' FHR values which, with one or two minor but complicated exceptions, indicated measured and valid, as opposed to interpolated, FHR data on a beat-by-beat basis. This second parameter provided the most precise assessment of data quality we could achieve for the 8040A and is that used in the results presented below (see Lawson *et al* (7) and Dawes *et al* (3) ).

The data collection time was controlled by the computer with storage to floppy disc taking place automatically after the first and second 15-minute periods comprising the 30-minute recording. After the recording, the data were recalled from disc and analysed in epochs of 5 minutes duration. This particular epoch length was chosen to facilitate comparison with data from Kariniemi *et al* (4,5).

The computer analysis gave the FHR parameters listed below. These were derived only from measurements indcated as 'valid' by the 8040A; i.e. data validation was primarily according to 8040A criteria and only secondary precautions (such as ensuring that rate differences were computed from truly adjacent heart periods) were included within the Apple computer programme.

Parameters calculated:
mean FHR
modal FHR (8 bpm running mean applied to rate histogram)
inter-quartile range of FHR (IQRR)
inter-quartile range of FHR differences (IQRRD)
mean absolute rate difference (MARD)
differential index (DI)(14).

Notes

1. FHR differences were obtained by successively subtracting one FHR value from the next.

2. Appropriate time-weighting of the FHR values was incorporated in the calculations to ensure that the true mean FHR was obtained and not simply the arithmetic mean of the recorded values. Similar precautions were taken when constructing the histogram from which the mode and inter-quartile range of FHR were derived.

3. Although the differential index was originally defined by Yeh *et al* (14) in terms of heart period measurements, it can equally well be calculated from instantaneous rate values. This can be seen by substituting $1/r$ for $t$ in the defining expression (14) where $r$ is the rate value corresponding to a heart interval $t$. Thus, it is a useful index for comparing beat-to-beat variation measurements made in terms of rate with those made in terms of period, although it suffers from being highly susceptible to the occasional, large artefact.

Graphical output from the computer for each epoch included the FHR waveform (so that any artefacts present in the data could be seen) and the histograms of rate values and rate differences from which some of the parameters were calculated by the programme.

On the fetal ECG side, custom designed equipment, incorporating on-line analogue subtraction to eliminate the maternal ECG, was used to process the fetal ECG signals recorded from the maternal abdomen (9,13). This particular system preserves all the fetal R-waves including those coincident with the maternal QRS and has facilities for continuously monitoring the signal-to-noise ratio of the fetal ECG and quantifying the precision of the measurements obtained (10). A chart recorder (Hewlett-Packard 8032A), similar to that incorporated in the 8040A, was used to display the FHR record derived from the fetal ECG. Because the computer could not handle the ultrasound and fetal ECG data simultaneously, the ultrasound measurements were processed on-line, whilst the fetal ECG signals were stored on analogue tape using a high quality instrumentation recorder (Tandberg 115D) running at 9.5 cm/second. The effect of the record/replay cycle on FHR data fidelity when using this type of recorder had been investigated previously (12), but was reassessed for this study and confirmed to be negligible compared with physiological variation and that due to unavoidable noise on the fetal ECG signal.

On replay from tape, the fetal ECG signals were subjected to an artefact rejection process employing an asymmetric and dynamic version of the more usual fixed heat-rate-change window (10) before being passed, as trigger pulses, to the ECG telemetry input of the 8040A operating in direct ECG mode. In this mode the 8040A does not use autocorrelation processing and thus it provided a convenient means of obtaining digitized FHR measurements from the fetal ECG signals and transferring them to the microcomputer. An important precaution, however, was to low-pass filter the trigger pulses to prevent aliasing errors arising from the digital sampling of them by the 8040A. A 3-pole, 40 Hz Low-Pass, Butterworth filter was used.

The computer analysis of the ECG data was identical to that performed on the ultrasound data.

In a further replay of the ECG signals from tape, the signal-to-noise assessment system (10) mentioned above was used to generate trigger pulses at the same mean heart rate (taken over the 30 minutes) as the actual fetal heart, but showing variation in rate due only to noise on the fetal ECG (i.e. no physiological variation). Analysis of these signals, again passed to the computer via the 8040A, gave measurements of the noise component of the observed heart rate variation plus that due to small measurement errors of the 8040A. This enabled an epoch-by-epoch assessment to be made of the accuracy of the measurements derived from the fetal ECG. Furthermore, the independent nature of the physiological and noise components of the variation meant that statistical correction of the measurements was possible by the principle of subtraction of variance (2). This was almost directly applicable to the DI measurements since this index is based on standard deviation, but allowance was made for possible differences in distribution shape when correcting the MARD and IQRRD measurements for noise. Noise errors were negligible for IQRR.

During each recording the patient rested on a bed with her trunk supported at an angle of approximately 45° to avoid supine hypotension. The Doppler ultrasound transducer was placed where the best signals were obtained and retained in position with an elastic belt. The four electrodes of the fetal ECG system were then applied after removing skin oil with an alcohol swab. 'Biolect-10' paste-less electrodes (MSB Ltd) were chosen for this study and were found to be more convenient to apply and more comfortable for the patient than conventional silver-silver chloride electrodes and there were no obvious drawbacks in terms of signal quality. Once the patient had settled, the tape and chart recorders were started, and the computer data collection initiated.

## Results

### Data quality

One of the 41 recordings attempted was discarded because of a fetal cardiac arrhythmia. The remaining 40 ultrasound records were all of good quality.

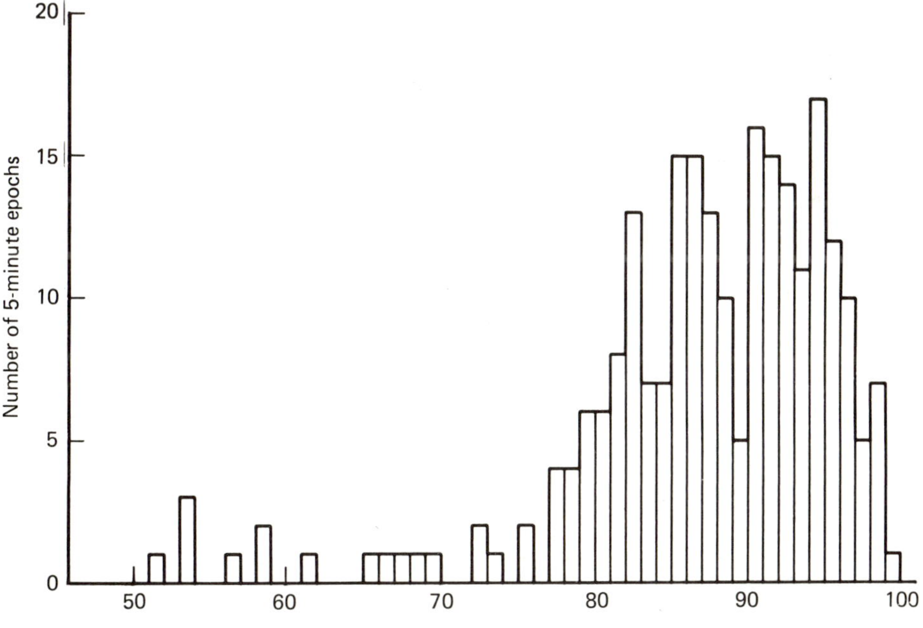


*Figure 1*. Ultrasound data quality. Frequency distribution of 239 5-minute ultrasound epochs by proportion of valid measurement time per epoch. Data from 40 recordings in 35 patients. Mean proportion of valid measurement time 87%

Figure 1 shows how the proportion of valid (flashed) measurement time in each of the 239 epochs analysed from the 40 records was distributed. No epoch contained less than 50% valid measurement time and the great majority (223/239) contained more than 75% valid measurement time.

On the other hand, only 25 satisfactory fetal ECG recordings (from 20 patients) were obtained. For the 135 epochs analysed, the mean proportion of valid measurement time was the same as for the ultrasound data (87%), but there were relatively more epochs with very high, and also low, proportions of valid data than in the ultrasound records. However, meaningful comparisons of this sort between the two methods were difficult because some ECG recordings were complete failures.

In the comparisons between measurements of heart rate variation from the two systems, only those epochs with more than 75% valid ECG measurement time were included. A few epochs were also excluded because they contained isolated artifacts which might have influenced the measurements. Thus the following results were obtained from 110 5-minute epochs of high quality data recorded from 20 different patients.

## Long-term variation

The inter-quartile range of rate over the 5-minute epoch was used as the measure of 'long term' heart rate variation. Figure 2 shows that the measurements obtained with the Hewlett-Packard ultrasound system agreed very closely with those derived from the fetal ECG.

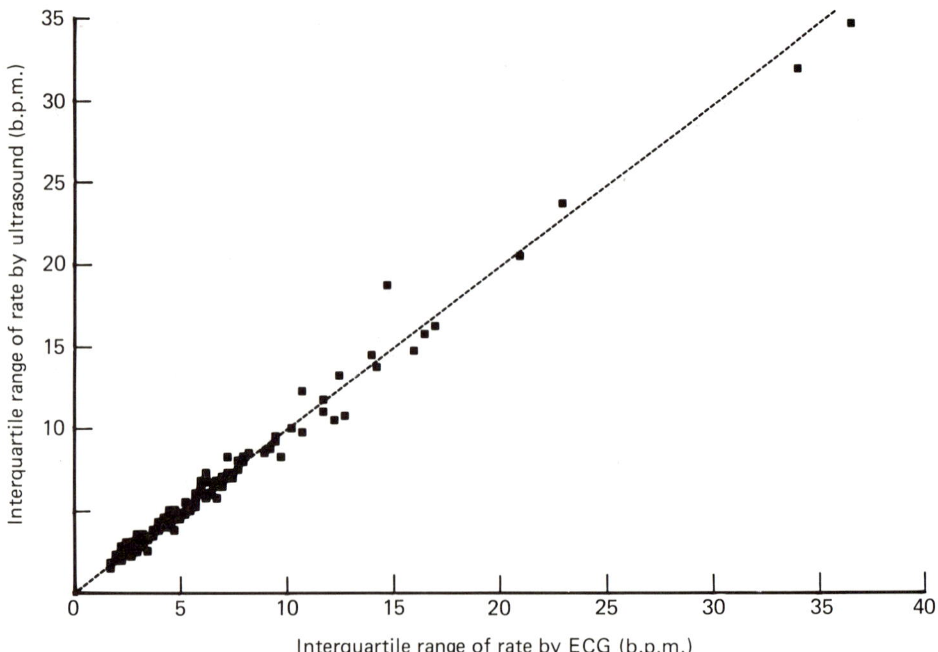


*Figure 2.* Long-term variation. Scattergram of IQRR by ultrasound versus IQRR by ECG; measurements in beats per minute. Each point represents one 5-minute epoch (n = 110). The line of equality is shown dashed. The regression equation of y on x is $y = 0.0875 + 0.968x$ with $r^2 \rangle 0.98$

### Short-term (beat-to-beat) variation

Three measures of beat-to-beat variation were computed. All showed appreciable disagreement between ultrasound and ECG methods. The results for the differential index (14) are plotted in Figure 3. Those for MARD and IQRRD were similar. It

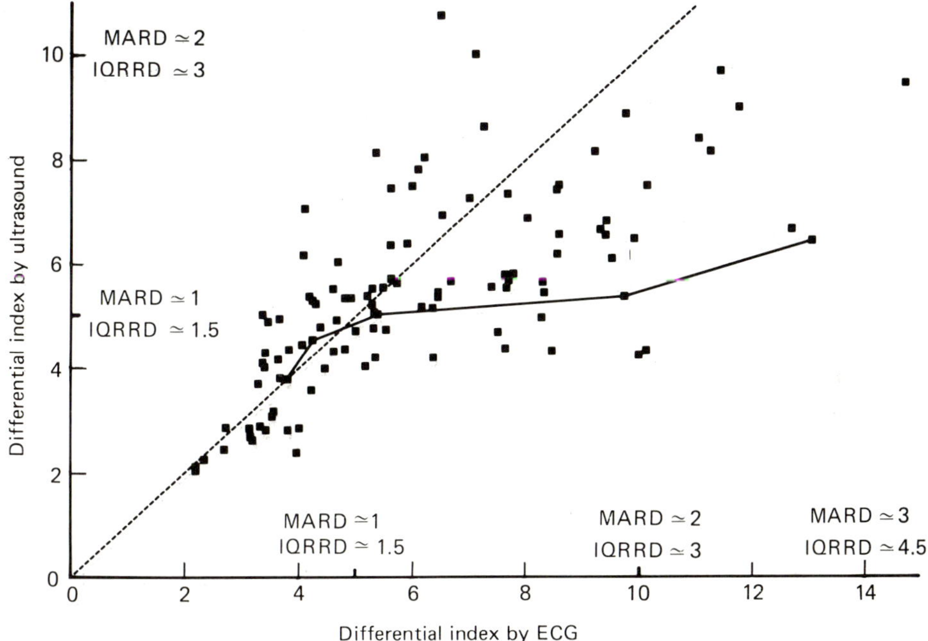


*Figure 3.* Short-term variation. Scattergram of DI by ultrasound versus DI by ECG. Each point represents one 5-minute epoch (n = 109). The line of equality is shown dashed. Approximately equivalent scale values for MARD (mean absolute rate difference) and IQRRD (inter-quartile range of rate differences) are given in beats per minute. The measurements linked by the solid line came from one 30-minute recording

can be seen that the ultrasound system was relatively accurate at low levels of beat-to-beat variation but that at high levels the true value tended to be under-estimated (by as much as 58% in one instance). In a few cases the ultrasound system overestimated the true variation (77% error in one case).

It was also observed that genuine large changes in beat-to-beat variation could occur within a 30 minute recording (illustrated by the six linked points in Figure 3).

## Discussion

This study has confirmed our initial impression that Doppler ultrasound FHR records produced by the Hewlett-Packard 8040A cardiotocograph are of high quality. Lawson *et al* (7) have also evaluated the 8040A and found a low level of data loss but, unfortunately, quantitative comparison with this study is not possible because of differences in methodology. The same Oxford group (Dawes *et al*(3)) previously assessed the quality of ultrasound records produced by the Hewlett-Packard 8030A cardiotocograph (which does not use autocorrelation) and found a mean failure time, i.e. that occupied by invalid heart intervals, of 40-45% over the last 10 weeks of gestation. This contrasts with the figure of 13% for the 8040A machine obtained by us, although it must be noted that the definition of invalid data used by Dawes *et al* (3) was their own and not that incorporated in the machine itself as in this investigation.

Given the low level of data loss, one would anticipate the accurate measurements of long-term variation found in this study. Lawson *et al* (7) also found good agreement between ultrasound measurements of long-term variation, made with the HP 8040A, and simultaneous direct ECG measurements.

The results for beat-to-beat variation were disappointing, although not altogether surprising. Hewlett-Packard have not claimed that the 8040A will measure beat-to-beat variation precisely, but we had nonetheless hoped that it might be sufficiently accurate to be useful. Whether or not this is so requires some discussion.

The few gross overestimates of beat-to-beat variation appeared to be due to poor ultrasound signals and the resulting 'jitter' on the FHR trace could be seen. Warning of this problem might be obtainable from the signal quality lights on the instrument whose status is also output with the other digital data. Perhaps this facility might be developed further in the context of beat-to-beat variation.

The consistent underestimation of high values of beat-to-beat variation was interesting and is well demonstrated in Figure 4. The FHR trace derived from the abdominal ECG clearly shows a high degree of beat-to-beat variation of the type known to be associated with fetal breathing (12), but this is absent from the ultrasound

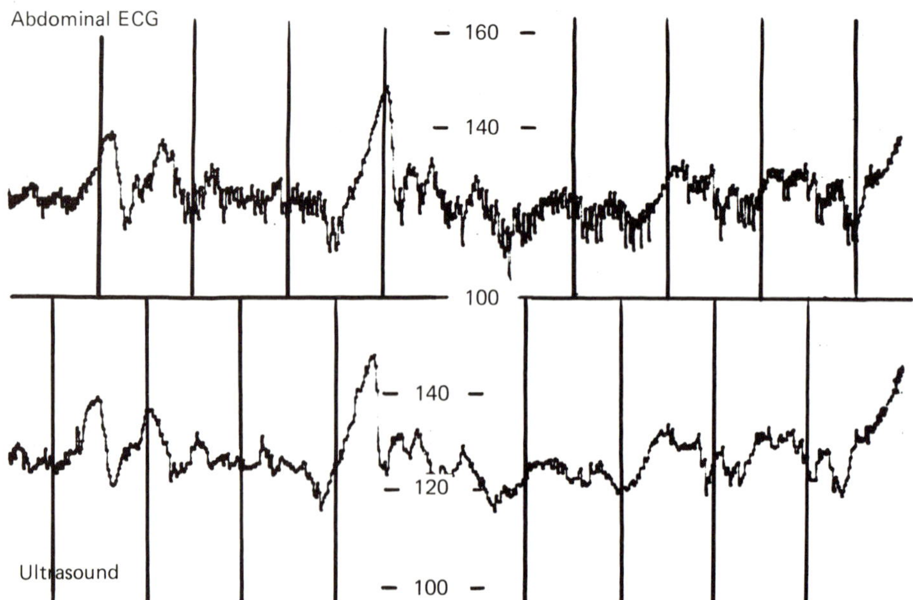


*Figure 4.* Example of a 5-minute epoch in which the ultrasound system failed to record the true beat-to-beat variation seen in the ECG record (heart rate given in beats per minute). The corresponding computer measurements were (U/S v ECG): IQRRD: 1.8 bpm v 3.7 bpm; MARD: 1.2 bpm v 2.5 bpm; DI: 6.5 v 13.1

trace. The time constant associated with the autocorrelation processing (which can vary between 320 ms and 1.2 s) has the effect of low-pass filtering the FHR pattern and is therefore likely to remove high-frequency variation of this type. However, the fact that the measurements appear to become more accurate at lower levels of variation gives some hope of being able to use ultrasound to monitor beat-to-beat variation in this clinically important range. Further technical refinement of the equipment to improve the accuracy of measurement may also be possible.

In their assessment of the 8040A, Lawson *et al* (7) also found that, on average, the ultrasound technique underestimated beat-to-beat variation, but by 35% compared with 12%, 15% and 20% respectively in our measurements of ID, MARD and IQRRD. (Each of these figures is based on the overall mean values from the two techniques.) The reason for this difference is not clear, but methodology and small patient numbers (20 in our case, 10 in theirs) may be responsible. The correlation coefficient of 0.95 found by Lawson *et al* (7) is much higher than the figure of 0.6 which is typical of our results for the three measures of beat-to-beat variation because their figure applies to 10 pairs of values each obtained over 64 minutes, whereas ours applies to more than 100 pairs of measurements over epochs of only 5 minutes.

Our measurements of beat-to-beat variation are also interesting in that they show disagreement in two further respects with the work of other groups. Kariniemi *et al* (5) claim that one 5-minute measurement of beat-to-beat variation (by DI) is representative and that measurements over longer epochs are unnecessary. However, we observed genuine large changes in our 5-minute values of beat-to-beat variation within individual 30-minute records, as indicated by the linked values of DI in Figure 3 (ranging from 3.7 to 13.1 in this case). Thus our data would suggest that a single 5-minute value is not necessarily representative.

Secondly, Lauersen *et al* (6) have estimated mean absolute beat-to-beat rate difference (MARD) from 32 'beat-pairs' within a 30-second sample of the heart rate trace recorded on paper at 25 mm/sec using a Roche ultrasound cardiotocograph. However, *all* the MARD measurements in this study fell *well below* their lower limit of normal of five beats per minute, implying that all the fetuses we studied were in jeopardy. In fact, by Lauersen *et al*'s own criteria (5-minute Apgar score of seven or greater and no fetal distress in labour) the great majority were born in good condition as expected. In view of this and the potential inaccuracy of their technique, the very high predictive values (positive 71%; negative 90%) found by Lauersen *et al* (6) for their measurements of beat-to-beat variation are remarkable.

## Acknowledgements

The 8040A cardiotocograph was kindly loaned by Hewlett-Packard GmbH and its workings patiently explained over many weeks by Erich Courtin and Martin Schraag of the same organization.

## References

1. Boylan P and Lewis P J. Fetal breathing in labor. *Obstetrics and Gynecology*, 56, 35-38 (1980).
2. Campbell R C. The normal distribution. In *Statistics for Biologists*, 153. Cambridge, Cambridge University Press (1974).

3. Dawes G S, Visser G H A, Goodman J D S and Redman C W G. Numerical analysis of the human fetal heart rate: the quality of ultrasound records. *American Journal of Obstetrics and Gynecology*, 141, 43-52 (1981).
4. Kariniemi V and Ämmälä P. Short-term variability of fetal heart rate during pregnancies with normal and insufficient placental function. *American Journal of Obstetrics and Gynecology*, 139, 33-37, (1981).
5. Kariniemi V, Siimes A and Ämmälä P. Antepartal analysis of fetal heart variability by abdominal electrocardiography. *Journal of Perinatal Medicine*, 10, 114-118 (1982).
6. Lauersen N H, Kurkulos M, Graves Z R and Lewin K. Reliability of antenatal testing: estriol levels versus nonstress testing. *Obstetrics and Gynecology*, 62, 11-16 (1983).
7. Lawson G W, Belcher R, Dawes G S and Redman C W G. A comparison of ultrasound (with autocorrelation) and direct ECG fetal heart rate detector systems. *American Journal of Obstetrics and Gynecology*, 147, 721-722 (1983).
8. Leventhal J M, Brown W U, Weiss J B and Alper M H. A new method of fetal heart-rate monitoring. *Obstetrics and Gynecology*, 45, 494-500 (1975).
9. Murrills A J, Shelley T and Wheeler T. The continuous precise measurement of fetal heart interval during pregnancy: a new technique using the abdominal fetal electrocardiogram. In *IERE Conference Proceedings no 34 - Applications of Electronics in Medicine*, 127-136, London, Institution of Electronic and Radio Engineers (1976).
10. Murrills A J and Wheeler T. Measurement of fetal heart rate variation from abdominal fetal ECG signals. In *Fetal and Neonatal Physiological Measurements*, edited by P Rolfe, 1-8, London, Pitman Medical (1980).
11. Wheeler T, Cooke E and Murrills A J. Computer analysis of fetal heart rate variation during normal pregnancy. *British Journal of Obstetrics and Gynaecology*, 86, 186-197 (1979).
12. Wheeler T, Gennser G, Lindvall R and Murrills A J. Changes in the fetal heart rate associated with fetal breathing and fetal movement. *British Journal of Obstetrics and Gynaecology*, 87, 1068-1079 (1980).
13. Wheeler T, Murrilis A J and Shelley T. Measurement of the fetal heart rate during pregnancy by a new electrocardiographic technique. *British Journal of Obstetrics and Gynaecology*, 85, 12-17 (1978).
14. Yeh S-Y, Forsythe A and Hon E H. Quantification of fetal heart beat-to-beat interval differences. *Obstetrics and Gynecology*, 41, 355-363 (1973).

Chapter 7

# Low antepartum fetal heart rate variability predicts late decelerations in labour of low risk pregnancies

**Veikko Kariniemi**

## Introduction

The differential index, DI (6), has been shown to predict fetal distress in labour of high risk pregnancies (1,2,3,5). The present study was undertaken to find out whether the antepartum DI has any value in screening low risk pregnancies for placental insufficiency. Any late decelerations in the intrapartum cardiotocograms were used as the end point of the evaluation.

## Subjects and methods

One hundred and eighty-one private patients volunteered for the study. A 5-minute analysis of fetal heart rate variability (FHRV) between weeks 20 and 43 of gestation was performed one to ten times (mean 4.1 ± 2.5) using a method which has been described previously (4) based on the abdominal fetal electrocardiogram (aFECG) as a triggering signal. One hundred and thirty-four of the fetuses were delivered vaginally and 47 abdominally (26%). Fifteen of the Caesarean sections were elective, thus 166 of the fetuses were monitored by cardiotocography during labour. The intrapartum cardiotocograms were evaluated visually: late and variable decelerations, as well as epochs of fixed baseline lasting longer than 5 minutes, were recorded. A fetal blood analysis was performed on eight fetuses and none had acidosis. The antepartum DIs and the findings in the intrapartum cardiotocograms were handled by the BMDP software analysis system. The comparison of means was performed by the Students *t* test in case of equal variances. The linear correlation of the measured parameters was computed. The frequencies were compared by the chi-squared test.

## Results

The material from 166 deliveries was divided into two groups according to the intrapartum cardiotocograms: one group with late decelerations (n = 37) and the other without late decelerations (n = 129). The former was considered to have a marginal and the latter a perfect placental function. The birthweights and the placental weights of the corresponding groups did not differ significantly. The DIs at

28 weeks' gestation were lower in the group with perfect placental function (Table 1).

**TABLE 1. Means of antepartum differential indices (DI) measured from abdominal fetal electrocardiogram of 166 fetuses serially at one to several week intervals in two groups of low risk pregnancies according to the presence of late decelerations in the intrapartum cardiotocograms.**

| | *Normal group* (n=129) | | | | *Intrapartum late decelerations* (n=37) | | | | |
|---|---|---|---|---|---|---|---|---|---|
| *Weeks of gestation* | *Mean DI* | *s.d.* | *s.e.m.* | *n* | *Mean DI* | *s.d.* | *s.e.m.* | *n* | *p* |
| 20 | 2.8 | 0.5 | 0.2 | 11 | 2.6 | 0.9 | 0.6 | 2 | NS |
| 21 | 2.8 | 0.6 | 0.2 | 14 | 2.6 | 0.7 | 0.4 | 3 | NS |
| 22 | 3.1 | 1.4 | 0.3 | 18 | 2.4 | 0.8 | 0.6 | 2 | NS |
| 23 | 3.3 | 0.6 | 0.2 | 14 | 2.8 | 0.7 | 0.5 | 2 | NS |
| 24 | 3.4 | 0.9 | 0.2 | 31 | 4.1 | 0.7 | 0.3 | 4 | NS |
| 25 | 3.6 | 1.3 | 0.3 | 23 | 4.2 | 1.1 | 0.5 | 5 | NS |
| 26 | 3.9 | 0.8 | 0.2 | 22 | 4.7 | 1.7 | 0.5 | 10 | NS |
| 27 | 4.5 | 0.9 | 0.2 | 18 | 3.9 | 0.6 | 0.2 | 6 | NS |
| 28 | 4.6 | 0.8 | 0.2 | 19 | 3.6 | 0.4 | 0.2 | 6 | 0.0059 |
| 29 | 5.2 | 1.7 | 0.5 | 12 | 3.6 | 0.9 | 0.4 | 5 | 0.0571 |
| 30 | 4.7 | 1.1 | 0.3 | 10 | 5.6 | 1.9 | 0.8 | 6 | NS |
| 31 | 5.4 | 1.5 | 0.4 | 12 | 4.7 | 1.3 | 0.6 | 5 | NS |
| 32 | 5.6 | 1.4 | 0.3 | 21 | 6.1 | 1.9 | 0.9 | 5 | NS |
| 33 | 6.5 | 1.9 | 0.4 | 22 | 6.1 | 1.7 | 0.7 | 6 | NS |
| 34 | 5.0 | 1.5 | 0.3 | 20 | 6.2 | 2.4 | 0.8 | 8 | NS |
| 35 | 6.0 | 1.6 | 0.3 | 32 | 6.2 | 0.9 | 0.3 | 9 | NS |
| 36 | 6.1 | 1.7 | 0.3 | 41 | 6.0 | 1.5 | 0.4 | 14 | NS |
| 37 | 6.0 | 1.8 | 0.3 | 39 | 6.5 | 1.7 | 0.4 | 17 | NS |
| 38 | 6.4 | 1.9 | 0.3 | 52 | 6.0 | 1.3 | 0.3 | 16 | NS |
| 39 | 6.4 | 2.0 | 0.3 | 61 | 6.4 | 2.0 | 0.5 | 20 | NS |
| 40 | 5.9 | 2.2 | 0.4 | 37 | 6.0 | 1.9 | 0.4 | 21 | NS |
| 41 | 6.2 | 2.6 | 0.6 | 18 | 5.8 | 2.2 | 0.6 | 13 | NS |
| 42 | 7.7 | 3.2 | 2.3 | 2 | 7.1 | 1.0 | 0.4 | 5 | NS |

At 29 weeks' gestation the difference was similar and almost significant. Otherwise, the DIs of the two groups did not differ. However, when DIs lower than 3.6 were observed after the 28th week, the relative risk of finding late decelerations in labour was 2.7 times that after higher antepartum DIs (Table 2).

**TABLE 2. Low differential index as a predictor of late decelerations in labour of 162 low risk pregnancies.**

| *Differential index* | *Late decelerations* *yes* | *no* | *Relative risk* |
|---|---|---|---|
| $<3.6$ | 15 | 18 | 2.7 ($p<0.001$) |
| $\geq$ | 22 | 107 | |

## Discussion

The present study suggests that antepartum DIs measured from aFECG may have value in selecting those pregnancies which later have problems with placental respiratory capacity. The previously presented cut-off level of the first lower percentile (Figure 1) of the antepartum DIs, which has been shown to be suitable in high risk pregnancies, might be too strict for screening purposes. Therefore, another normal limit, 3.6 after the 28th week (Figure 2), has been tested in the present study. The material presented here is too small for the end-point of severe asphyxia or fetal death (only one fetus died with two normal antepartum DIs), but it might be important also to detect those pregnancies which will have pathological patterns in intrapartum cardiotocograms. The antepartum DIs had no predictive value for variable decelerations.

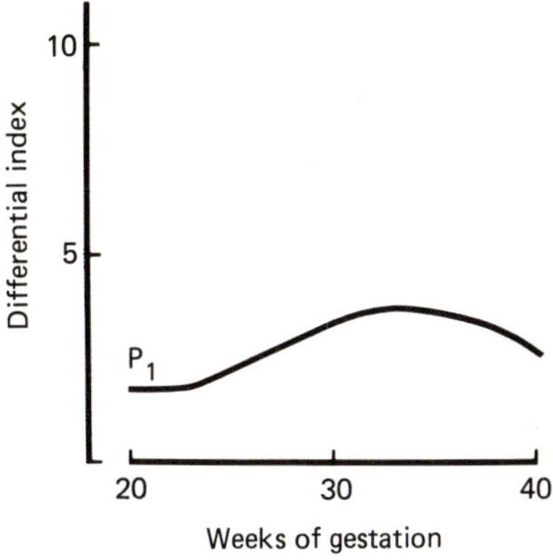


*Figure 1.* The first percentile limit of antepartal differential indices (DI) tested for high risk pregnancies and drawn from a reference material of 132 low risk pregnancies

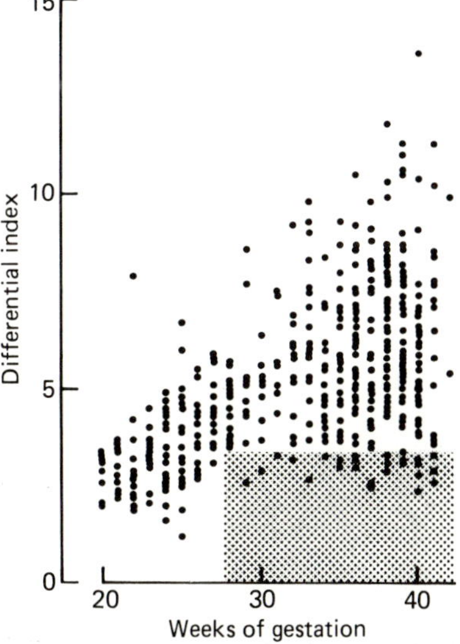


*Figure 2.* The scattergram of antepartal differential indices measured from 5-minute epochs of abdominal fetal electrocardiogram of 132 fetuses during normal pregnancy. The shaded area indicates the suggested abnormal range from the 28th week

## References

1. Ämmälä P and Kariniemi V. Short term variability of fetal heart rate in cholestasis of pregnancy. *American Journal of Obstetrics and Gynecology,* 141, 217 (1981).
2. Ämmälä P and Kariniemi V. Short term variability of fetal heart rate during pregnancies complicated by hypertension. *British Journal of Obstetrics and Gynaecology,* 90, 705 (1983a).
3. Ammala P and Kariniemi V. Short term variability of fetal heart rate in insulin-dependent diabetic pregnancies. *Journal of Perinatal Medicine,* 11, 97 (1983b).
4. Kariniemi V, Katila T, Laine H and Ämmälä P. On-line quantification of fetal heart rate variability. *Journal of Perinatal Medicine,* 8, 213 (1980).
5. Kariniemi V and Ämmälä P. Short term variability of fetal heart rate during pregnancies with normal and insufficient placental function. *American Journal of Obstetrics and Gynecology,* 139, 33 (1981).
6. Yeh S-Y, Forsythe A and Hon E H. Quantification of fetal heart beat-to-beat interval differences. *Obstetrics and Gynecology,* 41, 355 (1973).

Chapter 8

# The volumetric growth of the human placenta: a preliminary report of a computer-supported ultrasonographic study

**D Veersema, M Vossen, O Th Uttendorfsky and H J Hoogland**

## Introduction

Since Grannum and Hobbins (3) introduced their system of grading the placenta with use of ultrasonography, the literature has reflected an increasing interest in the use of ultrasound to study morphological aspects of the human placenta. In contrast, studies concerning biometrical aspects of the placenta are limited to a small number (1,2,4,5,6,7,8,9,11). However, since the relation of the weight of the fetus to the weight of its placenta is well known from postpartum studies (10), placentometry may very well contribute to the early detection of fetal growth retardation, a major issue in daily obstetrical practice.

Hoogland (6) used ultrasound to assess the placental surface area during pregnancy, and in fact he found a significant difference in placental size at a menstrual age of 150 days when he compared subsequent normal fetal growth to fetal growth retardation.

Unfortunately, available ultrasonic data on the volumetric growth of the placenta are controversial. Hellman et al (4) studied 207 pregnancies at various stages of gestation starting at 10 weeks' menstrual age, and found a continuously increasing placental volume until the end of gestation. A similar growth pattern was demonstrated by Vandenberghe (11). Bleker et al (1) published the results of a study in which 12 patients were included. Placental volume was assessed in each patient from 23 weeks' menstrual age until term at bi-weekly intervals. In this way individual growth curves could be produced which showed a maximal placental volume at the 34th week of pregnancy in most cases and a declining volume thereafter. Terinde and Kozlowski (9) in a study of placental growth in 157 gravidae, including patients with fetal growth retardation and diabetes, concluded that placental volume reached its maximum level at 34 weeks' menstrual age.

Most of these previous studies have used some form of (mathematical) model for the assessment of placental volume (4,1). The differences between these methods, as well as the variation of the pregnancies studied, e.g. including fetal growth retardation and diabetic patients, could explain the difference in the results.

## Material and method

Volumetric growth of the placenta was studied using a Philips Sono Diagnost B 7100 compound scanner with a grey-scale scan converter, connected to a Diagnostic Sonar echo-computer-lightpen-system. Serial sonograms of the placenta were obtained at 0.5 cm intervals in both transverse and longitudinal directions. In each sonogram placental area was determined using the computer-lightpen-system. Summation of all

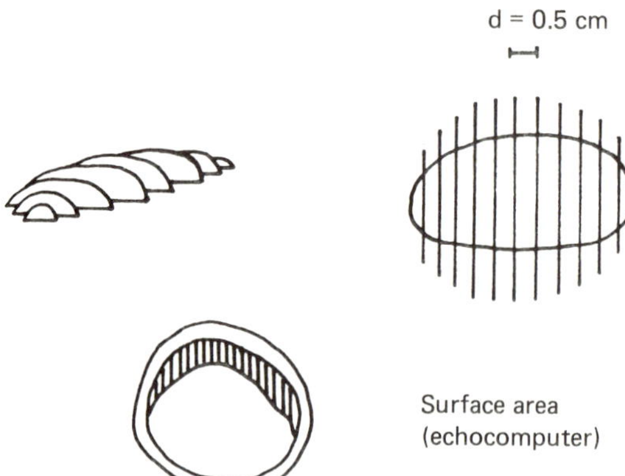


Figure 1. The experimental design of the study

placental areas multiplied by the sum of the intervals reflected placental volume in one direction. The average of the calculated volumes in both directions was recorded as the actual placental volume (Figure 1). In this way 14 pregnancies with normal fetal growth were studied from 10 weeks menstrual age until term. Ultrasonographies between 10 and 20 weeks were performed at weekly intervals, between 20 and 36 weeks at biweekly intervals and after 36 weeks again at weekly intervals. In five patients the placenta was located on the posterior wall of the uterus and could therefore only be studied until 20 weeks' menstrual age. The experimental design for calculating placental volumes was verified by comparing ultrasonographic results to a water-displacement technique when the placenta was ultimately delivered. The correlation between these methods was 0.98.

## Results

Table 1 gives a summary of the outcome of this preliminary study. A total of 224 measurements were performed, calculated from a total of 3010 sonograms. A curve

**TABLE 1. Mean placental volumes by gestational age.**

| | *Gestational age (lunar month)* | | | | | | | |
|---|---|---|---|---|---|---|---|---|
| | 3 | 4 | 5 | 6 | 7 | 8 | 9 | 10 |
| No. of observations | 59 | 72 | 36 | 19 | 11 | 10 | 10 | 7 |
| Mean volume (ml) | *30* | *95* | *163* | *321* | *460* | *548* | *631* | *668* |
| Standard deviation (ml) | 14 | 44 | 49 | 86 | 173 | 140 | 81 | 63 |
| Coefficient of variation (%) | 45 | 46 | 30 | 27 | 38 | 26 | 18 | 11 |

of the mean placental volume as shown in Table 1 plotted against the gestational age is shown in Figure 2.

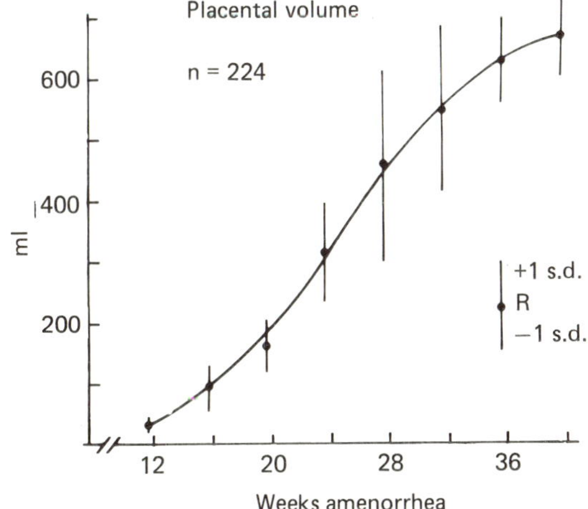


*Figure 2.* Composite placental growth curve from the 14 patients studied

The similarity of volume-calculations from both longitudinal and transverse placental sonograms showed a correlation of 0.99 and is presented in Figure 3.

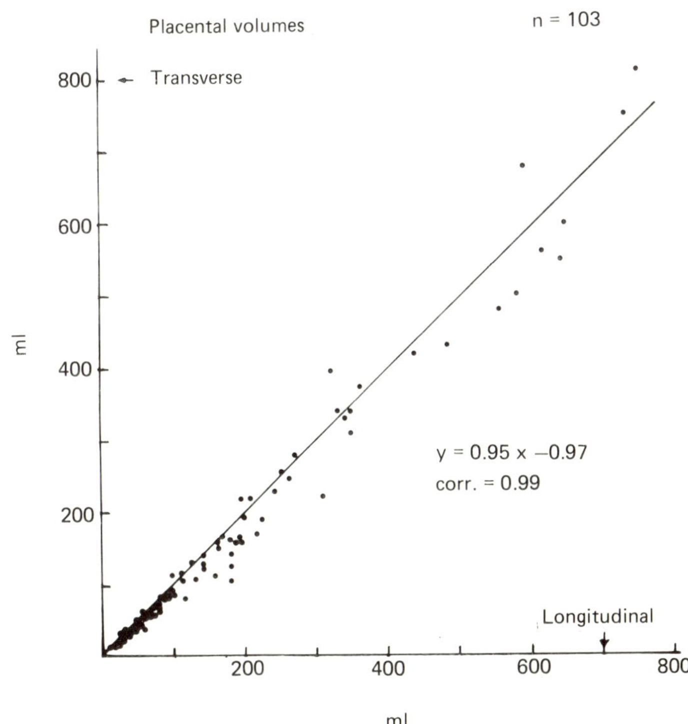


*Figure 3.* Comparison of longitudinal and transverse determination of placental volume

## Comment

In this preliminary report we have presented a relatively simple method of ascertaining placental volume throughout most of gestation. The method does not in any way compromise the shape of the placenta, which is illustrated by the good correlation of the method when applied postpartum and compared to the volume displacement in a waterbath. As demonstrated in Figure 2, and in agreement with the results of Hellman (4) and Vandenberghe (11), placental volume increased throughout pregnancy until term in the 14 patients studied. The average coefficient of variation of the mean placental volumes as shown in Table 1 and Figure 2 is 30%. This large relative standard deviation is somewhat smaller than the 37% reported by Hellman et al (4) and is in agreement with the extent of variability of fetal weight at the corresponding gestational age.

## Acknowledgement

This study was supported by a the Dutch Praeventiefonds.

## References

1. Bleker O P, Kloosterman G J, Breur W and Mieras D J. The volumetric growth of the human placenta: a longitudinal ultrasonic study. *American Journal of Obstetrics and Gynecology,* 127, 657 (1977).
2. Bleker O P and Hoogland H J. Ultrasound in the estimation of human intra-uterine placental growth. *Placenta,* 2, 275 (1981).
3. Grannum P A T and Hobbins J C. The ultrasonic changes in the maturing placenta and their relation to fetal pulmonic maturity. *American Journal of Obstetrics and Gynecology,* 133, 915 (1979).
4. Hellman L M, Kobayashi M, Tolles W E and Cromb E. Ultrasonic studies on the volumetric growth of the human placenta. *American Journal of Obstetrics and Gynecology,* 108, 740 (1970).
5. Hollander H J and Mast H. Intrauteriene Dickenmessungen der Plazenta mittels Ultraschall bei normalen Schwangerschaften und bei Rh-Incompatibilitat. *Geburtsh,* Frauenheilk, 28, 662 (1968).
6. Hoogland H J. Ultrasonic aspects of the placenta. *Thesis, University of Nijmegen,* (1980).
7. Hoogland H J, de Haan J and Martin Ch B. Placental size during early pregnancy and fetal outcome: a preliminary report of a sequential ultrasonographic study. *American Journal of Obstetrics and Gynecology,* 138, 441 (1980).
8. Schlensker K H. Plazentographie mittels Ultraschall-Schnittbild- Verfahren. *Gerburtsh, Frauenheilk,* 33, 879 (1971).
9. Terinde R and Kozlowski P. Placental growth and tissue characterization. In: *Dilemmas in Gestosis,* edited by H Janisch and E Reinold, 94-100, Stuttgart, Georg Theime Verlag (1983).
10. Thomson A M, Billewicz W Z and Hytten F E. The weight of the placenta in relation to birthweight. *Journal of Obstetrics and Gynaecology of the British Commonwealth,* 76, 865 (1969).
11. Vandeneberghe K. Ultrasonography of the placenta. *Journal of Perinatal Medicine,* 9 suppl. 1, 75 (1981).

Chapter 9

# Hypoxanthine, lactate, pH; indices of fetal hypoxia?

**D P Alexander, H G Britton, M Cooper, D Redstone and G D Ryan**

## Introduction

Hypoxia produces marked changes in fetal metabolism and it is commonly assumed that the biochemical markers for these changes will all behave similarly in hypoxia. This view tends to be reinforced by studies in which averaged data have been reported which show a general correlation between the parameters. It should be remembered, however, that these parameters are influenced by different aspects of hypoxia and there is no *a priori* reason why they should behave identically. Thus, hypoxanthine may be expected to be released from cells when the 'energy charge' is low (i.e. when rephosphorylation of ADP to ATP is reduced). This will not necessarily correspond with the onset of hypoxia since, in many cells, rephosphorylation of ADP may be expected to be maintained by glycolysis and, at least for a period, the energy charge will be maintained. Glucose levels may be important in this respect, to provide adequate substrate for glycolysis. In the whole fetus the concentration of hypoxanthine in the blood will depend on the contributions from the different tissues. Observations on arteriovenous differences would suggest that the liver and the heart are the major sources of hypoxanthine production but the placenta appeared to be a site of hypoxanthine uptake (6).

In contrast to hypoxanthine, the formation of lactic acid in tissues will occur when the oxygen supplies are inadequate to maintain oxidative phosphorylation. In the adult, some cells glycolyse under normal conditions of oxygenation and glycolysis occurs on a large scale during muscular exercise. To what extent these latter contribute to lactic acid production in the fetus is not known although in the sheep fetus there is an additional source of lactic acid from the placenta (2,3). However, it seems that there is at least the possibility that in the fetus elevation of lactic acid levels may on some occasions be due to factors other than hypoxia: for example muscular activity or a failure of the liver to take up lactate. In the presence of hypoxia one of the major sources of fetal lactic acid is the heart because of the glycogen depletion that occurs in this tissue (3,4). However, it would also seem that the fetal brain and perhaps liver may also make a substantial contribution (3). Skeletal muscle on the other hand, would not seem to contribute but may act as a 'sink' for lactic acid produced elsewhere. At high lactate concentrations the placenta takes up lactate although the amount removed is small (1).

The pH falls in hypoxia and this is commonly attributed to two factors namely a rise in $PCO_2$ and/or a rise in lactate. However, carbon dioxide has a high diffusibility in relation to oxygen and the shapes of the oxygen and carbon dioxide dissociation curves are such that placental insufficiency should produce only a modest rise in $PCO_2$ and a modest fall in pH. Further, if the umbilical flow were to be completely arrested the oxygen stores in the fetus are not large and only a small rise in $PCO_2$ and fall in pH would be expected from the utilization of these stores. Exact quantitation is difficult but the data would suggest that placental insufficiency with respect to gas exchange might produce a maximum rise of $PCO_2$ of the order of 10-15 mmHg (1.5-2.0 kPa) and a fall in pH of 0.1 units. It follows therefore that a substantial fall of pH in the fetus cannot be an indication of a simple failure of respiratory gas exchange by the placenta but, rather, must indicate the occurrence of glycolysis in the fetal tissues. Since it is conceivable that $CO_2$ may diffuse from cells more rapidly than lactic acid, it is possible that the pH in the blood may fall more rapidly than the rise in blood lactic acid. The change in blood pH for a given production of lactic acid will also depend upon whether any placental function is present. In the absence of placental function the rise in $PCO_2$ and the consequent impairment of the buffering action of the bicarbonate system will allow a much larger change in pH than if transfer of $CO_2$ across the placenta had taken place. It is often considered that a severe acidosis associated with a rise in $PCO_2$ is less harmful to the fetus than the same acidosis with a normal $PCO_2$ but, in reality, the converse may apply because a high $PCO_2$ implies very poor placental function. From the above it follows that a fall in fetal pH can be regarded mainly as an indicator of the accumulation of lactic acid in fetal tissues but that quantitatively the relationship may vary. Additionally, the fetal arterial pH may have a value of its own in indicating whether damaging hydrogen ion concentrations have been reached in the tissues. In this context, it should perhaps be emphasized that there is, at present, little informaton about the relation between the intracellular and extracellular pH in tissues. This is particuarly the case in the fetus since there is a large contribution of lactic acid from the heart to the fetal blood. It is difficult to know therefore whether the arterial pH closely reflects the intracellular pH or even the extracellular pH in, for example cerebral tissue.

From the above, it would seem that hypoxanthine, lactic acid, and pH are not to be regarded as similar indices for hypoxia in the fetus. The ideal index of hypoxia would give a clear indication of whether damaging conditions were present in neural tissue since this tissue seems most susceptible to damage. None of the indices, unfortunately, can be regarded as reflecting conditions in this tissue, nor even as indicating when the fetal state is such that neural damage is imminent. Because of these difficulties it was decided to adopt an empirical approach and to measure all of these parameters simultaneously in the experimental animal under various hypoxic conditions and in the subsequent recovery period. If parameters behaved similarly then the choice of the most suitable parameters would depend upon the convenience and accuracy of the measurement. If, on the other hand, the parameters varied independently, then measurement of all parameters would be desirable at least until more clear-cut information becomes available about the significance of each to fetal well-being.

## Methods

Near-term Shropshire Clun or crossbred ewes were anaesthetized with a spinal anaesthetic (nupercaine) having withheld food but not water for the previous 24 hours (1). The animal was maintained in a semi-supine (deck chair) position and the fetus delivered by hysterotomy. Fetal breathing was prevented by covering the head with a bag of warm saline and catheters were placed in the fetal femoral artery and dorsalis pedis of the mother under local anaesthesia for blood sampling and for blood pressure and heart rate recording. An aliquot from each blood sample was spun immediately for assay of lactate and hypoxanthine. Blood pH, $PCO_2$ and $PO_2$ were determined with an IL 613 blood gas analyser. Plasma lactate was measured with an Analox LM 2 lactate analyser. Plasma hypoxanthine was determined by oxygen consumption on 50 μl samples using xanthine oxidase and an Analox GM6 analyser. This procedure, which is based upon that of Saugstad (5), determines hypoxanthine and xanthine together.

Hypoxia was produced a) by the administration of gas mixtures low in $O_2$ to the mother (10-11% $O_2$ ); $CO_2$ (1.2-1.7%) was added to these gas mixtures to maintain the $PCO_2$ of the mother relatively constant or b) by intermittent total occlusion of the cord. Intermittent total occlusion was used instead of partial occlusion to avoid fetal blood pooling in the venous system of the placenta with the consequent disturbance of the fetal circulation. Typically the cord was occluded for 1-minute periods with 2-4 minute recovery periods.

## Results

In five animals hypoxia was produced by low oxygen mixtures given to the mother and in five animals the cord was occluded. After an initial control period hypoxia was

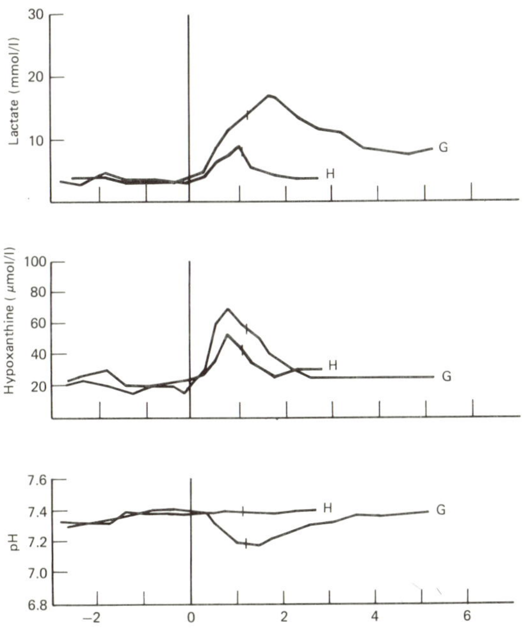


*Figure 1.* Plasma lactate and hypoxanthine, and blood pH values in exteriorized fetal sheep in which hypoxia was produced by intermittent cord occlusion. Five experiments were carried out. The data shown which were obtained from two of them (experiments G and H) were selected to illustrate specific points (*see text*). Hypoxia by intermittent cord occlusion commenced at the vertical line and terminated at the vertical bars in the individual records

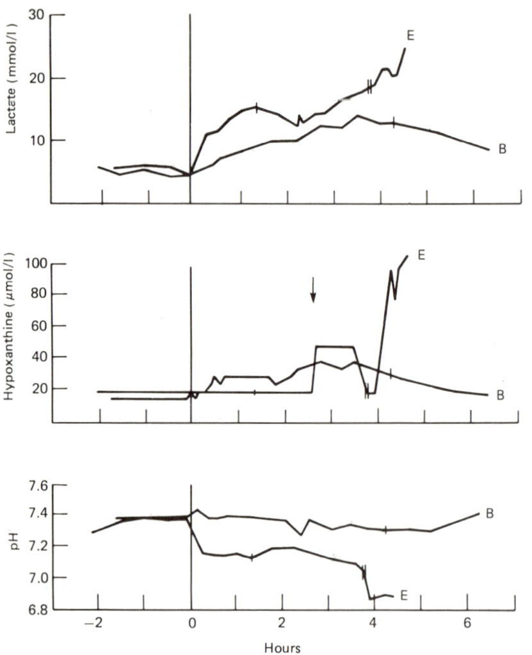


*Figure 2.* Plasma lactate and hypoxanthine, and blood pH in exteriorized fetal sheep that were submitted to hypoxia by administering gas mixtures low in $O_2$ to the mother. Five experiments were carried out. The data shown which were obtained from two animals (experiments B and E) were selected to illustrate specific points (*see text*). Hypoxia commenced at the vertical line and the termination of the hypoxia is indicated by the single vertical bars. The arrow on the record of experiment E indicates an infusion of hypoxanthine and the double bar indicates tying the cord

induced for a period which varied according to the condition of the preparation (1.3-3.1 h occlusion experiments; 0.9-1.3 h low $O_2$ experiments) and this was followed by a prolonged recovery period. A second gaseous hypoxia was then administered to some of the fetuses and in some the cord was tied.

In approximately one half of the experiments there was a reasonably good correlation between the behaviour of lactate, pH, and hypoxanthine although the plasma hypoxanthine returned to normal rather more rapidly than lactate after the termination of the hypoxia, as has been noted by others (6). To illustrate the general correlation that occurs, data from experiment G is shown in Figure 1. In the remaining experiments the parameters diverged from each other to a greater or less extent. Experiments showing a lack of correlation between the parameters were found both in the cord compression and low $O_2$ groups and there appeared to be no relationship to the method of inducing hypoxia.

A particular case in which lactate and pH were very poorly correlated is shown in experiment B (Figure 2). The moderately slow rise in lactate by about 9 mmol/l in this experiment was associated with virtually no change in pH. The failure of the pH to fall was not due to a concomitant fall in $PCO_2$ and must have been due to very effective buffering of the lactic acid produced. Since the rise in lactate took place over a period of 3.5 hours the possibility that some transplacental buffering may have taken place should be considered; this might possibly occur by a $Cl^-/HCO_3^-$ exchange mechanism. The converse, a relatively large change in pH with a relatively small change in lactate took place terminally in experiment E (Figure 2). This may be attributed to the relatively low $HCO_3^-$ at the time when the cord was tied and the lack of $CO_2$ transfer across the placenta which would impair the buffering by the bicarbonate system. The latter was reflected by a steep rise in blood $PCO_2$.

In five of the 10 experiments, lactate and hypoxanthine were well correlated in that both parameters rose together. However, there were considerable variations in the increment of hypoxanthine that was observed and in one experiment its concentration increased to over 200 μmol/l. In a sixth experiment (experiment C, Figure 2), there was no increment in hypoxanthine during the initial hypoxia despite a rapid increase in lactate and fall in pH. In this same experiment the converse was also shown, namely a rapid rise in hypoxanthine with relatively small rise in lactate, when the cord was tied terminally. This might have been due to the cessation of placental uptake of hypoxanthine. In the remaining four experiments the initial rise in hypoxanthine was not maintained and the concentration became constant or even fell while the lactate continued to rise. This is illustrated by experiment G (Figure 1).

Correspondingly, there was also a lack of correlation between pH and hypoxanthine in four of the 10 experiments. Extreme cases of this lack of correlation are shown in experiment H (Figure 1) and experiment E (initial hypoxia) (Figure 2). In the former there was a marked rise in hypoxanthine with no change in pH and conversely in the latter there was a marked fall in pH with no rise in hypoxanthine.

## Discussion

As discussed in the introduction, a substantial fall in fetal pH must indicate the occurrence of glycolysis in the fetal compartment but the magnitude of the fall in pH will depend upon whether $CO_2$ can cross the placenta and other factors. The relationship between pH and plasma lactate may also be affected by how rapidly lactic acid can leave the cells. A variable relationship between the fall of pH and the rise in lactate was therefore to be expected. However, the magnitude of the increase in plasma lactate that took place in some animals with little or no change in pH was unexpected. It may, as already discussed, indicate some transplacental buffering. From a practical point of view, however, it follows that in the fetal sheep lactate is a much more reliable and sensitive indicator of glycolysis than pH. Since lactate levels remain elevated for a long period after hypoxia, lactate also gives an indication of whether the fetus has suffered hypoxic episodes in the recent past. pH may possibly be of greater significance in determining whether damage to fetal tissues is occurring but, in the absence of definite information on this point, it might seem reasonable to assume that lactate levels substantially above control values (especially if rising) are an indication of conditions that are hazardous to the fetus.

If hypoxanthine is an indication that the 'energy change' is low in the fetal cells, then it might be expected that the rise in hypoxanthine would take place later than the rise in lactate. However, this was not the experimental finding. In about half the cases the rise in hypoxanthine followed the same pattern as lactate, although the magnitude of the rise in hypoxanthine was very variable and indeed in one animal there was no increase in the hypoxanthine. In the remaining experimental animals, the plasma hypoxanthine rose initially with the hypoxia but then failed to rise further or even fell despite a rising plasma lactate. Since hypoxanthine levels also fall more rapidly than lactate at the cessation of the hypoxia it would therefore appear that hypoxanthine is a less sensitive indicator of hypoxia than lactate. On the other hand hypoxanthine may have a particular significance in indicating serious depletion of ATP in the fetal cells. In this context it is possible that the fall in hypoxanthine that occurred in some of the animals despite a rising lactate was due to an elevation of glucose levels in the fetal circulation produced by the stress of the hypoxia. This could alleviate the depletion of ATP in the fetal cells thus leading to a fall in the hypoxanthine while the lactate levels would continue to rise.

From the above it seems clear that in a very substantial proportion of animals, the indices pH, lactate and hypoxanthine do not behave in the same way in hypoxia and that none of them can be regarded as an entirely satisfactory index of this condition. It seems probable that these general conclusions are also applicable to the human. In the management of fetal distress therefore it would seem desirable to monitor all of these variables and perhaps especially lactate. Nevertheless, it should be remembered that the placental structure in the human differs considerably from the sheep. If this should be reflected in differences in the permeability of the placenta to lactate, to buffers and perhaps hypoxanthine, there may be considerable quantitative differences between the species.

## References

1. Alexander D P, Beard R W, Britton H G, Fusi L, Redstone D and Walmsley M D. An evaluation of the tissue pH electrode for fetal monitoring using the fetal sheep as an experimental model. *American Journal of Obstetrics and Gynecology,* 140, 953-960 (1981).

2. Bird L I, Jones D M Jr, Simmons M A, Makowski E L, Meschia G and Battaglia F C. Placental production and fetal utilisation of lactate and pyruvate. *Nature,* 254, 710-711 (1975).

3. Britton H G, Nixon D A and Wright G H. The effects of acute hypoxia on the sheep fetus - some observations on recovery from hypoxia. *Biology of the Neonate,* 11, 277-301 (1967).

4. Dawes G S, Mott J C and Shelley H J. The importance of cardiac glycogen for the maintenance of life in foetal lambs and newborns animals during anoxia. *Journal of Physiology,* 146; 516-538 (1959).

5. Saugstad O D. The determination of hypoxanthine and xanthine with a $PO_2$ electrode. *Paediatric Research,* 9, 575-579 (1978).

6. Thiringer, K. Hypoxanthine as a measure of fetal asphyxia. University of Göteborg, Göteborg, Sweden (1982).

Chapter 10

# Apgar score and cord pH in relation to length of second stage

**S Alexander, F Cantraine and J Schwers**

## Introduction

For over a century (6), the second stage of labour has been considered to be a time of particular risk for the fetus. It has been shown (7) that perinatal mortality is increased when the duration of the second stage is long and, more recently, the importance of the gradual deterioration of fetal pH has been stressed (8,15). The aim of this study was to discover whether fetal heart rate recordings during the second stage could discriminate fetuses in jeopardy for those who do not require any assistance and for whom there is no benefit in intervention.

## Material and methods

During a 2-month period there were 172 deliveries of which 127, constituting a low risk group, were systematically investigated. These were term (37 to 41 completed weeks) singleton vaginal vertex deliveries with a normal course of pregnancy and normal first stage fetal heart rate recordings. Cases in which first stage fetal heart rate (FHR) showed decelerations, lack of reactivity or of variability were excluded.

FHR recordings during second stage were retrospectively analysed without knowledge of the patients' name or of the neonatal outcome. They were classified according to Melchior (11) (Figure 1). Normocardia (types 0 and 1) was considered normal. Bradycardia (types 2, 3 and 4) was considered pathological.

Cases were excluded if the trace was of poor quality or if the onset of second stage could not be defined (lack of vaginal examination describing full dilatation of the cervix when maternal urge to bear down began).

Cords were clamped immediately and umbilical arterial and venous samples were collected within 10 seconds in a heparinized syringe. They were immediately capped and immersed in crushed ice. Complete blood gas analysis was performed on a Corning 168 Blood Gas Analyser within less than 10 minutes. If the arteriovenous difference in pH was less than 2 mU the case was rejected.

This left 117 cases in the study and of these, 83 had normal second stage FHR (Melchior type 0 and 1) and 34 had pathological FHR (Melchior type 2, 3 and 4).

Apgar scores were carefully assessed by the midwives or paediatricians at 1, 5 and 10 minutes. There were no neonatal malformations, and in no case was the Apgar

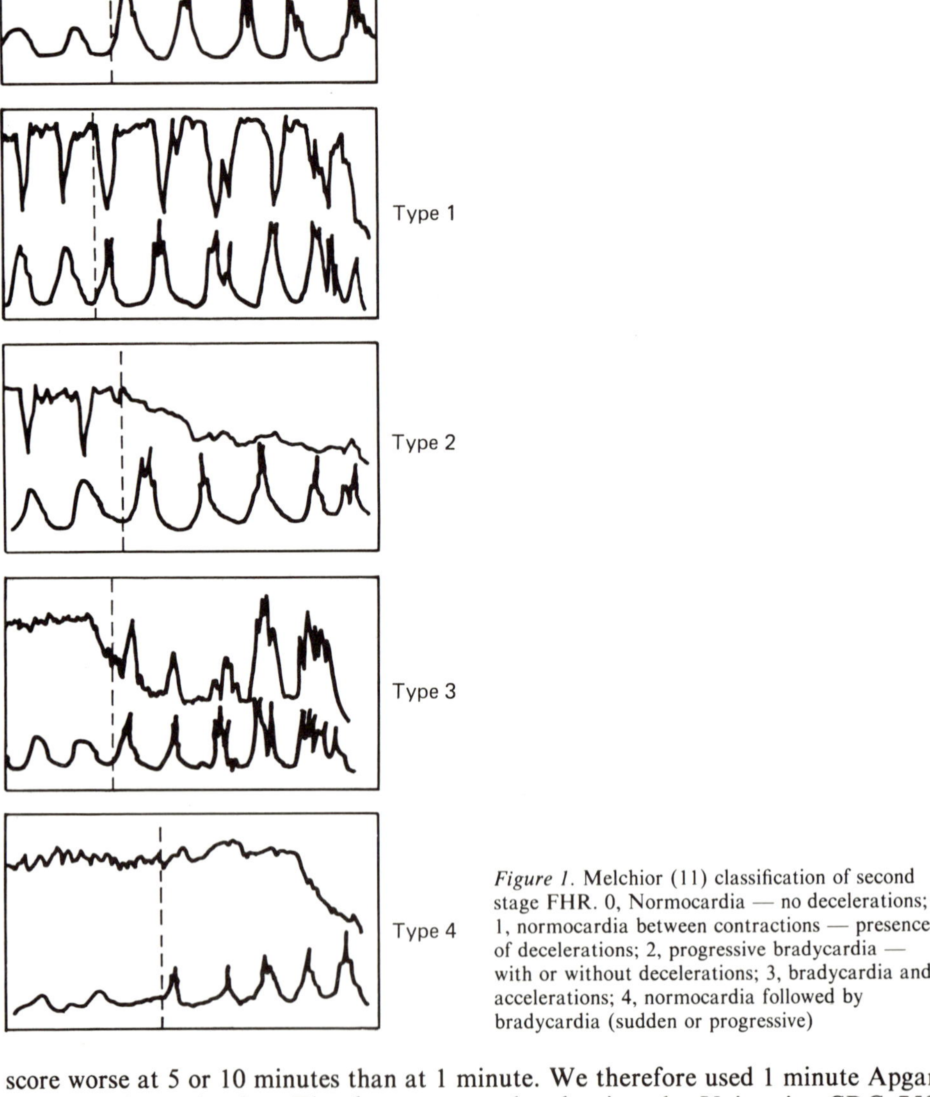


*Figure 1.* Melchior (11) classification of second stage FHR. 0, Normocardia — no decelerations; 1, normocardia between contractions — presence of decelerations; 2, progressive bradycardia — with or without decelerations; 3, bradycardia and accelerations; 4, normocardia followed by bradycardia (sudden or progressive)

score worse at 5 or 10 minutes than at 1 minute. We therefore used 1 minute Apgar scores in the evaluation. The data were analysed using the University CDC 759 computer and the SPSS package of the University of Brussels Computer Centre.

## Results

### Length of second stage

(Table 1) There was no difference between the two groups. All patients were pushing actively. The decision to accelerate second stage with instrumental extraction or

**TABLE 1. Analysis of second stage FHR according to Melchior (11) displayed two distinct groups in which fetal pH and the incidence of asphyxia were significantly different.**

| | *Group I* (n=83) *(normal FHR)* | *Group II* (n=34) *(pathological FHR)* | *Test* | *Significance* |
|---|---|---|---|---|
| Length of 2nd stage (minutes)* | 27±19 | 30±21 | t | NS |
| Arterial pH* | 7.26±0.6 | 7.21±0.7 | t | p=0.001 |
| Venous pH* | 7.31±0.6 | 7.27±0.7 | t | p<0.005 |
| Depressed neonates (Apgar<7 at 1 minute) | 8/83 | 9/34 | $X^2$ | p<0.005 |

*Results are mean ± s.d.
NS: not significant.

oxytocin was left to the discretion of the obstetrician. In a few cases, the second stage exceeded 90 minutes, although average duration was 27 ± 19 minutes in group I (normal second stage FHR) and 30 ± 21 minutes in group II (pathological second stage FHR).

## Cord blood pH

(Table 1) When FHR was abnormal, i.e. group II, both venous and arterial cord blood pH was lower than in group I. This difference was highly significant (p less than 0.001).

Umbilical artery pH was plotted against duration of second stage in the group with normal FHR: there was a weak (r=-0.22) but significant (p less than 0.05) negative correlation (Figure 2). The same negative correlation was observed between umbilical vein pH and duration of second stage. The correlation coefficient was again very low (r=-0.29) but significant (p less than 0.05). The slope of the regression line was 0.00078 for arterial pH and 0.00093 for venous blood pH. These weak correlation coefficients imply an average decrease in pH of 0.08 and 0.09 after 100 minutes.

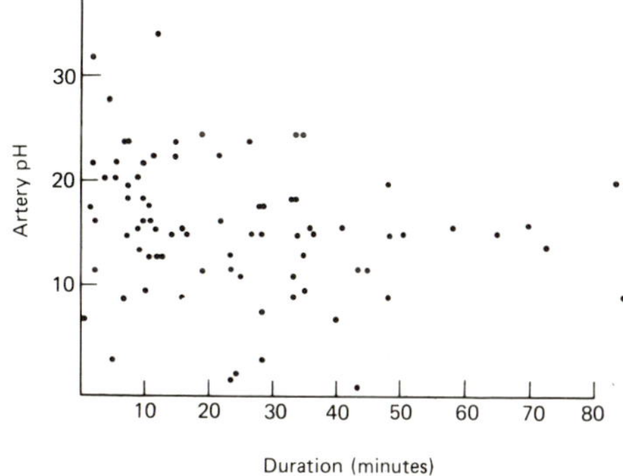


*Figure 2.* Scatter diagram of relation between duration of second stage and umbilical arterial pH in 83 patients with normal FHR. Two-tailed correlation test was performed: r = −0.22; p ⟨ 0.05; slope:−0.00078

In cases where fetal heart rate was abnormal (group II), there was no association between length of second stage and umbilical pH.

## Apgar score

Of the 83 neonates with normal second stage FHR, eight were born depressed (1 minute Apgar score less than 7), whereas of the 34 neonates with anomalies of second

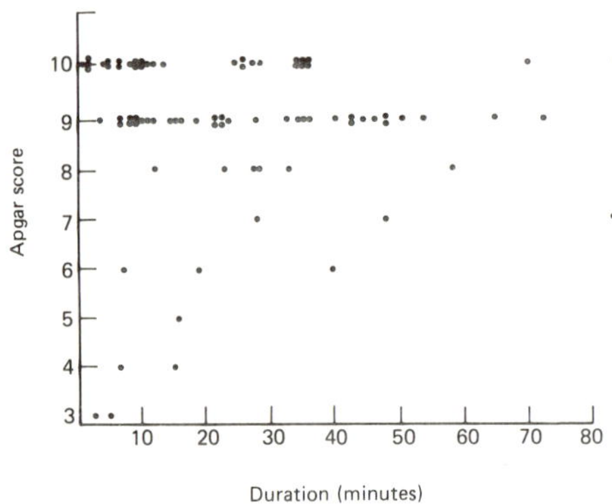


*Figure 3.* Scatter diagram of relation between duration of second stage and 1 minute Apgar score in 83 patients with normal FHR. No significant correlation was present

stage FHR, nine were depressed. The difference was significant ($\chi^2=4.2$, p less than 0.05).

Contrary to observations of pH, there was no tendency for Apgar score to decrease as the duration of second stage increased. No association was observed between length of second stage and Apgar score, whether traces were normal or pathological (Figure 3).

## Discussion

Although fetal heart rate has been extensively investigated during the first stage of labour, few reports have been specifically descriptive of the second stage. This may be partly due to the difficulty of defining the exact beginning of the second stage which has led certain authors to describe patterns during the last hour (3) or the last 10 minutes (5) before delivery.

There are also classification difficulties: 50-95% of recordings show decelerations of some kind (9); variability whether assessed clinically or with a computer, may be difficult to interpret and accelerations are often absent. Because of these problems, various authors, such as Gilstrap (5), Krebs (9), and Melchior (11) have suggested that second stage traces be classified according to the behaviour of the baseline. In this study we used Melchior's classification (Figure 1) because of its unambiguity in recognizing bradycardia with accelerations (type 3) from normocardia with decelerations (type 1).

As in other studies (3,5,9,11) the presence of fetal bradycardia was associated with increased risk of neonatal depression and asphyxia. In our group of low risk patients with normal first stage traces, there was no prediction of end stage deceleration and the likelihood of its appearing did not increase with duration of second stage.

There is much controversy concerning the length of the second stage and the necessity of speeding birth in the interest of the neonate. Arguments have been based on neonatal state as assessed by blood gas analysis or Apgar score. There has been agreement neither on the findings nor on their interpretation. A few prospective randomized studies have been performed, using cord blood pH as an indicator. Maresh (10) found no benefit for patients with epidural block in shortening the second stage. Other authors such as Wood (15) and Katz (8), in small series have concluded that there is a benefit in accelerating the second stage. Their main argument is the observation of a greater decrease in pH (difference between scalp pH at the beginning of second stage and cord artery pH) in the group with the longer second stage. Wood (15) describes a decrease in pH of 0.003 units/minute in his longitudinal study. In our transverse series of carefully selected patients, normal pregnancy, delivery and FHR trace, a slow decrease in pH was found in group I (normal second stage trace); although statistically significant, its clinical implication is highly questionable: a decrease in pH of 0.07 units after 100 minutes.

In group II (pathological second stage FHR traces), there was no association between length of second stage and neonatal condition; this may have been due to more frequent instrumental extraction or to the small number of patients in this group.

The exact significance of cord pH is not evident and although severe asphyxia is obviously to be avoided if possible, there are no arguments for believing that there is any advantage for a baby in being born with cord pH at 7.30 rather than 7.25.

Most follow-up studies have concentrated on the prognostic value of the Apgar score. Niswander (12) in a recent review of asphyxia and cerebral palsy in the fetus, suggests that chronic rather than acute asphyxia may be the culprit in causing brain injury.

Recent reports (13,14) have shown that neonatal asphyxia (low pH) has a poor relation to neonatal depression. This is in agreement with our findings.

No correlation was observed between Apgar score and length of second stage, neither in normal nor abnormal traces.

Our data are in good accordance with those reported by Cohen (4). In a survey of more than 4000 deliveries, he did not find an increase in perinatal mortality nor in low 1 minute Apgar score in long second stages with monitored patients. Furthermore, none of the prospective comparative studies (1,8,10,15) - whether they found a difference in pH between long and short pushers or not - has described a difference in Apgar score between their two groups.

The optimal management of second stage remains one of the most controversial issues in modern obstetric practice. Many publications which insist on shortening the second stage date from before modern methods of fetal monitoring and need to be reassessed. The more recent advocates of intervention at second stage mainly base their viewpoint on the decrease in pH as duration increases. This phenomenon has not been confirmed by all, but was observed in this investigation. Nevertheless it might simply reflect a similar decrease in maternal pH during expulsion (2) and its clinical and prognostic significance still remain to be investigated.

## References

1. Barnett M M and Humenick S S. Infant outcome in relation to second stage labour pushing method. *Birth*, 9, 221-228 (1982).

2. Benbassa A, Vinard J-L, Us seil C, Saien G, Minguet C and Malinas Y. Equilibre acido-base foetal et maternel pendant l'expulsion lors d'accouchements normaux. *Sociêtê Francaise de Mêdecine Pêrinatale*, 6, 369-372 (1976).

3. Bistoletti P, Lagercrants H and Lunell N-O. Correlations of fetal heart rate patterns with umbilical artery pH and catecholamines during last hour of labour. *Acta Obstetrica et Gynaecologica Scandinavica*, 59, 213-216 (1980).

4. Cohen W R. Influence of the duration of second stage labor on perinatal outcome and puerperal morbidity. *Obstetrics and Gynecology*, 49, 266-269 (1976).

5. Gilstrap L C III, Hauth J C and Toussaint S. Second stage fetal heart rate abnormalities and neonatal acidosis. *Obstetrics and Gynecology*, 63, 209-213 (1984).

6. Hamilton G. Classical observations and suggestions in obstetrics. *Edinburgh Medical Journal*, 7, 313-321 (1861).

7. Hellman L M and Prystowsky H. The duration of the second stage of labour. *American Journal of Obstetrics and Gynecology*, 63, 1223-1233 (1952).
8. Katz Z, Lancet M, Dgani R, Ben Hur H and Zalel Y. The beneficial effect of vacuum extraction on the fetus. *Acta Obstetrica et Gynaecologica Scandinavica*, 61, 337-340 (1982).
9. Krebs H B, Petres R E and Dunn L J. Fetal heart rate patterns in the second stage of labour. *American Journal of Obstetrics and Gynecology*, 140, 435-439 (1981).
10. Maresh M, Choong K-H and Beard R W. Delayed pushing with lumbar epidural in labour. *British Journal of Obstetrics and Gynaecology*, 90, 623-627 (1983).
11. Melchior J, Cavagna J-L and Bernard N. Le rythme cardial foetal pendant l'expulsion de l'accouchement normal. *Sociêtê Francaise de Mêdecine Pêrinatale*, 6, 225-232 (1976).
12. Niswander K R. Asphyxia is the fetus and cerebral palsy. *Year Book of Obstetrics and Gynecology*, 107-125 (1983).
13. Shaxted E J, Jenkins H M L and Maynard P V. Fetal pH. How accurate a guide to clinical condition? *Journal of Obstetrics and Gynecology*, 3, 247-248 (1983).
14. Sykes G, Molloy P M, Johnson P, Gu W, Ashworth F, Stirrat G M and Turnbull A C. Do Apgar scores indicate asphyxia? *Lancet*, 1, 494-496 (1982).
15. Wood C, Ng K H, Hounslow D and Benning H. Time - an important variable in normal delivery. *Journal of Obstetrics and Gynaecology of the British Commonwealth*, 80, 295-300 (1973).

Chapter 11

# *In vivo* observations on intravascular blood pressure in the fetus during mid-pregnancy

**B Castle, I Z Mackenzie**

## Introduction

Although erythroblastosis fetalis due to Rhesus iso-immunization has been considerably reduced by immunoglobulin prophylaxis, cases still occur. When severe in early pregnancy, treatment by intraperitoneal transfusions are usually unsuccessful. With the refining of fibreoptic equipment and the development of fetoscopy as a diagnostic and therapeutic tool, techniques of direct intravascular transfusion of the fetus have been explored with a view to improving prognosis for these severe cases (1,2,5). Experience to date of such techniques is limited but personal experience indicates that the response of the fetus to *in utero* intravascular transfusion is not predictable. This may be due to inappropriate techniques used in the transfusion procedure or due to fetal cardiovascular decompensation. In an attempt to advance development of *in utero* transfusions and to assess fetal condition, the basic physiological measurements of blood pressure during mid-pregnancy have been made.

## Patient details

Sixteen patients at 18-21 weeks' gestation admitted for induction of abortion with intra-amniotic prostaglandins have been studied. Thirteen terminations were for maternal reasons, in one the fetus was at risk of Duchenne's muscular dystrophy, one had Downs' syndrome and one had proven spina bifida. All patients gave informed signed consent to the investigation and support from the Local Hospital Ethical Committee had been given to the principle of fetoscopic research involving fetal blood sampling procedures.

Maternal pre-medication with papavaretum, 20 mg intramuscularly, was given 1-2 hours prior to fetoscopy and diazepam, 5 mg intravenously, was injected 5-10 minutes before instrumentation. Following ultrasound examination, local anaesthetic was infiltrated into the designated site in the anterior abdominal wall. Fetoscopy was performed using a Storz fetoscope, no 63200C with a 30° forward oblique viewing telescope. The fetal vessel was entered using a 350 mm long needle with a 21 gauge shaft and a 3 mm long 26 gauge tip (3). In all cases, the umbilical cord was located at a convenient place along its length and the umbilical vein and one of the umbilical arteries, in either order, were punctured. Once a free flow of blood was confirmed, the needle was cleared with 0.3 ml normal saline. The mean intravascular pressure was recorded on a heated-wire pen recorder (Devices), by connecting the needle to a fluid-filled catheter and pressure transducer (Type 4/422: Physiology pressure transducer, Bell and Howell, Basingstoke). Aliquots of the blood aspirated from the umbilical artery and/or vein were subsequently analysed for blood gas values (Mackenzie *et al*, see p 156) to confirm the correct designation of the vessel being studied.

In three cases following initial pressure recordings, small volumes of blood were injected into the fetal circulation (2) and a further pressure recording was made.

On completion of the clinical observations, prostaglandin $E_2$ was injected intra-amniotically via the fetoscope to induce abortion. In all instances a routine post-abortion fetal examination was performed and the fetus weighed. Where possible, the placental weight was recorded if expulsion had been spontaneous and complete.

## System validation

Prior to the clinical studies, a computerized analysis of the pressure and frequency response capability of the pressure recording system was made. The tip of the recording needle was inserted into a fluid-filled chamber with an oscillating diaphragm at the base generating the pressure signals. The chamber was connected to a stepped-down Quartz frequency generator and the response to a known frequency input was measured on both sides of the system.

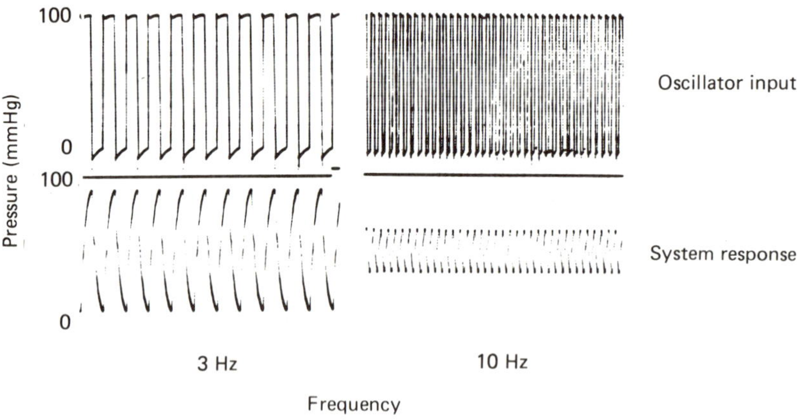


*Figure 1.* Pressure/frequency response capability of the pressure recording system

Figure 1 illustrates the generated waveform and the wave response recorded through the needle. The computerized plot of the waveform characteristic was good. Calculated attenuation was 16% at 3 Hz rising to 30% at 10 Hz. In spite of this limited bandwidth, the system is clearly capable of measuring mean blood pressure.

## Results

Table 1 lists the mean corrected arterial and venous pressures together with the range. (Corrected = intravascular pressure - intra-amniotic pressure.) Also shown are the

**TABLE 1. Cord arterial and venous pressures and intra-amniotic pressures measured during mid-pregnancy.**

| | *Mean (±s.d.)* | *Range* | *n* |
|---|---|---|---|
| Corrected arterial pressure* (mmHg) | 15.2±6.0 | 6.5–26.5 | 13 |
| Corrected venous pressure* (mmHg) | 2.2±1.7 | 0–5.0 | 15 |
| Intra-amniotic pressure (mmHg) | 6.7±3.8 | 2–15 | 16 |
| Gestational age (weeks) | 19.1±0.8 | 18–21 | 16 |
| Fetal weight (g) | 235±79 | 144–424 | 16 |

*See text.

mean, standard deviation, and ranges for intra-amniotic pressures. In 12 cases when both arterial and venous pressures were recorded, the mean AV ratio was 2.7 (range 1.9 - 4.4). In all but one case, the venous pressure was 0.5 - 5 mmHg above the intra-amniotic pressure; in one instance the two values were identical. Figure 2 illustrates a typical series of pressure recordings made in one subject at 19 weeks' gestation. There was no significant correlation between gestation and arterial pressure (r = 0.3657, 10 d.f., p = 0.167) or venous pressure (r = 0.4521, 13 d.f., p = 0.091). Similarly, there was no correlation between fetal weight and arterial pressure (r = 0.186, 10 d.f., p = 0.563) and venous pressure (r = 0.389, 13 d.f., p = 0.151). In eight cases where placental weight was available, there was no correlation with intravascular pressures.

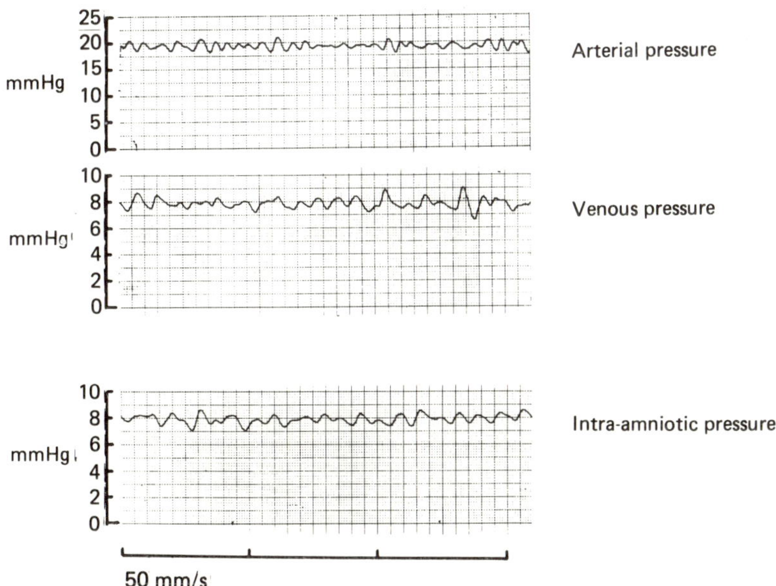


*Figure 2.* Umbilical arterial and venous pressures and intra-amniotic pressures at 19 weeks' gestation

In the three fetuses subjected to direct intravascular transfusion, marked rises in pressures occurred. Intra-arterial transfusion of 10 ml blood at 1 ml per minute into a 424 g fetus with an estimated circulating blood volume of 69 ml (4) (a 14.5% increase in volume) produced a 30% rise in mean arterial pressure (20 to 27 mmHg). The second fetus transfused intra-arterially with 10 ml of blood weighed 179 g with an estimated circulating volume of 29 ml (a 34.5% increase in volume). This produced a 120% rise in mean arterial pressure (9 to 20 mmHg). In the only fetus transfused intravenously, 10 ml of blood was transfused into a 187 g fetus with an estimated circulating blood volume of 30 ml (a 33% volume increase), producing a rise of 170% in intravenous pressure (5 to 13.5 mmHg).

## Discussion

The *in vitro* validation of the system for recording intravascular pressures suggested that the technique was capable of achieving reliable reproducible results for mean blood pressure measurement. The precise effect that the resting uterine (intra-amniotic) pressure has upon the intravascular pressure in vessels in the umbilical cord is not certain. In chronically catheterized animal models, electronic subtraction of the intra-amniotic pressure from the intra-arterial pressure is performed to give the corrected arterial pressure. Owing to the limitations of the technique used in the present study, this could not be done. However, subtraction of the intra-amniotic from intravascular pressures that were measured will give an indication of the true intravascular pressures. This does, however, indicate that cord venous pressures in the present study were generally less than 5 mmHg which is lower than might be expected in the absence of changes in fetal intrathoracic pressures.

The pressure measurements obtained in the current work are lower than those extrapolated from neonatal values recorded following both term and preterm delivery (7). Similarly, they are lower than the values reported in the human during fetal exteriorization at hysterotomy at similar gestational ages (6). There must, however, be some doubt as to the legitimacy of extrapolation of blood pressure recordings made in the neonate following delivery, since parturition in most instances results in conversion from a fetal to adult circulation. Also, in many cases, values recorded in preterm neonates would, in general, be associated with the presence of some pathology which either precipitated the need for preterm delivery or necessitated blood pressure monitoring. Of equal importance is the influence of the intact fetal circulation including the placental circulation in our mid-pregnancy observations which no longer exists following birth. It is probable that the placenta contains half the fetoplacental circulating blood volume and additionally, it may act as a large arterio-venous shunt. Similar doubts exist as to the effect upon the blood flow and blood pressure of the exteriorization of the fetus at hysterotomy (6). One final consideration is the difference in pressure recording sites which could influence results; in the present series pressures were measured in the umbilical vessels compared with carotid artery pressures measured in the exteriorized hysterotomy cases, while in the neonate catheterization of a central vessel such as the aorta is generally used.

Changes in blood pressure associated with intravascular transfusions indicate that the immediate effect is to produce a rise of 30 - 170% in intravascular pressures in the cord, the increase depending upon the volume transfused according to fetal size and circulating blood volume. There does not appear to be any difference in response whether the umbilical vein or an umbilical artery is used for transfusion. The resultant intravascular pressure changes produced by direct intravascular transfusion indicate that there are considerable circulatory disturbances produced. Relative to fetal size, however, the volumes transfused were large and the transfusion rate was rapid, probably causing acute fluid overload. It is uncertain what part the placental bed plays in circulatory volumetric compensation *in utero* . We have only observed acute changes rather than any chronic adaptation and with such small numbers, our conclusions are as yet very preliminary.

With the collection of data on the fetus *in utero* under minimally disturbed conditions, it may now be possible to assess more accurately the state of the fetus during pregnancies complicated by various conditions such as erythroblastosis fetalis. Further, it may allow a more logical approach to *in utero* transfusions of the fetus with resulting improved survival chances.

## Acknowledgements

The authors acknowledge the expert nursing care and technical assistance provided by Sister Jane Ferguson and the post-abortal examinations by Dr Jean Keeling and Miss Sheila Moore.

## References

1. Bang J, Beck J and Trolle D. Ultrasound-guided fetal intravenous transfusion for severe rhesus haemolytic disease. *British Medical Journal*, 284, 373-374 (1982).
2. MacKenzie I Z *et al.* Midtrimester intrauterine exchange transfusion of the fetus. *American Journal of Obstetrics and Gynecology*, 143, 555-559 (1982).
3. MacKenzie I Z and MacLean D A. Pure fetal blood from the umbilical cord obtained at fetoscopy. Experience of 125 consecutive cases. *American Journal of Obstetrics and Gynecology*, 138, 1214 (1980).
4. Morris J A, Hustead R F, Robinson R G and Haswell G L. Measurement of feto-placental blood volume in the human pre-viable fetus. *American Journal of Obstetrics and Gynecology*, 118, 927 (1984).
5. Rodeck C H *et al.* Direct intravascular fetal blood transfusion by fetoscopy in severe rhesus iso-immunisation. *Lancet*, 1, 625-627 (1981).
6. Rudolf A M, Heyman M A, Teramo K A W *et al.* Studies on the circulation of the pre-viable human fetus. *Paediatric Research*, 5, 452 (1971).
7. Versmold H T, Kitternan J N, Phibbs R H, Gregory G A and Tooley W H. Aortic blood pressure during the first 12 hours of life in infants with birth weight 610-4220 g. *Pediatrics*, 67, 607-613 (1981).

Chapter 12

# Interpretation of amniotic fluid measurements by means of some multivariate methods

**R Martino, C Velussi, P Grella, V Martino, G de Toffoli Konishi**

## Introduction

The variations which occur in physiological conditions in the amniotic fluid towards the end of pregnancy (weeks 30-40) are better known and studied than are those of the first half of pregnancy. This is because samples of amniotic fluid (amniocentesis) are taken mostly in order to check the maturation of the fetus, maturation that quite obviously is attained near the conclusion of intrauterine life.

However, the ever-increasing use of amniocentesis to assess the presence of congenital malformations in the fetus in the second quarter of pregnancy now makes it possible to observe variations in the composition of amniotic fluid in this period, and these variations may be assessed to see if they have a clinical significance. There are many variables which can be investigated, some of which are intrinsic (related to the composition and structure of amniotic fluid) and others extrinsic (parameters related to sample-taking and the women under examination). The study has to take into account all of these variables in order to detect reliably those which indicate significant variations with the growth of the fetus, and which may therefore be useful as indicators of fetal evolution.

The univariate statistical approach cannot be used with these dynamic properties of amniotic fluid and we therefore adopted the multivariate approach (1,3,4,5).

## Materials

The amniotic fluid was obtained by a transabdominal amniocentesis in 35 pregnant women, between weeks 16 and 28 of pregnancy. The procedure was performed because there was a suspicion of congenital malformation. However, in all cases there was no such malformation observable at birth. In other words, all the newborns were in fact normal.

The average volume of amniotic fluid collected was 25 ml. In some cases the fluid was contaminated by the presence of maternal blood but in no case by fetal blood. The contamination is in itself considered as a descriptive variable (even though the variation is minimal). The sample of amniotic fluid was maintained at -20°C until the physical analysis was finally performed. The period of time at -20°C was also entered as 'input datum'.

# Methods

The physical variables considered in our work included density, surface tension, refractive index, osmolality and alpha-fetoproteins. These are discussed below.

### Density

This was determined by means of: (a) a picnometer with an internal volume of 5 $cm^3$ because of the low quantity of amniotic fluid available; (b) a thermostatic bath; and (c) a precision balance.

All measurements were carried out at 37°C, with weighing of the picnometer: (a) full of air; (b) full of distilled water; and (c) full of amniotic fluid.

### Surface tension

The surface tension was determined, after having thermostated the samples at 37°C, by means of a Cenco-Du Nouy Interfacial Tensiometer mod. 70545 which was housed on an antivibration table. This instrument uses a thin torsion wire to apply the necessary force required to pull a platinum-iridium ring (6 cm in diameter) from the surface of the test liquid. Attached to the torsion head is a graduated dial with a vernier which permits a direct reading of the applied force with a resolution of 0.1 dyne. The containers had a 4.5 cm diameter and the liquid filled them to a level of approximately 6 mm (10 $cm^3$). Because we noticed that the apparent surface tension indicated on the tensiometer's scale differed from that obtained with an absolute method (for example with a stalagmometer), we applied a correction factor to the results obtained. This correction factor was calculated using the Zuidema and Waters formula (8).

### Refractive index

The instrument used to measure the refractive index was a Bertuzzi-Unirefrax refractometer. The instrument was connected to a thermostating apparatus set at 37°C and exposed to a yellow monochromatic light source (sodium vapour lamp).

This instrument is constructed from a system of Abbe's prisms and of a scale which is graduated in thousandths from nD 1300 to nD 1700. There was the possibility of estimating to a few fractions of thousandths. In order to determine the refractive index it is merely necessary to place a few drops of amniotic fluid, at 37°C, on the inferior prism of the apparatus and to close the prism carrier. The reading which follows is fast, easy and precise.

### Osmolality

The instrument used to determine the osmolality was a Vogel Digital Micro-osmometer. This apparatus gives the osmolality of biological fluids using the cryoscopic method, that is by measuring the freezing point of a solution. This method is simpler, faster and more precise than others (such as the determination of vapour tension or a membrane's osmotic pressure) provided that one operates within a rather short range of values. The sample (100 $\mu$l) was placed in a plastic cuvette which is cooled by means of a Peltier element. During the cooling, the temperature is accurately measured because the cuvette is an integral part of the measuring head. During the first phase the sample reaches an 'overcooling' temperature without freezing, and at this stage a cold needle is introduced into the sample which initiates the freezing process. This technique has good reproducibility because the freezing process is almost instantaneous; it is also preferable to other systems which utilize shakers (agitators). Furthermore, the digital display allows a direct reading of the measurements in Osm/kg $H_2O$ since there is a linear relationship between the osmolality and the lowering of the freezing point (6).

## Alpha-fetoproteins

The quantitative determination of alpha-fetoproteins in the amniotic fluid was conducted with the radio-immunological method after standard sample dilution (1 to 100) by means of a Biodata Kit (7).

**TABLE 1. Primary data matrix.**

| | *PWAGE* | *PWEEK* | *AFSAG* | *DENS* | *R.IND* | *OSM* | *SURFT* | *αFPC* | *AFSCO* |
|---|---|---|---|---|---|---|---|---|---|
| S01 | 44 | 19 | 15 | 1.001394 | 1.3343 | 270 | 47.43 | 6367.199 | 4 |
| S02 | 47 | 18 | 8 | 1.002814 | 1.3343 | 270 | 54.15 | 17865 | 1 |
| S03 | 23 | 26.5 | 1 | 1.003035 | 1.334 | 243 | 49.07 | 1039 | 1 |
| S04 | 39 | 16 | 1 | 1.002434 | 1,334 | 274 | 51.31 | 30391 | 1 |
| S05 | 41 | 17.5 | 46 | 1.003047 | 1.335 | 266 | 54.34 | 8669 | 1 |
| S06 | 30 | 17.5 | 39 | 0.997309 | 1.3352 | 295 | 53.29 | 22422 | 1 |
| S07 | 29 | 18 | 39 | 1.002987 | 1.3351 | 256 | 53.36 | 18281 | 2 |
| S08 | 29 | 21.5 | 82 | 1.00018 | 1.3353 | 256 | 49.08 | 7968.797 | 2 |
| S09 | 32 | 16 | 39 | 1.003666 | 1.3353 | 270 | 54.64 | 16211 | 1 |
| S10 | 32 | 20 | 82 | 1.00148 | 1.3362 | 266 | 54.16 | 8671.898 | 1 |
| S11 | 38 | 18 | 25 | 1.00574 | 1.3352 | 266 | 52.28 | 11113 | 1 |
| S12 | 24 | 17 | 18 | 1.00215 | 1.3351 | 269 | 51.12 | 10010 | 1 |
| S13 | 31 | 16 | 11 | 0.999688 | 1.335 | 274 | 53.47 | 17656 | 1 |
| S14 | 31 | 18 | 63 | 1.001183 | 1.3358 | 258 | 54.25 | 5410 | 3 |
| S15 | 39 | 16 | 11 | 1.003166 | 1.3358 | 273 | 50.73 | 13594 | 1 |
| S16 | 39 | 19 | 63 | 1.001622 | 1.336 | 271 | 52.98 | 13594 | 2 |
| S17 | 41 | 16 | 9 | 1.001123 | 1.3353 | 276 | 53.37 | 8847.699 | 1 |
| S18 | 27 | 17 | 2 | 1.002322 | 1.336 | 262 | 52.59 | 18984 | 1 |
| S19 | 29 | 28 | 16 | 1.00098 | 1.3358 | 260 | 52.98 | 14961 | 1 |
| S20 | 41 | 17 | 9 | 1.000064 | 1.3353 | 276 | 54.26 | 12617 | 1 |
| S21 | 41 | 21 | 16 | 1.002391 | 1.3363 | 273 | 47.81 | 2418 | 3 |
| S22 | 24 | 17 | 2 | 1.000666 | 1.3358 | 267 | 53.28 | 11406 | 1 |
| S23 | 24 | 21 | 7 | 1.001967 | 1.336 | 269 | 49.46 | 5800 | 2 |
| S24 | 25 | 20 | 78 | 0.999984 | 1.3353 | 245 | 55.93 | 22656 | 1 |
| S25 | 42 | 18 | 7 | 1.000967 | 1.3356 | 269 | 55.04 | 10859 | 1 |
| S26 | 39 | 17 | 16 | 1.00099 | 1.3353 | 272 | 55.04 | 11406 | 2 |
| S27 | 38 | 18 | 30 | 1.000031 | 1.3353 | 228 | 56.12 | 11797 | 1 |
| S28 | 38 | 22 | 3 | 1.001967 | 1.336 | 276 | 52.39 | 3672 | 2 |
| S29 | 44 | 18 | 24 | 1.001567 | 1.3356 | 273 | 55.72 | 10527 | 1 |
| S30 | 42 | 17 | 24 | 1.001087 | 1.3356 | 278 | 56.81 | 12031 | 1 |
| S31 | 40 | 17 | 30 | 1.000651 | 1.3356 | 266 | 55.83 | 12246 | 1 |
| S32 | 39 | 17 | 3 | 1.001487 | 1.3356 | 270 | 54.35 | 11875 | 1 |
| S33 | 40 | 17 | 3 | 1.001667 | 1.3363 | 257 | 55.53 | 10586 | 1 |
| S34 | 44 | 19 | 23 | 1.00071 | 1.336 | 267 | 53.76 | 11133 | 1 |
| S35 | 39 | 18.5 | 9 | 1.001371 | 1.336 | 272 | 51.71 | 14961 | 1 |

PWAGE = Pregnant woman age (years)
PWEEK = Pregnancy week
AFSAG = AF sample ageing (days)
DENS = Density
R.IND = Refractive index
OSM = Osmolality (mOsm/kg)
SURFT = Surface tension (dyne/cm)
αFPC = α-fetoprotein concentration (ng/ml)
AFSCO = AF sample contamination (dimensionless)

## Multivariate statistical approach

In order to determine whether or not the structural variations of amniotic fluid relate to the gestational period, we have used two groups of amniotic fluid samples, sufficiently separate from a chronological point of view (about week 16 and week 22 of pregnancy).

From the primary data matrix (Table 1) we have chosen rows S04, S09, S12, S13, S15, S17, S18, S20, S22, S26, S30, S31, S32, and S33 for the first group (G1 or I), related to the amniotic fluid samples of week 16 or 17 of pregnancy and rows S03, S08, S10, S19, S21, S23, S24 and S28 for the second group (G2 or II), related to

**TABLE 2. Standard Student's test result.**

| *Variables* | *Sizes* | *Means* | *s.e.* | *Groups* |
|---|---|---|---|---|
| 1 PWAGE | 14 | 35.5714 | 1.75635 | <17 Weeks |
| | 8 | 30.125 | | >20 Weeks |
| | DF=20 | T=1.872 | p~0.0729 | |
| 2 PWEEK | 14 | 16.6428 | 0.13289 | <17 Weeks |
| | 8 | 22.5 | 1.07321 | >20 Weeks |
| | DF=20 | T=−7.182 | p~0 | *** |
| 3 AFSAG | 14 | 12.7142 | 3.09631 | <17 Weeks |
| | 8 | 35.625 | 13.3295 | >20 Weeks |
| | Df=20 | T=−2.138 | p~0.0428 | * |
| 4 DENS | 14 | 1.00151 | 3E-04 | <17 Weeks |
| | 8 | 1.0015 | 3.8E-04 | >20 Weeks |
| | Df=20 | T=0.02 | p~1 | |
| 5 R.IND | 14 | 1.33543 | 1.4E-04 | <17 Weeks |
| | 8 | 1.33561 | 2.7E-04 | >20 Weeks |
| | DF=20 | T=−0.653 | p~0.5275 | |
| 6 OSM | 14 | 270.285 | 1.55284 | <17 Weeks |
| | 8 | 261 | 4.3589 | >20 Weeks |
| | DF=20 | T=2.417 | p~0.024 | * |
| 7 SURFT | 14 | 53,7378 | 0.49008 | <17 Weeks |
| | 8 | 51.36 | 1.027 | >20 Weeks |
| | DF=20 | T=2.367 | p~0.0266 | * |
| 8 αFPC | 14 | 14132.9 | 1468.79 | <17 Weeks |
| | 8 | 8398.33 | 2555.18 | >20 Weeks |
| | DF=20 | T=2.101 | p~0.0461 | * |
| 9 AFSCO | 14 | 1.07143 | 0.07143 | <17 Weeks |
| | 8 | 1.625 | 0.26305 | >20 Weeks |
| | DF=20 | T=−2.549 | p~0.0182 | * |

*=Simple significance ($p<0.05$); **=High significance ($p<0.01$); ***=Very high significance ($p\ll0.01$).

PWAGE = Pregnant woman age (years)
PWEEK = Pregnancy week
AFSAG = AF sample ageing (days)
DENS = Density
R.IND = Refractive index
OSM = Osmolality (mOsm/kg)
SURFT = Surface tension (dyne/cm)
αFPC = α-feto-protein concentration (ng/ml)
AFSCO = AF sample contamination (dimensionless)

samples of weeks 20, 21 and 28. The standard Student's *t* test applied to these groups gave the results shown in Table 2. We have compared the two groups by simple linear discriminant function analysis, which consists of finding a transform which gives the minimum ratio of the difference between a pair of group multivariate means to the multivariate variance within the two groups.

By using four variables (labelled OSM, SURFT, $\alpha$FPC and AFSCO) we obtained a very strong separation between the two multivariate means (expressed in units of the pooled variance). With six variables (DENS, R.IND and the previous four) we obtained only good separation, but a more precise classification (Figure 1). The Andrew's plotting procedure, preceded by principal component analysis, demonstrated that members of group II have stronger variability than those in group I (Figure 2).

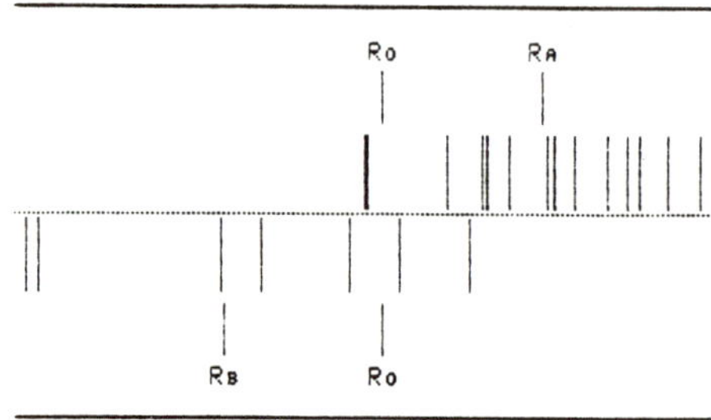


Group I, 16th – 17th week
Group II, 20th – 28th week
Variables : OSM, SURFT, $\alpha$FPC, AFSCO

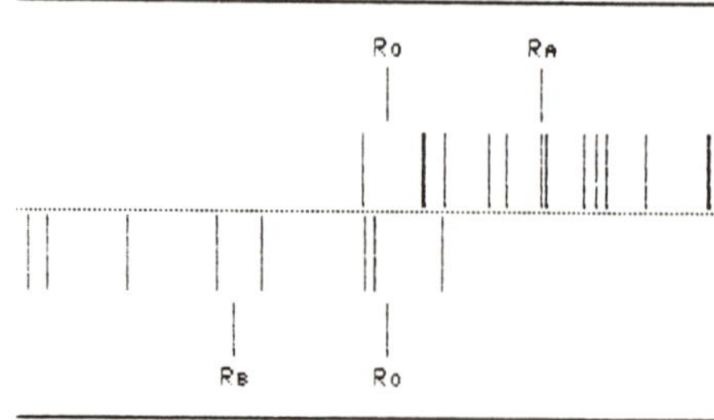


Group I, 16th – 17th week
Group II, 20th – 28th week
Variables : DENS, R.IND, OSM, SURFT, $\alpha$FPC, AFSCO

*Figure 1*. Projection of samples (group I and II) onto discriminant function line. $R_A$ = projection of multivariate mean of group I; $R_B$ = projection of multivariate mean of group II

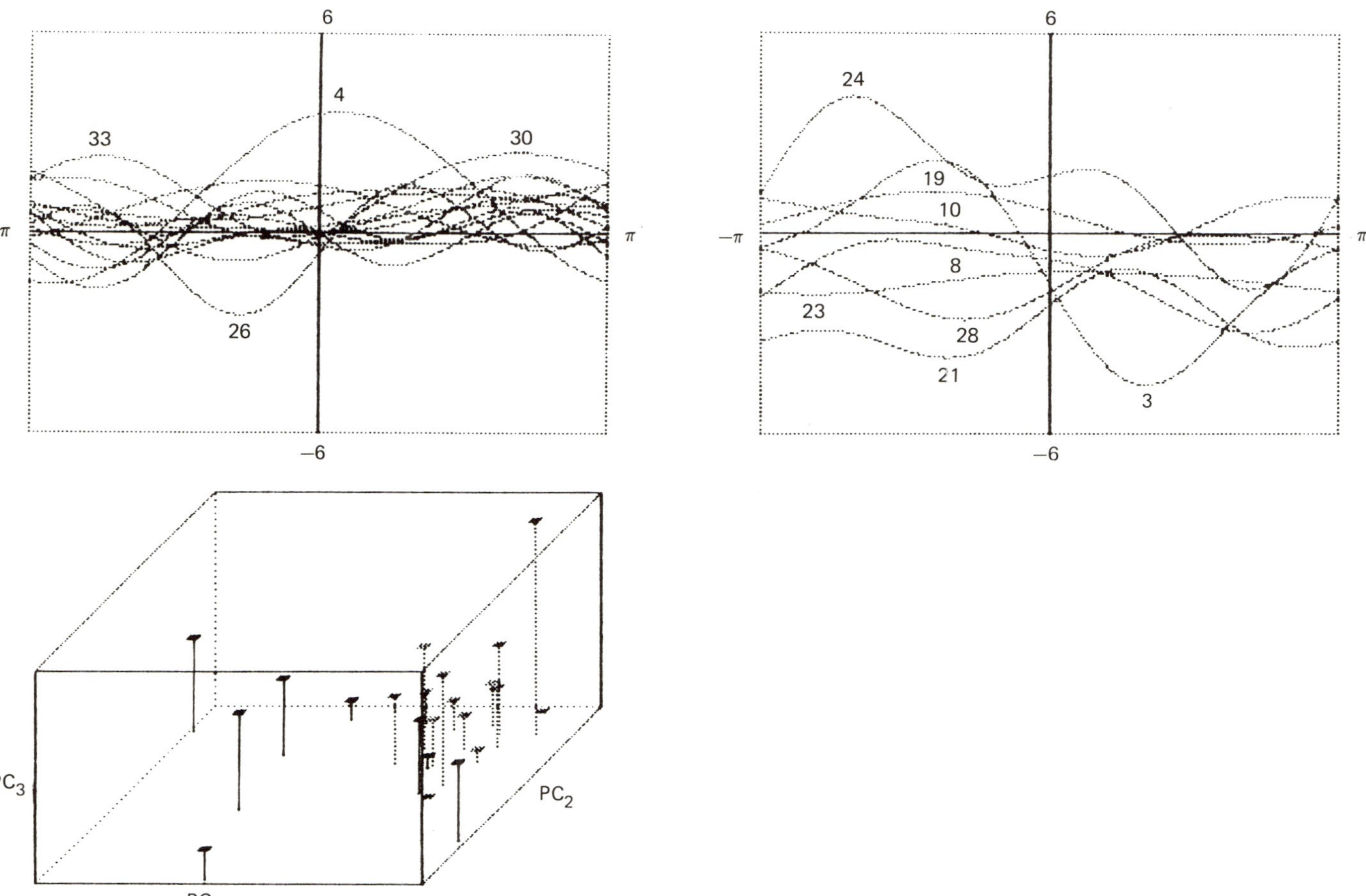


*Figure 2.* Andrews' diagrams: left, for group I (⟨17 weeks); right, for group II (⟩ 20 weeks). Cartesian space of the first 3 principal components (PC) relative to input data (variables: OSM, SURFT, $\alpha$FPC, AFSCO). Grey symbols, elements of group I, black symbols elements of group II

This fact only confirms what was to be expected, because in later phases of the gestational period the differentiation mechanisms greatly accentuate themselves.

## Discussion and conclusions

Our work demonstrates that it is useful to perform physical measurements on the amniotic fluid, because, first, the measurements are fast, easy, precise and inexpensive, and, secondly, they are able to give us a satisfactory picture of the fetal evolution through the detectable variations of amniotic fluid composition and structure. We were rather sceptical as to the possibility of the amniotic fluid giving any relevant information because earlier work based only on viscosity measurement gave poorly discriminating results (2). However, the above-mentioned quartet (OSM, SURFT, $\alpha$FPC and AFSCO) appears to be a promising indicator of fetal maturation and we now intend to use the same or similar technology for normal and pathological groups.

## References

1. Andrews D F. Plots of high-dimensional data. *Biometrics*, 28, 125-136 (1972).
2. Bauer R, Martino R and Velussi C. Low-shear rotational rheometry for special biofluids. In Proceedings of the International Conference, *Applications of Physics to Medicine and Biology*, Miramare, Trieste, IAEA, UNESCO (1982).
3. Davies R G. *Computer Programming in Quantitative Biology*, London, Adademic Press (1971).
4. Marriott F H C. *The Interpretation of Multiple Observations*, London, Academic Press (1974).
5. Martino R, Velussi C, Bettini V and Zampirollo P. Plots of 5-dimensional haemorheological data and statistical considerations. *Clinical Haemorheology*, 3, 248 (1982).
6. Natelson S, Scommegna A and Epstein M B. *Amniotic Fluid*. New York, John Wiley (1974).
7. Sandler M (editor). *Amniotic Fluid and its Clinical Significance*, New York and Basel, Marcel Dekker (1981).
8. Zuidema and Waters Formula. *Industrial and Engineering Chemistry*, 13, 312 (1941).

Chapter 13

# Fetal head compression during the second stage of labour: a new measuring method

**Leif Svenningsen and Øystein Jensen**

## Introduction

Fetal head compression resulting in elevated intracranial pressure has been considered by several authors as an important factor in cerebral birth trauma (1, 4, 5, 8-11, 14). Measurement of the *de facto* intracranial pressure cannot be performed in the human fetus, but measurement of the compressing forces on the fetal head during its passage through the birth canal provides an indirect means of estimating the fetal stress.

Electronic methods for measuring the compression and traction forces of instrumental delivery have been described (5, 11) and a transducer device that measures the cervix-to-head pressure during the first stage of labour has been presented (7, 8), but for measurement during the second stage of labour we have found no suitable device described. We present here a new compression transducer which gives reliable information about the compressive force on the fetal head as labour progresses, and which withstands all the strains of the second stage of labour.

## Materials and methods

### The compression measuring system

The 6.5 mm thick and 18 mm diameter compression transducer assembly shown in Figure 1 is built around a special version of a pressure transducer manufactured by Aksjeselskapet Mikro-elektronikk (AME), Horten, Norway. The silicone rubber encapsulated transducer element functions as a load-cell measuring deflection of its membrane due to load application on the silicone rubber top. The deflection is converted to a resistance variation in two piezo-resistive elements buried in a silicon beam linked to the membrane through a sapphire-tipped screw. A Wheatstone bridge is completed by two external passive resistors. A differential voltage signal proportional to the applied load (force or pressure) can thus be read from the bridge. The low-level signal is amplified in a special purpose amplifier and recorded on a conventional strip-chart recorder.

Referring to the lettered parts of Figure 1, the pressure transducer element (h) is glued to the polished brass backplate (f), which is rounded with a 50 mm radius. The sensitive side of the assembly is encapsulated in a silicone rubber top (g) (type Tait, manufactured by Jotun, Sandefjord, Norway). Several experimental designs have

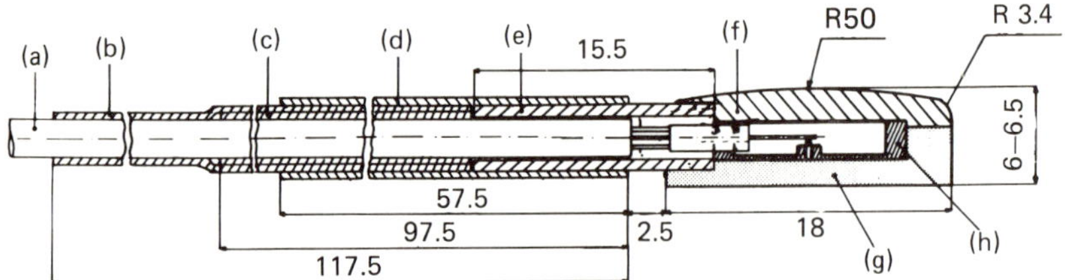


*Figure 1.* Longitudinal section of the compression transducer. The pressure sensitive element (h) is encapsulated between a silicone rubber top (g) and a rounded brass backplate (f). The design is further described in the text

shown that the selection of silicone rubber type is highly critical with respect to backplate adhesion, even when the brass surface has been treated with an etching primer prior to encapsulation. The cable (a) is led out of the transducer through a piece of 12G steel cannula tubing (e) which has been silver-soldered to the backplate. The cable is fastened by three layers of heat-shrinkable tubing (c), (d) and (e), which also functions as distance markings from the transducer centre at 60 mm, 100 mm and 120 mm respectively.

When the compliant top of the compression transducer is brought into planar contact with the fetal head during labour, the recorded bridge voltage is proportional to the *force* acting from the maternal tissues to the fetal head. However, to facilitate comparison with the commonly measured intrauterine amniotic pressure, the fetal head compression is presented in units of pressure. As the connection between force, the area which force is acting on and the equivalent pressure is described by the simple formula Pressure = (Constant) x (Force/Area), the actual relation between the physical units measured and the transducer's dimensions can be deducted to be:

Pressure (mmHg) = 29.4 x Force (N)

The special-purpose amplifier has a facility to display the transducer loading in either force or pressure units, as well as to display the highest value recorded during a session. The maximum non-linearity and hysteresis of the complete compression transducer to a uniform (force) loading over an equivalent range of 0-200 mmHg (0-26.7 kPa) is less than 2 mmHg (0.27 kPa). Zero point stability over a period of four months of use was better than 3 mmHg (0.40 kPa), and the calibration factor stability was better than 0.5% over the same period. The overload capability of the compression transducer is determined by the load-cell's membrane and is at least 1400 mmHg (187 kPa). The compression transducer withstands a continuous, ready-for-use storage in a 2% glutaraldehyde cold-sterilizing solution.

## Clinical application

In a pilot series of measurements, the compression transducer was applied during a total of 19 deliveries to record the fetal head compression pressure versus time as labour progresses.

In all our recordings the transducer was inserted to a position as shown in Figure 2 when the cervix was effaced and open for 8 cm or more. The fetal head was at the ischial spine, or higher, and the sagittal suture usually in the oblique or sagittal position. The transducer was introduced through the vagina and placed on the parietal

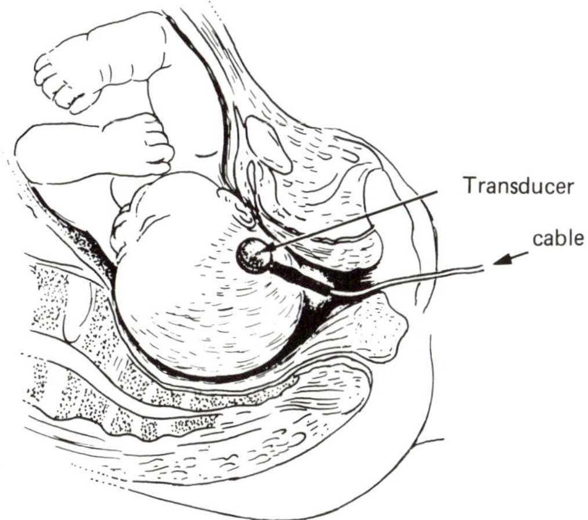


*Figure 2.* The transducer's standard position on the fetal parietal bone. The transducer is positioned when the cervix is effaced, according to distance markings on the transducer's cable

bone near the ear. The distance markings on the transducer cable were used for positioning. The polished rounded backplate of the transducer and its compliant and adhering silicone rubber surface facilitates a steady application relative to the head and a movement relative to the birth canal wall. The compression transducer was finally delivered with the birth of the head.

In eight deliveries, the intra-amniotic fluid pressure was recorded simultaneously with the compression pressure, using a conventional fluid-filled system (Hewlett Packard model 14099C Intrauterine Pressure Monitoring Kit and an external transducer) or a new miniature fibreoptic catheter-tip pressure transducer described by Svenningsen *et al* (see p.15).

All the parturients had single fetuses with flexed vertex occiput anterior presentations. The gestational age at delivery varied from 39 to 42 weeks. Fourteen of the parturients were primiparas. Six of the primiparas were given continuous lumbar epidural analgesia. The indications for epidural block were either severe pain or protracted first stage of labour. All the others were given conventional analgesia, i.e. pethidine 100 mg intramuscularly, $N_2O$ and pudendal block. One parturient had no analgesia. The neonates weighed between 2980 g and 4400 g, with a mean of 3804 g. One-minute Apgar scores were all between 8 and 10. Head circumference was between 34 and 38 cm. None of the parturients had clinical evidence of obstruction to vaginal delivery (contracted pelvis).

## Results

A typical recording of simultaneous intra-amniotic pressure (IAP) and head compression pressure (HCP) is shown in Figure 3, and is discussed further below. The eight patients in whom we monitored both IAP and HCP made 13 ± 6 pushing efforts before bearing down, developing a mean maximum HCP = 153 mmHg ± 93 mmHg (20.4 kPa ± 12.4 kPa) and a mean maximum IAP = 120 mmHg ± 53 mmHg (16.0 kPa ± 7.1 kPa).

The HCP versus time for a selected subgroup of patients is shown in Figure 4. The HCP as well as the necessary number of pushing efforts varied widely among the patients. We had only one para 3 patient, and she developed significantly lower

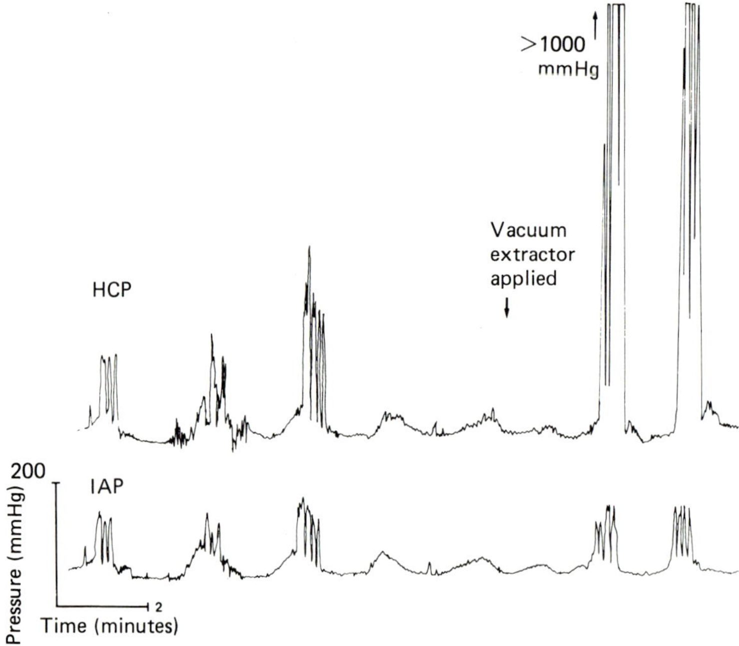


*Figure 3*. Simultaneously recorded intra-amniotic pressure (IAP) and fetal head compression pressure (HCP). The IAP was measured with the miniature fibreoptic catheter-tip pressure transducer described in Svenningsen et al. (see p.000)

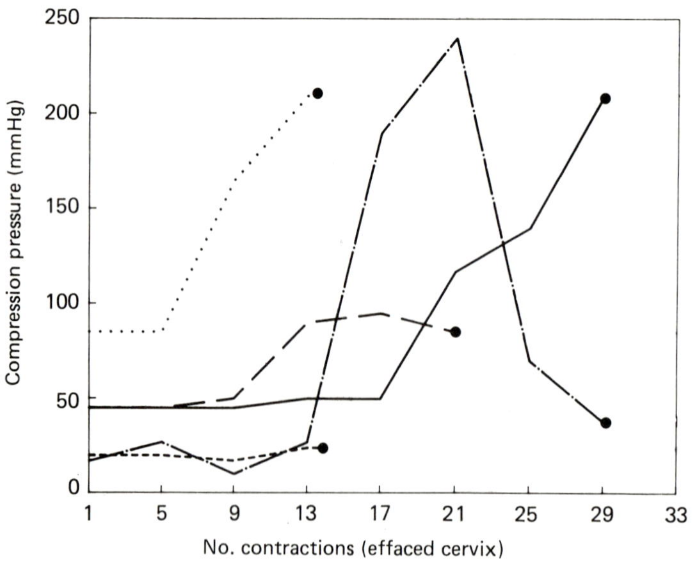


*Figure 4*. Fetal head compression versus time as labour progresses for five selected, typical patients. Bearing down is indicated by •. Note that the para 3 patient is bearing down with only 14 pushing efforts and with a small head compression pressure. Note also the wide variation in maximum recorded head compression pressure among the patients. — AGT, para 1; . . . . . VKB, para 2; --- SA, para 3; ——AHG, para 1; —•— AMT, para 1

maximum HCP than the others. The total group of 19 patients produced 11 ± 8 pushing efforts before bearing down, developing a mean maximum HCP = 160 mmHg ± 80 mmHg (21.3 kPa ± 10.7 kPa). The maximum HCP recorded in any normal session was 720 mmHg (96 kPa).

## Discussion

It is well known that the conventional intrauterine pressure-measuring systems have serious inherent deficiencies, and that the unknowns of the physiological system and the exogenous effect of performing a measurement often have a greater impact on the result than has the accuracy of the measuring system (2, 12, 13). As the accuracy of the transducer itself is within a few millimetres of mercury, the validity and interpretation of the data obtained with the compression transducer are limited by factors determined by the application of the measuring device to the fetal head.

The method described here relies on an assumption that the transducer is in planar contact with the fetal parietal bone. If the head is modelled as a 'fluid' contained in a distensible semi-rigid container, then the aplanation principle applies; shear forces will be cancelled and the force (i.e. equivalent to pressure when area is known) acting on both sides of the wall will be equal. The pressure within the fetal head would then be proportional to the compression pressure. If, on the other hand, the head is modelled as a solid sphere, the compression transducer will detect an artefactually increased load due to the central portion being more deeply stressed. Due to this effect one can compute by standard geometry formulas that a 3 cm radius solid sphere will give a recording nearly three times that of an 8 cm radius sphere when both are pressed with the same force on to the silicone rubber top. Very often, extensive moulding of the fetal head occurs; and so the head is delivered as an oblate spheroid and not like a solid sphere. It is really not possible to answer theoretically to what extent the fluid head model is correct, but perhaps additional simultaneous measurements of head compression pressures, forces and mechanical dimensions in an animal model could clarify this matter.

The insertion of the transducer between the head and the birth canal increases the canal wall tension due to distension. Even if the head were a solid sphere with a typical radius 5 cm, the insertion of the transducer would increase the circumference less than 2%. The distending pressure in a (closed) distensible hollow object is a function of the two principal radii of curvature of the object (law of Laplace). It is disputable whether the law of Laplace is applicable when the membranes are ruptured, but in a cylindrical approximation to the birth canal the radial pressure changes proportional to tension. A 2% circumferential increase will thus lead to a 2% radial pressure increase; i.e. the insertion of the transducer itself contributes only to a very small pressure increase even if the head is modelled as a solid sphere. This effect will probably not be noticeable at all in the fluid head model because the transducer will share the distension between the wall and the head.

The interpretation of the results further relies on the assumption that the compression transducer does not slide on the fetal head during the pushing efforts. There is no way that this can be guaranteed unless a rigid mounting bracket of some kind is inserted. For obvious reasons, the clinical application to routine births dictates a minimum of extra devices, i.e. at the expense of being able to define the exact position.

The amount of compression of the fetal head is modified by several factors, including the size of the baby, the coefficient of friction of the maternal tissues, a roomy or a tight pelvis, and the forced expulsive effort. Owing to the high maternal tissue strain and the relatively small area of contact between the fetal head and the birth canal, the wall-to-head pressure must be greater than the intra-amniotic pressure. Generally the fetal head will be subjected to greater forces along the largest circumference (the contacting circle) than the intrauterine expulsive forces. The findings in our pilot study are in accordance with various recordings by other workers (3, 6, 7, 8, 14) who have shown that the *cervical pressure* on the fetal head is two and a half to four times the amniotic fluid pressure when the head is engaged in the pelvis, and that the wall-to-head pressure is greatest at the largest circumference of the head.

Instrumental delivery methods such as forceps or vacuum extractors (as well as fundal pressure applied by the midwife) increase the total expulsive force to overcome the fetal/ maternal friction, but the forces or pressures acting on the fetal head must then inevitably increase. This is clearly demonstrated in the last part of Figure 3. The labour of this patient was induced because of pre-eclampsia. She had epidural analgesia and the contractions were stimulated by oxytocin. After 14 hours a vacuum extraction was tried as an aid to delivery. As is evident, there was a tremendous rise in HCP during this (unsuccessful) procedure. The fetus had to be delivered later by caesarean section.

The head is the most vulnerable part of the fetus during labour as it is the least compressible and pliable part. The region of the skull which presents in labour depends on the degree of flexion of the head, and the area involved can be correlated to the diameter of that region. Owing to the mobility of the bones within their membranous covering, the shape of the head can be modified to enable it to mould into the pelvis and to distribute the pressure. According to this analysis, the pressure of the pelvic floor acts about equally on both parietal bones, distributing the compression pressure to the fetal intracranial volume. Our material does not yet allow general conclusions to be made about fetal head compression during the second stage of labour. Our predominant hypothesis that the increased compressive force on the fetal head in the pelvic region measured by this compression transducer reflects the fetal intracranial pressure will be further investigated. The primary purpose of this paper has been to present an experimental method for the investigation of compressive forces and basic pressure relations on the fetal head in the second stage of labour. The transducer design described is very simple to use and rugged enough to withstand an accidental drop on the floor. It presents no danger whatever to the fetus or the parturient in terms of mechanical damage or infection.

## Acknowledgements

We are grateful to the company A/S Mikro-elektronikk, Horten, Norway, for their kind co-operation during the development of the transducer.

## References

1. Basell G M, Humayun S G and Marx G F. Maternal bearing down efforts - another fetal risk? *Obstetrics and Gynecology,* 56, 39-41 (1980).

2. Csapo A. The diagnostic significance of the intrauterine pressure. I. *Obstetrics and Gynecology Survey,* 25, 403-435 (1970).

3. Hashimoto T, Kokuho K and Furuya H. Pressures on the human fetus during labour. *Acta Neonatologica Japonica,* 15, 345-350 (1979).

4. Kelly J V. Compression of the fetal brain. *American Journal of Obstetrics and Gynecology,* 85, 687-694 (1963).

5. Kelly J V and Sines G. An assessment of the compression and traction forces of obstetrical forceps. *American Journal of Obstetrics and Gynecology,* 96, 521-537 (1966).

6. Lindgren L. The lower parts of the uterus during the first stage of labour in occipito-anterior vertex presentation: studies by means of intrauterine tocography. *Acta Obstetrica et Gynaecologica Scandinavica,* 34, suppl., 1-79 (1955).

7. Lindgren L. The engagement of the fetal head in the uterus when the vertex presents. *Acta Obstetrica et Gynaecologica Scandinavica,* 51, 37-45 (1972).

8. Lindgren L. The influence of pressure upon the fetal head during labour. *Acta Obstetrica et Gynaecologica Scandinavica,* 56, 303-309 (1977).

9. Maltau J M and Egge K. Epidural analgesia and perinatal retinal haemorrhages. *Acta Anaesthesiologica Scandinavica,* 24, 99-101 (1980).

10. Mann L I, Carmichael A and Duchin S. The effect of head compression on FHR, brain metabolism and function. *Obstetrics and Gynecology,* 39, 721-726 (1972).

11. Moolgaoker A S, Ahamed S O S and Payne P R. A comparison of different methods of instrumental delivery based on electronic measurements of compression and traction. *Obstetrics and Gynecology,* 54, 299-309 (1979).

12. Neuman M R, Jordan J A, Roux J F and Knoke J D. Validity of intrauterine pressure measurements with transcervical intra-amniotic catheters and an intra-amniotic miniature pressure transducer during labour. *Gynecological Investigation,* 3, 165-175 (1972).

13. Neuman M R. Pressure measurements in obstetrics. In *Indwelling and Implantable Pressure Transducers,* edited by D G Fleming, W H Ko and M R Neuman, 85-95, Cleveland, Ohio, CRC Press (1977).

14. Schwarcs R L, Strada-Saenz G *et al* . Pressure exerted by uterine contractions on the head of the human fetus during labour. *Perinatal Factors Affecting Human Development,* 115, Washington DC, Pan American Health Organization (1969).

Part 2

# Fetal Monitoring

Chapter 14

# Measurement of heart rate variation in the human fetus

G S Dawes, C W G Redman

## Introduction

In 1973 we installed a small multi-user minicomputer (Nova 1200) in the laboratory. This had a priority interrupt which could be allocated to any of the eight ports. We took the opportunity to start measurements of fetal heart rate variation in lambs, using an ECG from electrodes implanted on the fetal chest (1). The results led to the clinical developments described in this chapter. First, we found a large increase in heart rate variation with gestational age. Second, there were periodic changes in fetal electrocortical activity and episodes of fetal breathing. There were also other long term biological rhythms which caused an increase in the standard deviation of pulse intervals, as well as diurnal variation. Third, we found that fetal heart rate became more variable in acute hypoxia, e.g. isocapnic hypoxia in which the fetal $PaO_2$ was reduced from 23 to 15 mm Hg (3.1 to 2 kPa) without metabolic acidaemia.

There were some features of this investigation on fetal lambs which differed from the generally accepted view of fetal heart rate variation in the human fetus *in utero*, this view being based on visual analysis. So, in 1978, we started to record human fetal heart rate patterns quantitatively. The technical details of the developments of analysis on line at the bedside, have been described elsewhere (13). Measurement of pulse intervals to an accuracy of 1 ms is sufficient for practical clinical purposes.

## Detection of heart rate

One of the important issues is the choice of the antenatal heart rate detector. Fetal electrocardiograms of reasonable quality can be obtained from electrodes placed carefully on the maternal abdomen, but only in selected patients and after 34 weeks' gestation (e.g. 4, 12). Many of the problem cases in which a good quality record is required are at a gestational age earlier than this. The range of phonocardiograph detectors available 5 years ago were less satisfactory, largely because they used a narrow band pass filter and a peak detector. We were left with Doppler ultrasound, and found that the instruments available before 1982 had limitations, with a signal loss which *averaged* more than 20% (5). This signal loss increased during episodes of high heart rate variation, and also at lower gestational ages. If signal loss was detected by passing the pulse intervals through a simple error algorithm, adequate samples of reasonable quality could be achieved in the majority of records. It was evident that visual analysis of records was fraught with difficulties (10,11).

Recent advances have substantially improved the accuracy and reliability of Doppler ultrasound systems in measuring fetal pulse intervals, by the use of a range gate to reduce noise, or by auto-correlation to make the maximum use of the signals available (8,9). Yet it is still essential to record signal loss and to be aware of its consequences. Even in the most reliable hands, episodes of signal loss occur through fetal movements, or with auto-correlation, during episodes of hiccoughs. During episodes of high signal loss, the measured heart rate variation is substantially and artefactually reduced.

The practical use of heart rate monitors for research, and indeed for clinical practice antenatally, is greatly enhanced by analysis using a microcompter on line. This enables a baseline to be fitted, using digital filters (2). Brief accelerations and decelerations can then be measured by the microcomputer from this baseline. And episodes of high or low variation can be detected and measured for size and duration. It is still not widely appreciated that there are episodic chages in human fetal heart rate variation, probably associated with changes in fetal electro-cortical activity as in sheep near term. This cyclical activity normally persists into labour.

## Recent technical developments

With this background, we now outline recent developments, first instrumentally. Our original specification for a fetal heart rate microcomputer for use at the bedside on-line was based on the NASCOM II, interfaced to a slave microcomputer (6502, Mos Technology Inc with 1 kb RAM and 3 kb EPROM). The latter was used for collecting fetal pulse intervals, tocodynamometer measurements and fetal movements, with data reduction over 1/16 minute. The pulse intervals were passed through an error algorithm. The data were collected into a 16 bit word (10 bits for pulse interval and 5 for extrauterine pressure) and transferred to the NASCOM, which analysed the complete time series every 5 minutes. The data and a summary of the results were filed on floppy discs, whence the previous observations on a patient were automatically recalled to provide a sequential analysis of progress over days or weeks. This has proved a useful asset in the care of high risk pregnancies over the past 2 years. We have four such machines in use on several research projects, at a cost of about £2700 (1984 prices + VAT) for components, including disc drives and an Adcomp X80SP printer, for each machine, which takes a technician about 3 months to assemble.

These instruments have limitations. The nine programmes for data collection, analysis, recall and display are written in Basic, with machine code subroutines, and occupy 63 kbytes. The analysis programme takes 4 minutes to deal with 60 minutes data, because interpretive Basic is slow. The graphics display available when the system was designed was crude. The system cannot readily be made available to obstetric colleagues because specialist knowledge is required for instrumental assembly.

The programmes have now been rewritten in PASCAL for use on a Sage II 16-bit microcomputer. This is fast so that data collection can continue from a Hewlett-Packard 8040A pulsed Doppler monitor, via a clock driven priority interrupt, during analysis. The fetal heart rate, baseline, movements and the tocodynamometer output are plotted in different colours, together with episodes of high or low heart rate variation (presented as a bar graph) against time. The data are filed on and can be recalled from disc. Analysis is fast (less than 15 s) so that the baseline can be automatically refitted where necessary, and a further analysis executed. This is necessary when the fetal heart rate trace is flat. The cost (microcomputer, VDU, colour graphics, monitor, disc drives and printer, totalling about £6500) is more, but no assembly is required.

The essential features of both pieces of equipment are, first that they interact with the nurse and patient to optimize the record and minimize the recording time. Second, they provide hard copy records and analyses of uniform quality. And third the data are stored for easy retrieval, either on individual patients or for research. As to the latter, there is one important consideration. The incidence of abnormal fetal heart rate traces is low, since changes in the heart rate (and blood pressure) are relatively late manifestations of fetal ill health, in man as in sheep. Hence attention has to be directed to the accumulation of many hundreds of records, whence the lowest fifth centile, say of the frequency distribution of some variable, can be determined (3,9). In other words, such research must necessarily be long term.

## Recent findings

What have we found? First, that the new range of fetal heart rate Doppler ultrasound monitors are more accurate and reliable, with a tenth of the signal loss of their predecessors (7). Second, there is a large effect of gestational age, with a sharp increase in heart rate variation and number of accelerations (of defined size and duration) near term. The episodes of high and low fetal heart rate variation are already established by 28 weeks' gestation and persist into labour. Third, the frequency distribution of heart rate variation is wider than supposed (3). At 32 weeks' gestation 3% of the clinic population have a low fetal heart rate variation and yet deliver normal babies at term (9). Even in babies delivered by Caesarean section for abnormally flat traces (suboptimal or decelerative) there is no evidence of persistent acidaemia as judged by umbilical cord blood samples compared with a control group of elective sections (6). We still lack an adequate physiological explanation for the natural and the pathological occurrence of persistent flat fetal heart rate traces (i.e., with a mean range in pulse interval less than 25 ms, corresponding to about 8.5 b.p.m.).

Finally we need to consider the use of fetal heart rate analysis in relation to other indices of health. It has long been evident from work on fetal lambs that gross cardiovascular changes, in blood pressure or heart rate, are a late indication of ill-health. Recent qualitative and quantitative (9) analyses of human antenatal records agree with this conclusion; large antenatal screening programmes are not justified. However, fetal heart rate records are still, with fetal movement measurements, the only indicator of impending fetal death. So they will continue to have a place in the management of high risk pregnancies. They may be useful in determining those patients who should be monitored throughout labour.

One final point should be made. It is difficult for the nursing staff and junior hospital doctors to acquire the expertise to discriminate the occasional fetal heart-rate trace of sinister significance from those within the range of normality. This problem is accentuated by the presence of episodic rhythms of heart rate variation, associated with behavioural (sleep) patterns of brainstem activity. A microcomputer can be programmed to retain the background information derived from a study of thousands of records. It is better at identifying the abnormal or sinister tracing. It is more reliable.

## Acknowledgements

We are indebted to our clinical colleagues, without whose enthusiastic collaboration the clinical studies described would not have been possible, and to Mr R. Belcher and Miss M. Moulden for able technical assistance. We also acknowledge with gratitude grants from the Medical Research Council.

## References

1. Dalton K J, Dawes G S and Patrick J E. Diurnal respiratory and other rhythms of fetal heart rate in lambs. *American Journal of Obstetrics and Gynecology*, 127, 414-424 (1977).
2. Dawes G S, Houghton C R S and Redman C W G. Baseline in human fetal heart rate records. *British Journal of Obstetrics and Gynaecology*, 89, 270-275 (1982).
3. Dawes G S, Houghton C R S, Redman C W G and Visser G H A. Pattern of the normal human fetal heart rate. *British Journal of Obstetrics and Gynaecology*, 89, 276-284 (1982).
4. Dawes G S, Visser G H A, Goodman J D S and Levine D H. Numerical anlysis of the fetal heart rate: modulation by breathing and movement. *American Journal of Obstetrics and Gynecology*, 140, 535-544 (1981).
5. Dawes G S, Visser G H A, Goodman J D S and Redman C W G. Numerical analysis of the human fetal heart rate: the quality of ultrasound records. *American Journal of Obstetrics and Gynecology*, 141, 43-52 (1981).
6. Henson G L, Dawes G S and Redman C W G. Antenatal fetal heart-rate variability in relation to fetal acid-base status at Caesarean section. *British Journal of Obstetrics and Gynaecology*, 90, 516-521 (1983).
7. Lawson G W, Belcher R, Dawes G S and Redman C W G. A comparison of ultrasound (with auto correlation) and direct ECG fetal heart rate detector systems. *American Journal of Obstetrics and Gynecology*, 147, 721-722 (1983).
8. Lawson G W, Dawes G S and Redman C W G. A comparison of two fetal heart rate ultrasound detector systems. *American Journal of Obstetrics and Gynecology*, 3, 840-842 (1982).
9. Lawson G W, Dawes G S and Redman C W G. Analysis of fetal heart rate on-line at 32 weeks gestation. *British Journal of Obstetrics and Gynaecology*, in press (1984).
10. Lotgering F K, Wallenberg H C S and Schouten H O A. Interobserver and intraobserver variation in the assessment of antepartum cardiotocograms. *American Journal of Obstetrics and Gynecology*, 144, 701-705 (1982).
11. Trimbos J B and Keirse M J N C. Observer variability in assessment of antepartum cardiotocograms. *British Journal of Obstetrics and Gynaecology*, 85, 900-906 (1978).
12. Visser G H A, Goodman J D S, Levine D H and Dawes G S. Diurnal and other cyclic variations in human fetal heart rate near term. *American Journal of Obstetrics and Gynecology*, 42, 535-544 (1982).
13. Wickham P J D, Dawes G S and Belcher R. Development of methods for quantitative analysis of the fetal heart rate.*Journal of Biomedical Engineering*, 5, 302-308 (1983).

Chapter 15

# The correlation of maternal and fetal heart rates - an important aspect of CTG interpretation

**Joachim H Nagel**

## Introduction

Although cardiotocography (CTG) is the most commonly used method in perinatal monitoring, there are still some difficulties surrounding its interpretation. In many cases an unequivocal diagnosis is not possible without additional physiological information. The reasons may be either physiological or due to shortcomings of existing instrumentation. A typical example is shown in Figure 1, where the CTG reveals no reason for the acceleration of the fetal heart rate (FHR). Uterine activity is completely absent, and no fetal movement is detectable. Considering, however, the maternal heart rate (MHR), the acceleration becomes intelligible as a result of feto-maternal coupling.

A most serious situation is documented in Figure 2. There is a quite normal CTG, no uterine activity and an FHR curve of rather good quality that reveals no abnormalities. But the simultaneously recorded fetal ECG shows severe arrhythmia. Probably no existing fetal monitor would have been able to detect this condition. We were able to recognize the arrhythmia because we monitored not only the fetal but also the maternal heart rate, which was found to be markedly abnormal. Our interpretation of the feto-maternal coupling indicated that a direct influence on the fetal cardiac system was to be expected, so we recorded the fetal ECG in order to check the inconspicuous FHR curve.

## Interaction between maternal and fetal heart rate

### Oxygen availability

The question arises as to whether or not the correlation between FHR and MHR represents a random event. We feel sure that there is a systematic dependence. Fetal oxygen availability is a direct function of maternal cardiac output and oxygen saturation, as well as of placental sufficiency. It is well known that a reduction in available oxygen usually influences the fetal heart rate through the action of the cardiac regulatory system, which tends to compensate for the oxygen deficit by accelerating the heart to ensure an adequate supply to fetal tissues. As a consequence, both placental insufficiency and changes in maternal blood supply may influence FHR.

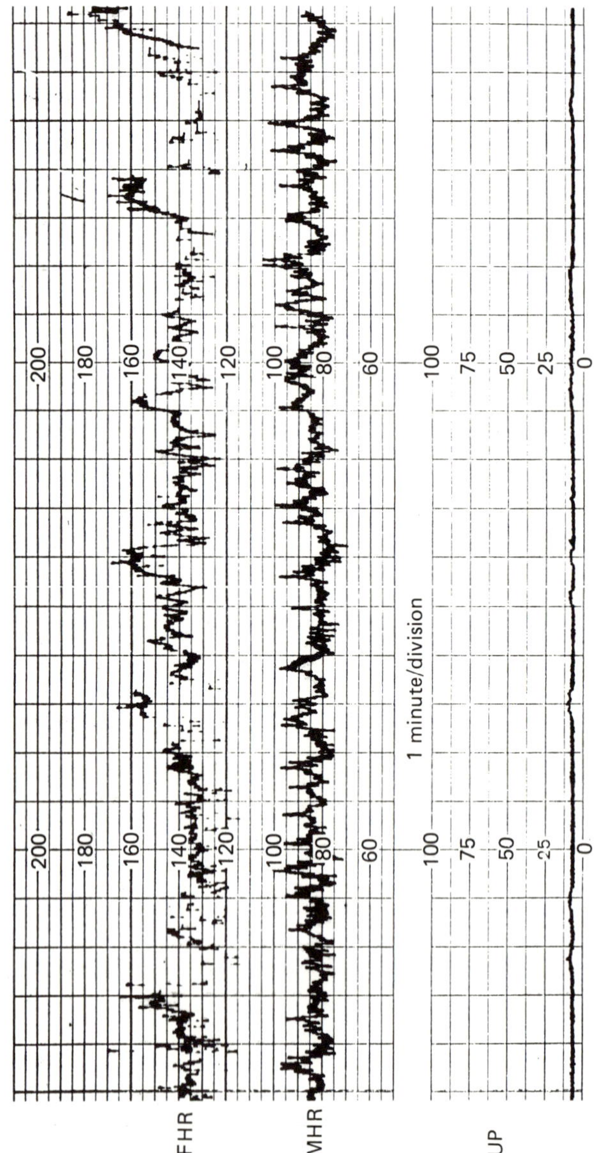


*Figure 1*. CTG showing large fluctuations of FHR and MHR with no uterine activity

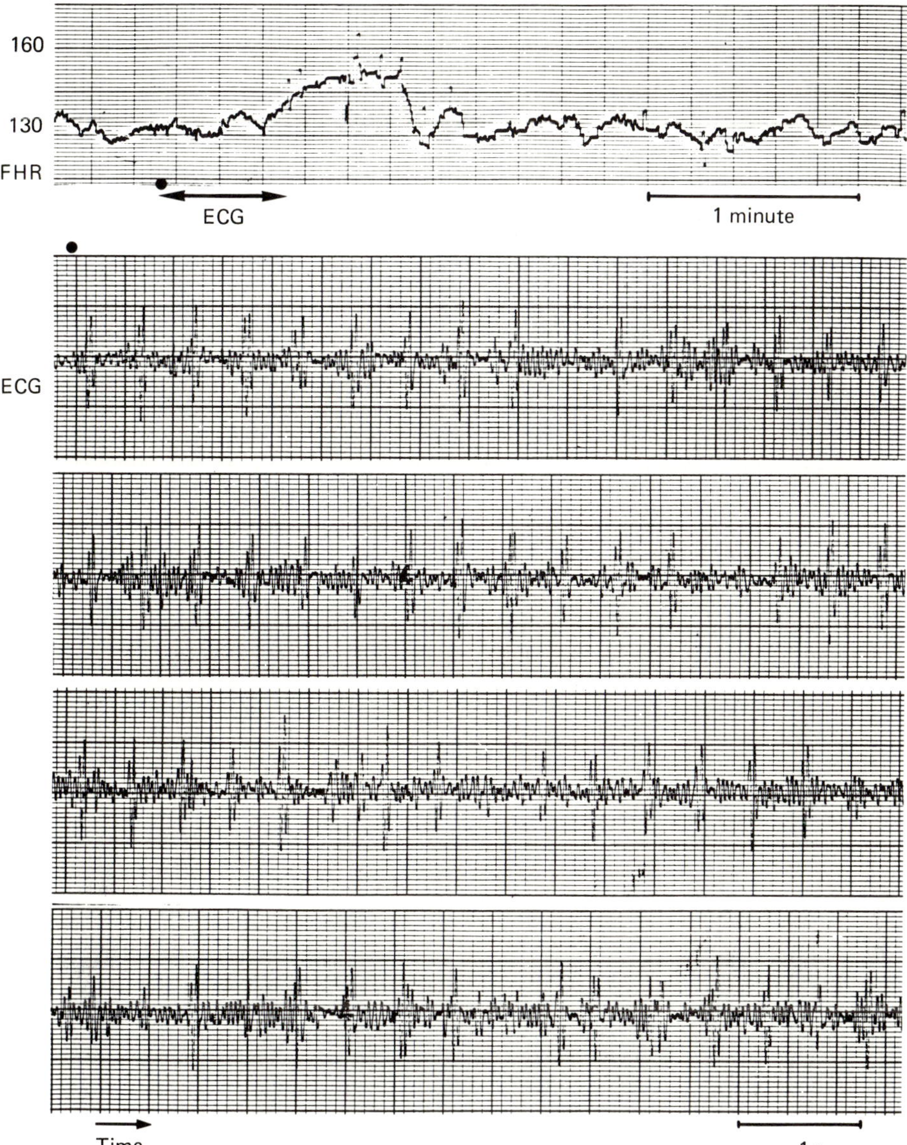


*Figure 2.* Fetal arrhythmia hidden by an inconspicuous FHR curve

This reasoning is not new, but what is important is to draw the right conclusions. CTG interpretation is usually based on correlations between FHR and uterine pressure. But what is to be done in the absence of pressure changes, or if an abnormal pattern presents during labour? Can we be sure that the increasing uterine pressure is the reason for heart rate variations in every case? And what influence has the maternal cardiovascular system?

Let us consider the physiological situation. Labour activity represents a stress not only for the fetus, but also for the mother, resulting in maternal heart rate variations

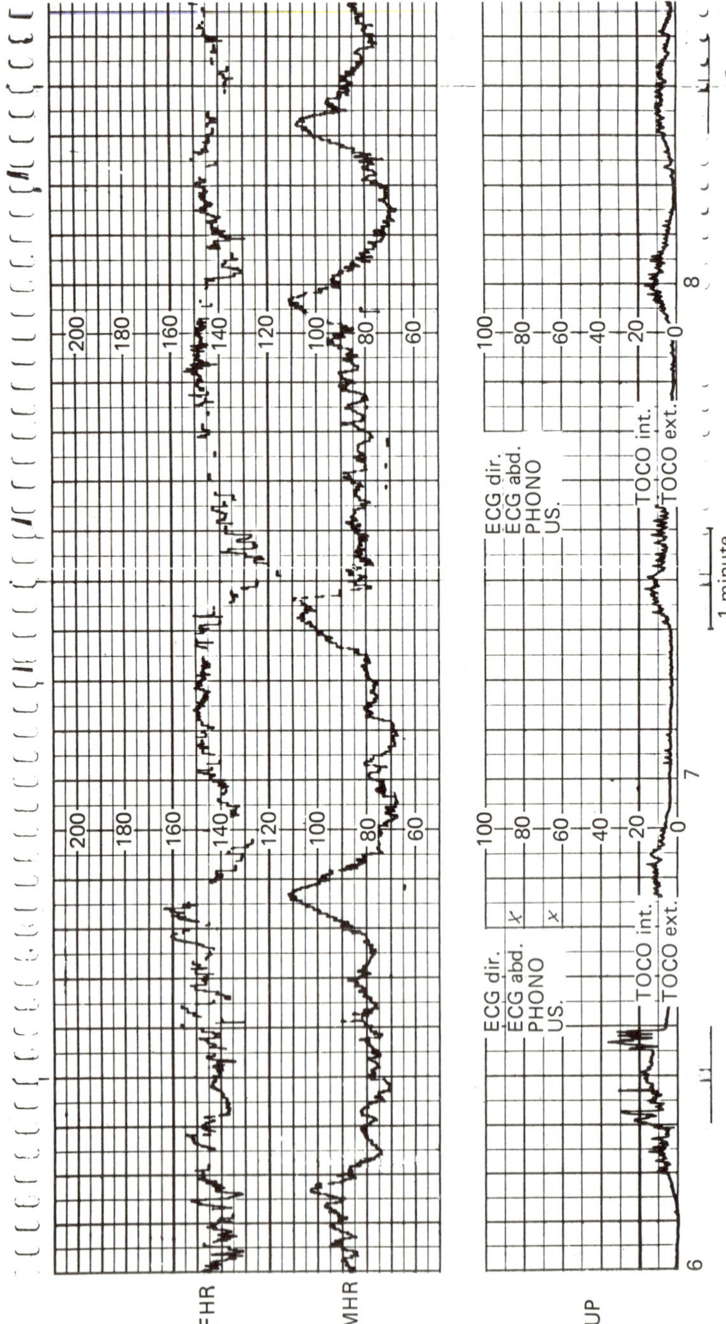


*Figure 3.* Simultaneous recording of CTG and MHR showing the predominant influence of MHR on fetal heart rate

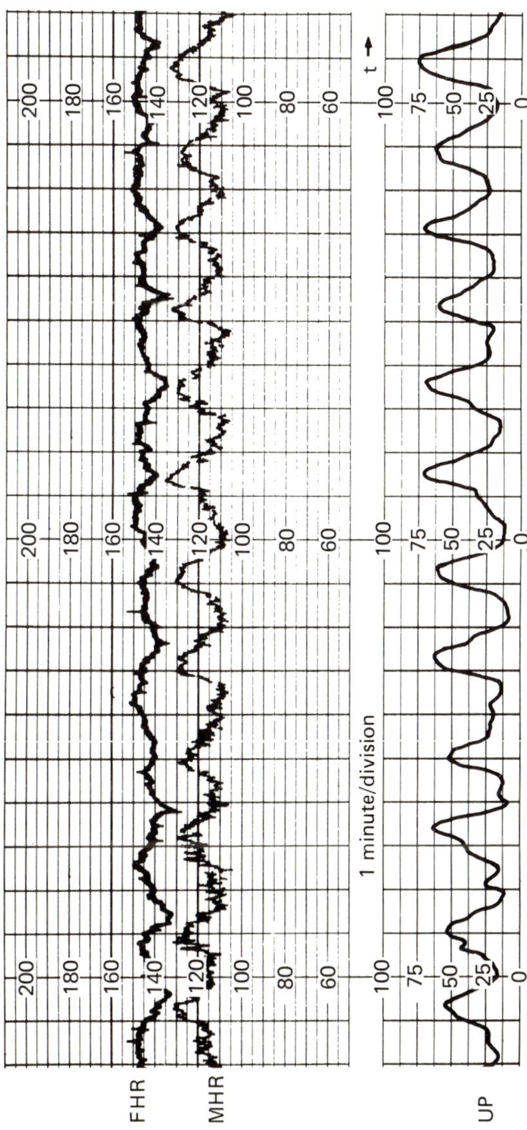


*Figure 4.* Simultaneous recording of MHR and CTG

and intensified respiration. Some authors have already demonstrated an augmented $PO_2$ during labour. With normal maternal cardiac output and placental sufficiency this means an increase in the fetal oxygen supply. The physiological reaction will be a deceleration of fetal heart rate, as is, indeed, observed. On the other hand, fetal stress caused by uterine compressions would, as a normal physiological reaction, result in an acceleration comparable to that of the maternal heart. Obviously there are two opposing regulatory processes. So should we not logically attribute the commonly observed decelerations to the maternal cardiovascular system rather than to uterine pressure? An obvious case is shown in Figure 3. The normal reaction to labour activity is an accleration of MHR and a 'dip' in the FHR. The first contraction shown in Figure 3 does not produce a maternal response, and thus there is no deceleration of FHR.

**Interpretation of the timing of FHR 'dips'**

A second point of interest is the interpretation of the onset of the 'dips'. If the previous statement holds, then we must also relate it to the changed conditions of the maternal cardiovascular system. Again, the consequences are quite surprising. With the onset of a uterine contraction we first detect a maternal reaction, expressed as a change in the heart rate. The associated increase in $PO_2$ results in fetal heart rate deceleration. But there must be a delay vis-à-vis the acceleration of the maternal heart because the passage of oxygen through the placenta takes a certain time, which will depend upon placental efficiency. In common with umbilical cord compression, placental insufficiency retards the increase in fetal $PO_2$ and thus heart rate deceleration. So we will detect a late deceleration. But the essential point is that late decelerations should not automatically be interpreted as placental insufficiency or any other disorder, since we have to take into account a second time constant, namely the time delay in the maternal response to uterine contraction, which may be increased without any consequences for fetal well-being. This accords with the experience of other authors who have found, without knowing the physiological reason, that a late 'dip' should not be interpreted as a sign of risk provided the FHR oscillations remain within their normal range. Therefore, we believe that the unequivocal interpretation of 'dips' would be considerably improved by a knowledge of the maternal condition.

Figures 3 and 4 show the simultaneous recording of both maternal and fetal heart rates together with uterine pressure. There is a remarkable conformity between FHR and MHR, but with an inverse relationship. Detailed analysis of the correlation between FHR and MHR, which is very simple to perform, provides important information. The correlation coefficient is highest when the maternal heart rate is delayed vis-à-vis the FHR for about 30-40 seconds. This is the response time of the placenta and the fetal regulatory system. In other words, if the maternal oxygen supply changes, it will take about 30 seconds for the FHR to respond. This is an important fact which permits an assessment of placental sufficiency by following up this time delay. Insufficiency will increase the delay and reduce the correlation.

## Conclusions

The heart rate is a rather poor indicator of the physiological condition both in the fetus and in the mother. Even such simple measurements as maternal blood pressure recording can provide additional information (Figure 5). However, for an accurate

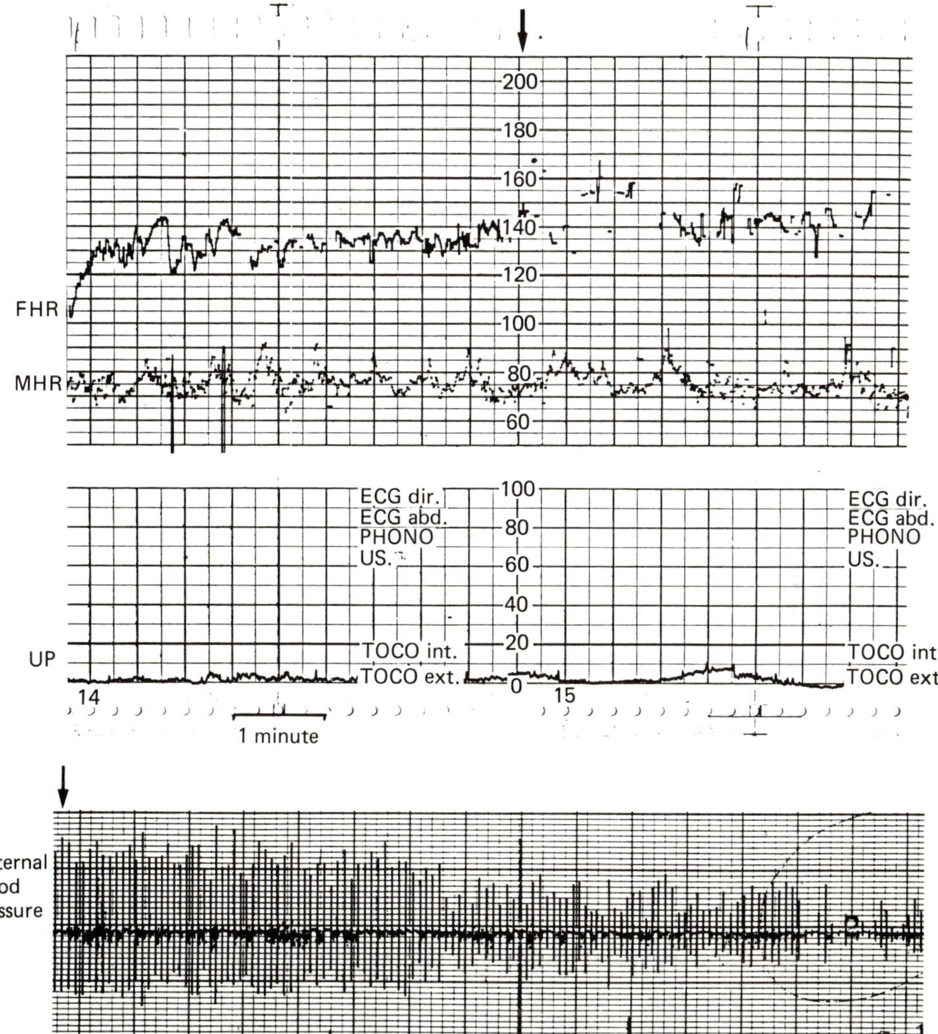


*Figure 5.* Fetal arrhythmia caused by a breakdown of maternal blood pressure

analysis of the feto-maternal coupling at least cardiac output and maternal oxygen saturation should be monitored. Nevertheless, our investigations have shown that for routine use even the MHR provides sufficient information to improve the interpretation of the CTG quite considerably. The correlation analysis of fetal and maternal heart rates facilitates diagnosis, particularly in borderline cases, and may help to prevent misinterpretation of the CTG. Since the provision of an additional MHR channel in perinatal monitors is very simple and inexpensive, future systems should not be without one.

Chapter 16

# Heart rate variation and movement incidence in growth-retarded fetuses with decelerative heart rate patterns: correlations with fetal acid-base status

**D J Bekedam, G H A Visser**

## Introduction

With progressive deterioration of the fetal condition in utero, both heart rate variation and fetal movements decrease. Just before fetal death, the baseline variability is decreased to less than 5 beats/minute, with no accelerations and with late decelerations - the terminal pattern (2). This condition is strongly associated with fetal acidaemia.

Predicting the condition at birth of intrauterine growth retarded fetuses (IUGR) having heart rate patterns with a lesser degree of abnormality has never succeeded with any precision. As heart rate variation in IUGR fetuses, in the absence of late decelerations, is usually within normal limits (12), reduction of variation has to be considered as a rather late sign of compromise. On the other hand, variation is already reduced before fetal acidaemia develops (3).

The same problem arises with the incidence of fetal movement. From 'subjective' records of fetal motility kept by pregnant women, it is known that , in most instances, fetal death is preceded by a sudden cessation of fetal movements - fetal movement alarm signal (8,11). However, decreased fetal movements are found in IUGR fetuses days or even weeks before delivery or before intrauterine death (6, 9).

The physiological mechanisms behind this reduction of fetal activity and heart rate variation are poorly understood. The aims of the present study are twofold. First, to gain more insight into when heart rate variation and movements decrease in IUGR fetuses. Second, to examine their relationship to the acid-base status at delivery. In this paper we present the first results obtained from 18 IUGR fetuses from whom combined recordings of fetal heart rate (FHR) and fetal motility were obtained shortly before Caesarean section.

## Patients and methods

The study group consisted of 18 patients with decelerative antenatal FHR traces, who were delivered by Caesarean section between 28 and 39 weeks' gestation. All patients were admitted to the obstetric ward with the clinical diagnosis of IUGR. Twelve patients had mild to severe toxaemia, four of whom were treated with antihypertensive drugs. No other drugs were used. Patients were recorded in bed, lying in a semi-recumbent position, slightly tilted to the left. All recordings were made within 24 hours before Caesarian section, 70% within 6 hours. FHR recordings, each of 1 hour's duration, were obtained with a Hewlett Packard cardiotocograph (8030A).

Fetal pulse intervals were derived from an abdominal electrocardiographic signal or from a phonomagnetic signal and were stored on a minicassette after having been pre-processed by a microcomputer. The data were analysed using a computer programme of which a detailed description has previously been published (1). The baseline variation was calculated as the root mean square (RMS), after exclusion of accelerations and decelerations in excess of 40 ms (14 beats/minute). Only heart rate records with a fail time less than 70% were used in the study, and three heart rate records had to be rejected for this reason. Earlier published data from uncomplicated pregnancies were used as a control (13).

Fetal movements and breathing movements were observed using a linear array scanner (Searle or Aloka 256SD). The transducer was held in a parasagittal plane so that the fetal chest and head were visible. Fetal body movements (and breathing movements) were recorded digitally by means of an event marker and encoded onto the same tape as the fetal pulse intervals. Since data were subsequently analysed in 3.75 second epochs, only one fetal body movement was accepted each 3.75 seconds, irrespective of the frequency of activating the event marker. Data from 100 1-hour records, obtained in normal pregnancies between 28 and 40 weeks' gestation, were used as controls. In only one of these recordings was the incidence of body movements less than 6.5%. Therefore, this value was used to define the lower limit of normal fetal movement incidence.

All patients were delivered under general anaesthesia. At delivery the umbilical cord was clamped and umbilical arterial and venous blood was analysed immediately for pH, $PCO_2$, $PO_2$ and base excess using an automatic pH/blood gas analyser (RVL 940).

The blood gas values of 30 infants delivered by elective Caesarean sections at 37 to 40 weeks' gestation were used as controls. All infants had normal antenatal fetal heart rate records. Caesarian sections were performed for indications other than asphyxia and/or IUGR. The indications were breech presentation (n = 10), cephalo-pelvic disproportion (n = 18) and poor obstetrical history (n = 2).

## Results

All 18 infants had a birthweight below the tenth percentile according to the Dutch curves of Kloosterman (n = 10, 2.3rd centile; n = 4, fifth centile).

Assessed visually according to the criteria of Visser and Huisjes (14), three heart rate patterns were 'terminal' and 15 decelerative. Two of the fetuses with a terminal FHR pattern died in utero.

Baseline heart rate variation was reduced in 12 out of 15 cases (80%; see Figure 1). The fetal movement incidence was reduced in 14 cases out of 18 (78%; see Figure 2). The lowest movement incidence was found in the three fetuses with 'terminal' heart rate patterns.

The umbilical artery pH (pHua) was less than 7.20 in seven of the 16 liveborn fetuses (44%). Only one pH was less than 7.15. The base deficit exceeded 10 mmol/l

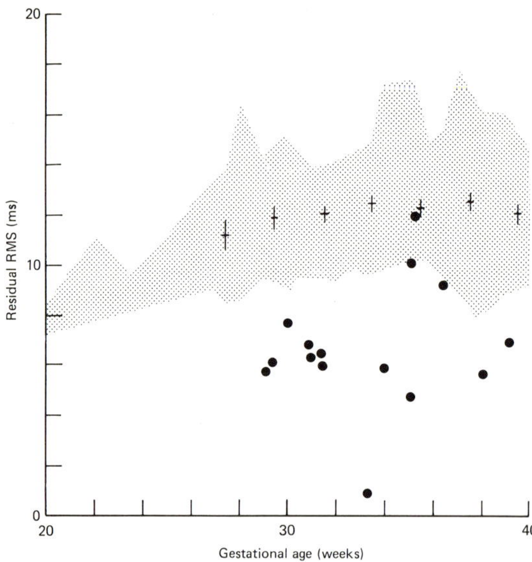


*Figure 1.* Long-term baseline heart rate variation (RMS) in 15 growth-retarded fetuses with decelerative heart rate patterns. The grey background indicates the values found in normal pregnancies

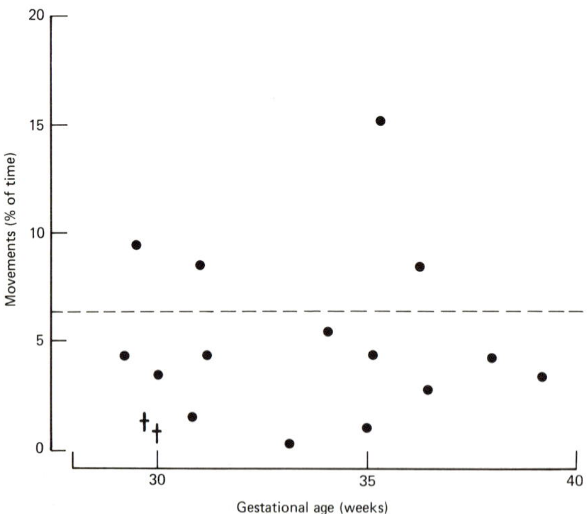


*Figure 2.* Movement incidence (% of time) in 1-hour records from 18 growth-retarded fetuses with decelerative heart rate patterns. The dotted line indicates the lower limit of normality. † = intrauterine death within 24 hours

in five cases. The mean pHua (±s.d.) was 7.20 ± 0.057, which was significantly lower than that in the control group (7.27 ± 0.06; see Table 1). There was also a significant difference in umbilical artery $PO_2$ values between the study group and the control group (1.63 kPa ± 0.45 vs. 2.92 kPa ± 0.72; see Table 1). As this difference may be partly due to the Bohr effect, arterial $PO_2$ values of IUGR fetuses with a pHua between 7.20 and 7.28 were compared with those of the control group with a

**TABLE 1. pH and $PO_2$ from umbilical arterial blood from the growth-retarded infants (IUGR) and control group (mean and s.d.)**

| | *IUGR* (n=16) | *Control group* (n=30) |
|---|---|---|
| pHua | 7.20 (±0.057) | 7.27 (±0.06)* |
| $PO_2$ (kPa) | 1.63 )±0.45) | 2.92 (±0.72)** |
| Infants with pHua 7.20–7.28 | n=9 | n=12 |
| $PO_2$ kPa | 1.48 (±0.48) | 2.55 (±0.52)** |

Student's *t* test * p 0.05 2-tailed
** p 0.001 2-tailed

control group with a pHua in the same range (see Table 1). Again a significant difference in $PO_2$ was found between the groups.

The movement incidence was significantly correlated with the pHua ($r = 0.53$; $p < 0.05$, two-tailed). Its relationship with FHR variation was not significant ($r = 0.47$; $0.05 < p < 0.1$, two-tailed). (Note: inclusion of more recent study group observations also produced a significant correlation between the latter two measures.)

## Discussion

Although the IUGR group consisted of highly compromised fetuses, according to the antenatal FHR tracings, only one of the liveborn infants had a pHua lower than 7.15. This finding confirms earlier studies showing that only terminal heart rate records are associated with fetal acidaemia (15). Eight of the infants had a pHua greater than 7.20 and yet, in the group, 80% had a reduced baseline variability. This result confirms the findings of Henson *et al* (3), that the initial reduction of heart rate variation is not caused by fetal acidaemia. Hypoxia, on the other hand, may play a role as umbilical arterial $PO_2$ values were significantly lower than in the control group. From experimental studies in growth retarded fetal sheep, it is known that low arterial $PO_2$ values precede acidaemia (10). A further indication for the role of hypoxia is the fact that reduction of heart rate variation apparently coincides with the occurrence of late decelerations, the latter being thought to indicate hypoxaemia (4, 5).

As for the body movement incidence, there is a weak relationship with the umbilical artery pH and this might become more evident if more fetuses in a 'terminal' condition can be included in the study group. However, with reduced movement incidence most fetuses had a pH greater than 7.15. It is therefore doubtful whether reduced fetal movement incidence can be ascribed only to acidaemia. Chronic hypoxaemia may be associated with this reduction. To some extent this is supported by the experimental study of Natale *et al* (7), who found a reduction in forelimb movements of fetal sheep during hypoxia.

Further research is required to ascertain the particular effects of low $PO_2$ values, or preferably of accurately measured oxygen saturation. If the possible sources of error, such as the effects of general anaesthesia and surgical intervention on blood gas values in both control and growth-retarded groups, are taken into account, then the study of the effect of low $PO_2$ values on heart rate variation and movement incidence could prove rewarding.

It is concluded, that:

1 Hypoxaemia may play a larger role in the initial reduction of baseline heart rate variation and movement incidence than acidaemia.
2 Fetal movement incidence and heart rate variation decline before acidaemia develops; the movement incidence is, however, related to the pHua.
3 Baseline heart rate variation usually only falls below normal when late decelerations are present. This is based on the present and on an earlier study (12).

## Acknowledgements

This research was supported by the Dutch Princess Beatrix Foundation.

## References

1. Dawes G S, Visser G H A, Goodman J D S and Redman C W G. Numerical analysis of the human fetal heart rate: the quality of ultrasound records. *American Journal of Obstetrics and Gynecology,* 141, 43-52 (1981).
2. Emmen L, Huisjes H J, Aarnoudse J G, Visser G H A and Okken A. Antepartum diagnosis of the 'terminal' fetal state by cardiotocography. *British Journal of Obstetrics and Gynaecology,* 82, 353-359 (1975).
3. Henson G L, Dawes G S and Redman C W G. Antenatal fetal heart-rate variability in relation to fetal acid-base status at caesarean section. *British Journal of Obstetrics and Gynaecology,* 90, 516-521 (1983).
4. Itskovitz J, Goetzman B W and Rudolph A M. The mechanism of late deceleration of the heart rate and its relationship to oxygenation in normoxemic and chronically hypoxemic fetal lambs. *American Journal of Obstetrics and Gynecology,* 142, 66-73 (1982).
5. Myers R E, Mueller-Heubach E and Adamsons K. Predictability of the state of fetal oxygenation from quantitative analysis of the components of late deceleration. *American Journal of Obstetrics and Gynecology,* 115, 1083 (1973).
6. Mor-Yosef S, Sadovsky E, Brzezinski A, Levinsky R and Ohel G. Fetal movements and intrauterine growth retardation. *International Journal of Gynecology and Obstetrics,* 21, 315-318 (1983).
7. Natale R, Clewlow F and Dawes G S. Measurement of fetal forelimb movements in the lamb in utero. *American Journal of Obstetrics and Gynecology,* 140, 545-551 (1981).
8. Pearson J F and Weaver J B. Fetal activity and fetal wellbeing. An evaluation. *British Medical Journal,* 1, 1305 (1976).
9. Roberts A B, Little D, Cooper D and Campbell S. Fetal activity in normal and abnormal pregnancies. *Proceedings of the 5th Fetal Breathing Conference, Nijmegen 1978,* The Netherlands, Ed T Eskes.
10. Robinson J S, Kingston E J, Jones C T and Thorburn G D. Studies on experimental growth retardation in sheep. The effect of the removal of endometrial caruncles on fetal size and metabolism. *Journal of Developmental Physiology,* 1, 45-64 (1979).
11. Sadovsky E and Yaffe H. Daily fetal movement recording and fetal prognosis. *Obstetrics and Gynecology,* 41, 845-849 (1973).
12. Visser G H A. Antenatal cardiotocography in the evaluation of the fetal well-being. *Australian and New Zealand Journal of Obstetrics and Gynaecology,* (in press) (1984).
.13 Visser G H A, Dawes G S and Redman C W G. Numerical analysis of the normal human antenatal fetal heart rate. *British Journal of Obstetrics and Gynecology,* 88, 792-802 (1981).
14. Visser G H A and Huisjes H J. Diagnostic value of the unstressed antepartum cardiotocogram. *British Journal of Obstetrics and Gynaecology,* 84, 5, 321-326 (1977).
15. Visser G H A, Redman C W G, Huisjes H J and Turnbull A C. Nonstressed antepartum heart rate monitoring: implications of decelerations after spontaneous contractions. *American Journal of Obstetrics and Gynecology,* 138, 429-435 (1980).

Chapter 17

# Cycles of fetal heart rate variability in spontaneous and induced labour

**J A D Spencer, P Johnson**

## Introduction

Continuous recordings of the normal fetal heart rate (FHR) during the antepartum period exhibit consecutive episodes of high and low variability (22,23). There is increasing evidence that such cycles of FHR variability occur with fetal behavioural state changes (11,16,21). Mature fetal behavioural state changes have been shown to occur after 38 weeks' gestation in man when there is a stable association, for prolonged periods, between changes in fetal body movements, fetal eye movements and fetal heart rate variability (16). Cycles of each of these variables are present prior to 36 weeks, but periods of coincidence occur by chance.

Antenatal studies have shown the duration of episodes of low FHR variability to be between 15 minutes and 22 minutes, with ranges of 6-50 minutes, and total cycle lengths of 76-92 minutes. These compare favourably with similar episodes of low and high heart-rate variability in the newborn (4,10,20). Periods of quiet sleep in the newborn can be identified by episodes of low heart-rate variability (4,7,21). The implication of the normality of episodes of low FHR variability during antenatal monitoring has led to the recognition that monitoring should last longer than the duration of such quiet episodes (20).

Fetal heart rate variability is subject to modification by fetal breathing movements; periods of fetal breathing produce an increase in FHR variability (6,24). Fetal breathing is not a parameter of fetal behavioural state, but episodes of breathing may occur simultaneously with fetal body movements and episodes of high FHR variability (9,18). Fetal breathing is significantly reduced prior to the onset of labour (3), and virtually ceases during active labour (18). Fetal body movements decrease in labour but may not disappear entirely (18). Episodes of low and high FHR variability have been shown to continue after induction of labour (9,18). Therefore, cycles of FHR variability may be the best guide to fetal behaviour during labour.

The effect of episodes of low FHR variability on the interpretation of the cardiotocograph (CTG) during labour may be important because conventional analysis of the FHR presumes that a reduction in variability signifies fetal asphyxia. In view of the lack of information on this possibility, we decided to quantify the occurrence of cycles of FHR variability in labour in a preliminary study to see how often and how long a questionable reduction of variability might occur. A further hypothesis was that such cycles of FHR variability are more likely to occur after the interruption of late pregnancy by induction of labour than after the onset of spontaneous labour.

## Method

Over a 19-week period all first-stage CTG traces of 6 hours' duration or longer were visually analysed for evidence of cycles of FHR variability. Each episode was identified by a change of at least 5 beats per minute (long-term variability) sustained for a minimum of 5 minutes' duration. All episodes were measured by working backwards through the recording from the end of the first stage. The last epoch was not included as part of a cycle. A complete cycle required consecutive epochs of high and low FHR variability with changes before and after. Two complete cycles were necessary before a CTG was considered to show evidence of fetal behavioural state changes. The analysis was performed without knowledge of the details of labour, and the information coded for computer analysis. The relevant details concerning the labours were subsequently collected and coded. Only term labours were included in the study, and only the first twin of twin labours was included. Ninety-two traces (30%) were assessed independently by a second observer.

## Results

Ninety-four spontaneous and 207 induced labours at term had first-stage CTGs of 360 minutes or longer (mean duration 549 minutes, range 36-1320 minutes). The derivation of the study group is illustrated in Figure 1. The length of CTGs was significantly longer in induced labours (mean 568 minutes, s.d. 195 minutes) compared with spontaneous labours (mean 508 minutes, s.d. 157 minutes) ($p = 0.005$). Table 1 shows that the incidence of cycles of FHR variability was significantly greater in induced labour compared with spontaneous labour, and particularly so in CTGs of less than 9 hours' duration.

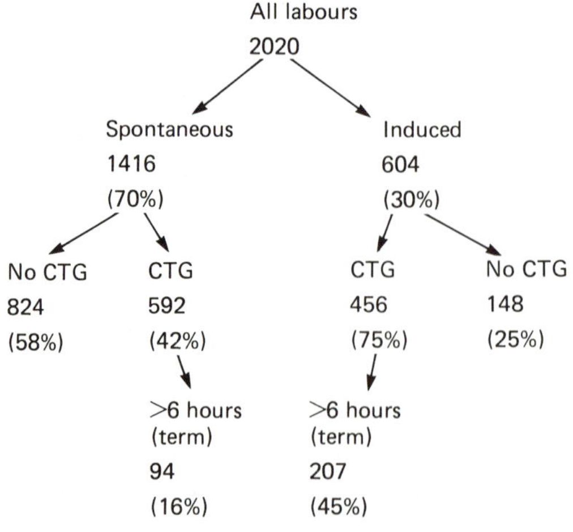


*Figure 1.* Total labours during study period (19 weeks)

**TABLE 1. Cycles of FHR variability in spontaneous and induced labour.**

| | *All CTGs (no.)* | *Cycles* *Yes* | *No* | *6–9 hours Cycles* *Yes* | *No* | *>9 hours Cycles* *Yes* | *No* |
|---|---|---|---|---|---|---|---|
| Spontaneous labour | 94 | 36 | 58 | 15 | 45 | 21 | 13 |
| Induced labour | 207 | 140 | 67 | 62 | 39 | 78 | 28 |
| Chi square | | p<0.0001 | | p<0.0001 | | NS | |

NS: Not significant.

**TABLE 2. Labour length and cycles of FHR variability.**

| | *Total length of first stage CTG* | | | | | |
|---|---|---|---|---|---|---|
| | *All labours* | | *Spontaneous* | | *Induced* | |
| | *Mean* | *s.d.* | *Mean* | *s.d.* | *Mean* | *s.d.* |
| CTGs with cycles (176) | 594 | 203 | 585 | 182 | 596 | 209 |
| CTGs without cycles (125) | 487 | 134 | 460 | 118 | 510 | 144 |
| Student *t*-test | p<0.001 | | p=0.001 | | p=0.001 | |

Durations in minutes.

Table 2 shows that CTGs with cycles were significantly longer than those without in both spontaneous and induced labours. The durations of mean cycle length and mean quiet and active episodes were not significantly different in spontaneous and induced labours, as shown in Table 3.

**TABLE 3. Durations of FHR variability cycles in labour.**

| | *Total labours* (n=176) *Mean* | *s.d.* | *Min.* | *Max.* | *Spontaneous* (n=36) *Mean* | *s.d.* | *Induced* (n=140) *Mean* | *s.d.* | *t-test* |
|---|---|---|---|---|---|---|---|---|---|
| No. cycles | 3.7 | 1.7 | 2 | 11 | 3.7 | 1.5 | 3.7 | 1.7 | NS |
| Complete cycles | 92 | 32 | 47 | 202 | 95 | 36 | 91 | 31 | S |
| Quiet episodes | 25 | 11 | 12 | 93 | 28 | 11 | 25 | 11 | NS |
| Active episodes | 66 | 31 | 22 | 180 | 67 | 35 | 66 | 29 | NS |
| First quiet | 25 | 13 | 7 | 90 | 27 | 15 | 24 | 12 | NS |
| First active | 64 | 39 | 12 | 250 | 63 | 39 | 64 | 40 | NS |

Durations in minutes.
NS: not significant.

The cumulative frequency of the durations of first quiet epoch is plotted in Figure 2 to show the duration of CTG recording necessary to include increasing percentages of quiet episodes. Tables 4 and 5 show that intrapartum events and outcome were not significantly different in labour with and without cycles of FHR variability. The

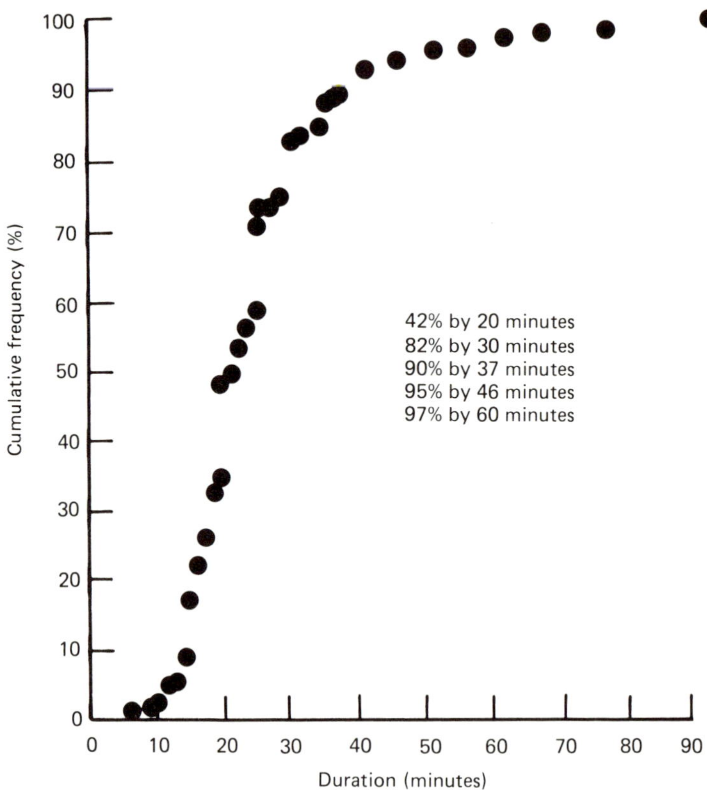


*Figure 2.* Cumulative frequency of first quiet episodes of intrapartum FHR variability

**TABLE 4. Intrapartum events and cycles for FHR variability.**

| | *Oxytocic* | | *Membranes* | | *Analgesia* | |
|---|---|---|---|---|---|---|
| | *None* | *SYNT/PG* | *SROM* | *ARM* | *None* | *PETH/EPI* |
| CTGs with cycles (176) | 13 | 163 | 32 | 144 | 17 | 159 |
| CTGs without cycles (125) | 15 | 110 | 34 | 91 | 8 | 117 |
| Chi square | NS | | NS | | NS | |

SYNT: syntocinon; PG: prostaglandin; SROM: spontaneous rupture of membranes; ARM: artificial rupture of membranes; PETH: pethidine; EPI: epidural analgesia.
NS: not significant.

**TABLE 5. Labour outcome with and without cycles of FHR variability.**

| | *Type of delivery* | | | *1-minute Apgar* | | *5-minute Apgar* | |
|---|---|---|---|---|---|---|---|
| | *SVD* | *IVD* | *C/S* | 0–4 | 5–9 | 0–4 | 5–9 |
| CTGs with cycles (176) | 80 | 70 | 26 | 15 | 161 | 0 | 176 |
| CTGs without cycles (125) | 56 | 51 | 18 | 9 | 116 | 1 | 124 |
| 1-Chi square | NS | | NS | | NS | | |

SVD: spontaneous vaginal delivery; IVD: instrumental vaginal delivery; C/S: Caesarian section.
NS: not significant.

agreement between assessments of 30% of the CTGs by two different observers was 88%.

## Discussion

Interobserver agreement over FHR variability is high (8), whereas correlation between visual assessment and on-line computed indices is poor. Cycles of FHR variability are readily appreciated by visual assessment in the majority of cases in which they are present. The similarity between previously reported quiet episodes and the duration of these episodes in labour strongly suggests that fetal behavioural changes continue in many labours, and more so in induced labours. Although episodes of low FHR variability may well relate to quiet 'fetal sleep' periods, high FHR variability cannot distinguish between active fetal sleep and awake states.

The presence of normal baseline FHR variability has always been felt to be indicative of a fetus in good condition (1,17). Reduced FHR variability is regarded as a sign of fetal distress during labour, requiring further investigation (5,19). However, decreased or absent variability has been shown to occur with equal frequency in the presence or absence of acidosis (15).

Apart from fetal behavioural changes, other factors are known to affect the fetal baseline variability during labour. Yeh's 'Interval Index' of long-term variability is temporarily but significantly decreased following pethidine (12), but it is not affected by oxytocin (13). The use of bupivacaine for epidural analgesia causes a significant increase in variability (14). In this study there were no differences in the use of these drugs between labours with and without cycles of FHR variability.

Recently, increased short-term variability has been correlated with increased fetal scalp noradrenaline levels in the absence of fetal acidosis (2). It may be that increased levels of catecholamines are associated with an activated fetal state although the accepted view is that raised noradrenaline in labour is an early indication of fetal distress.

This study found episodes of high and low FHR variability in 58% of monitored term labours over 6 hours' duration. It appears there is a greater decrease in such cycles in spontaneous labour and this may be related to factors governing the onset of labour. Five per cent of the first quiet episodes in this study were between 45 and 90 minutes' duration, and in these cases other tests such as fetal stimulation or fetal blood sampling may be needed to differentiate physiological from pathophysiological changes in baseline FHR variability.

## Acknowledgements

We thank Mrs P Yudkin for advice and the Medical Research Council for financial support.

## References

1. Beard R W, Filshie G M, Knight C A and Robert G M. The significance of the changes in the continuous fetal heart rate in the first stage of labour. *Journal of Obstetrics and Gynaecology of the British Commonwealth*, 78, 865-881 (1971).
2. Bistoletti P, Lagercrantz H and Lunell N-O. Fetal plasma catecholamine concentrations and fetal heart rate variability during first stage of labour. *British Journal of Obstetrics and Gynaecology*, 90, 11-15 (1983).

3. Boddy K. Fetal circulation and breathing movements. In *Fetal Physiology and Medicine,* edited by R W Beard and P W Nathanielz, 302-328. W B Saunders Co Ltd, London (1976).
4. Carse E A, Wilkinson A R, Whyte P L, Henderson- Smart D J and Johnson P. Oxygen and carbon dioxide tensions, breathing and heart rate in normal infants during the first six months of life. *Journal of Developmental Physiology,* 3, 85-100, (1981).
5. Cibils L A. Clinical significance of fetal heart rate patterns during labour. *American Journal of Obstetrics and Gynecology,* 125, 290-305 (1976).
6. Dawes G S, Visser G H A, Goodman J D S and Levine D H. Numerical analysis of the human fetal heart rate: modulation by breathing and movement. *American Journal of Obstetrics and Gynecology,* 140, 535-544 (1981).
7. DeHaan R, Patrick J, Chess G F and Jaco N T. Definition of sleep state in the newborn infant by heart rate analysis. *American Journal of Obstetrics and Gynecology,* 127, 753-758 (1977).
8. Escarcena L, McKinney R D and Depp R. Fetal baseline heart rate variability estimation. *American Journal of Obstetrics and Gynecology,* 135, 615-621 (1979).
9. Greene K R, Natale R and Harrison C Y. Heart period variation and gross body movements after amniotomy in the human fetus. In *Fetal and Neonatal Physiological Measurements,* edited by P Rolfe, 250-255, Pitman Medical, Tunbridge Wells (1980).
10. Junge H D. Behavioural states and state-related heart rate and motor activity patterns in the newborn infant and fetus antepartum - a comparative study. *Journal of Perinatal Medicine,* 7, 85-148 (1979).
11. Junge H D and Walter H. Behavioural states and breathing activity in the fetus near term. *Journal of Perinatal Medicine,* 8, 150-157 (1980).
12. Kariniemi V and Ämmälä P. Effects of intrapartum pethidine on fetal heart rate variability during labour. *British Journal of Obstetrics and Gynaecology,* 88, 718-720 (1981).
13. Kariniemi V, Paatero H and Ämmälä P. The effects of oxytocin on the fetal heart rate variability during labour. *Journal of Perinatal Medicine,* 9, 251-254 (1981).
14. Lavin J P, Samuels S V, Miodovnik M, Holroyde J, Loon M and Joyce T. The effects of bupivacaine and chlorprocaine as local anaesthetics for epidural anesthesia on fetal heart rate monitoring parameters. *American Journal of Obstetrics and Gynecology,* 141, 717-722 (1981).
15. Low J A, Cox M J, Karchmar E J, Panchani S R and Piercy W N. The prediction of intrapartum fetal metabolic acidosis by fetal heart rate monitoring. *American Journal of Obstetrics and Gynecology,* 139, 299-305 (1981).
16. Nijhuis J G, Prechtl H F R, Martin C B and Bots R S G M. Are there behavioural states in the human fetus? *Early Human Development,* 6, 177-195 (1982).
17. Paul R H, Snidan A K, Yeh S-Y, Schifrin B S and Hon E H. The evaluation and significance of intrapartum baseline FHR variability. *American Journal of Obstetrics and Gynecology,* 123, 206-210 (1975).
18. Richardson B, Natale R and Patrick J. Human fetal breathing activity during electively induced labour at term. *American Journal of Obstetrics and Gynecology,* 133, 247-255 (1979),
19. Thomas G and Blackwell R J. The analysis of continuous fetal heart rate traces in the first and second stages of labour. *British Journal of Obstetrics and Gynaecology,* 82, 634-642 (1975).
20. VanGeijn H P, Jongsma H W, deHaan J, Eskes T K A B and Prechtl H F R. Heart rate as an indicator of the behavioural state. *American Journal of Obstetrics and Gynecology,* 136, 1061-1066 (1980).
21. Visser G H A, Carse E A, Goodman J D S and Johnson P. A comparison of episodic heart rate patterns in the fetus and newborn. *British Journal of Obstetrics and Gynaecology,* 89, 50-55 (1982).
22. Visser G H A, Goodman J D S, Levine D H and Dawes G S. Diurnal and other cyclic variations in human fetal heart rate near term. *American Journal of Obstetrics and Gynecology,* 142, 535-544 (1982).
23. Wheeler T and Murrills A. Patterns of fetal heart rate during normal pregnancy. *British Journal of Obstetrics and Gynaecology,* 85, 18-27 (1978).
24. Wheeler T, Gennser G, Lindvall R and Murrills A J. Changes in the fetal heart rate associated with fetal breathing and fetal movement. *British Journal of Obstetrics and Gynaecology,* 87, 1068-1079 (1980).

Chapter 18

# The effect of noise on the accuracy of the determination of fetal heart rate variability

M C Carter

## Introduction

It is often assumed that the variability of the fetal heart rate (FHR) trace produced from the fetal electrocardiogram (FECG) by commercially available electronic fetal monitors (EFM) accurately measures a physiological effect. The accuracy with which an EFM measures the intervals between successive FECG complexes and displays this information on a chart-recorder may affect the appearance and clinical interpretation of the FHR trace. Because 16-20% of the interval differences of the human FHR are less than 1 ms (6), the 'ideal' EFM should be able to resolve the interval to less than 1 ms. However, at this resolution the signal-to-noise ratio of the processed FECG signal can have a large effect on the accuracy of the FHR determination.

The unwanted noise signal present on the FECG recording is the combination of electromyographic signals from the mother and fetus, electrode interface effects, noise from the electronic amplifiers and electromagnetic interference from external sources such as electric motors and 50 Hz mains interference. EFMs usually detect the prominent QRS complex of the FECG waveforms to calculate the FHR from the interval between successive QRS complexes. The accuracy with which the same point in each cardiac cycle is detected has a direct effect on the precision of the calculated FHR. A noise signal will disturb the QRS-wave both in amplitude and temporally. Amplitude changes will affect the accuracy of detection of the correct trigger point if threshold-detecting devices are used. Peak-detecting devices will be affected by the temporal shift which may cause a peak to be detected either before or after the true cardiac event (Figure 1). The major difficulty in measuring the beat-to-beat variation in the human FHR is the restricted precision with which the fetal R-wave trigger point can be determined. As part of an EFM evaluation project the effect of noise signals on the accuracy of the FHR determination was investigated.

## Materials and methods

In the first part of the study the signal-to-noise ratio of the FECG waveform was measured. Using these data, the ability of four EFMs to reject noise signals and to calculate an accurate FHR was measured. The four monitors studied were: Corometrics 112 (112), Hewlett Packard 8040A (8040A), Kranzbuehler 5005 (5005) and

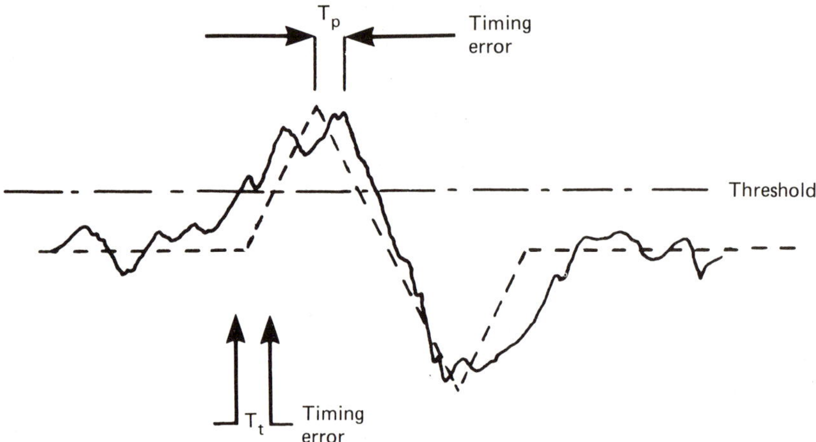


*Figure 1.* Timing-errors caused by the perturbation of the FECG signal by noise. Dotted lines represent a simulated FECG with no noise signal. Full lines represent the same simulated FECG perturbed by noise. Tp is the timing-error generated by a peak detector. Tt is the timing-error generated by a fixed threshold detector

Sonicaid FM3R with ECG (FM3R ECG) and abdominal ECG modules (FM3R AbdECG).

## Part 1: Levels of noise signals present with the FECG signal

The FECGs of 23 fetuses were recorded on a frequency modulated tape recorder (Store 4, Racal Recorders Ltd). The length of recording varied between 15 minutes and 4 hours. All recordings were made from a Copeland electrode (A W Showell (Surgicraft) Ltd) attached to the fetal scalp. The recordings were made with an ECG amplifier which had a flat response from 0.1 Hz to 150 Hz (-3dB points).

One hundred FECG complexes and the intervals between them were superimposed on top of each other on a variable persistence storage oscilloscope. The peak-to-peak amplitude of the noise measured in the interval between FECG complexes was expressed as a percentage of the peak-to-peak amplitude of the QRS complex (Figure 2). One hundred and eighteen measurements were made at 15-minute intervals throughout the recordings.

## Part 2: The effect of noise on FHR determination

The accuracy of the detection of the R-wave and subsequent calculation of FHR was determined by applying a simulated FECG to the ECG input of an EFM. The period, controlled by a crystal oscillator, between successive intervals was varied to give, at the chart-recorder input, an FHR which alternated between 115 and 120 beats per minute (b.p.m). The interval between the peak of the simulated FECG and the resultant FHR output was measured with a resolution of 25 ms. This interval was measured for 65 280 periods and displayed on a histogram as a time-error distribution.

The effect of noise on the accuracy of the FHR determination was measured by adding a random noise signal, of the same bandwidth as that found with the FECG signal, to the simulated ECG. Time-error distributions were obtained for levels of noise corresponding to the upper-limit, lower-limit and mean level of noise measured

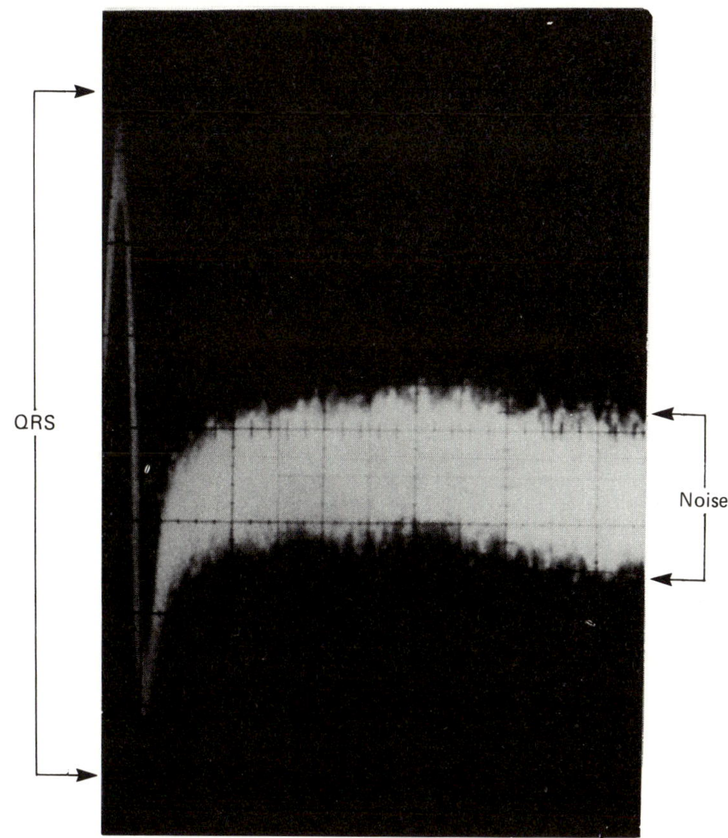


$$\% \text{ Noise} = \frac{\text{Noise}}{\text{QRS}} \times 100$$

*Figure 2.* The signal-to-noise ratio of FECG is defined as the peak-to-peak amplitude of noise expressed as a percentage of the peak-to-peak amplitude of the QRS-wave of 100 FECG complexes

in part 1 of the study. The standard deviation of the time-error distribution was plotted against the level of input noise for each monitor. These measurements were made with the 112, 5005 and FM3R ECG and FM3R AbdECG. The 8040A does not produce a signal which can be used to measure the time-error because the output FHR signal has no fixed temporal relationship to the input signal. In this case, the digital signal representing the FHR was obtained from the 8040A and the variation in FHR for each noise level was measured at 120 and 180 b.p.m.

## Results

### Part 1

The frequency distribution of the amplitude of the noise signals obtained from the recordings of the FECG is shown in Figure 3. The distribution is approximately

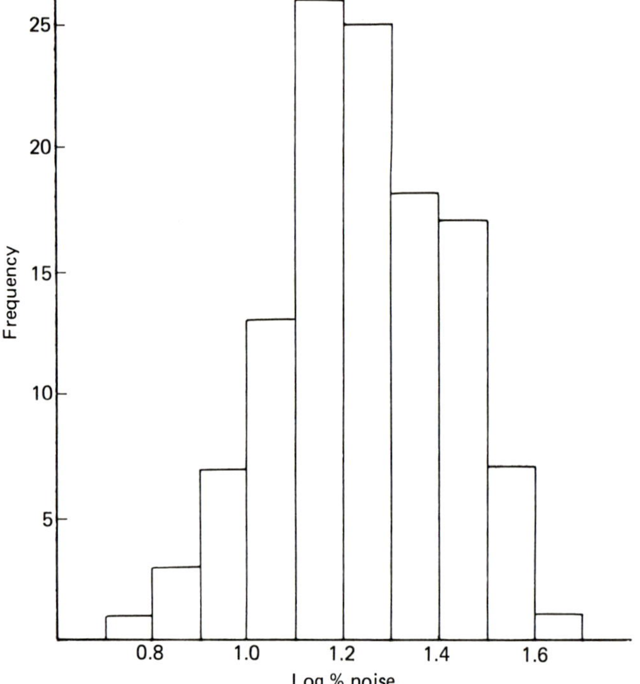


*Figure 3.* Frequency distribution of the signal-to-noise ratio of the FECG

lognormal with a noise level of 17% ± (log x) = 0.17 (mean ± s.d.). The upper and lower limits of the normal range were 38.9% and 7.8% respectively.

### Part 2

Figure 4 shows the standard deviation of the time-error distributions plotted against the level of noise. The upper-limit, lower-limit and mean levels of noise derived in part 1 of the study are indicated.

At the lower-limit the range of timing-errors due to noise was 0.2-0.78 ms. The timing-error at the upper-limit of the normal noise range increased to 1.53 ms for the most accurate EFM studied whilst the least accurate EFM had a timing-error of 5.2 ms.

## Discussion and conclusions

Commercially available EFMs have a timing-error of less than 0.5 ms and will give an accurate determination of FHR when there is no noise present. However, noise signals are always present when recordings are made from biological systems. The mean level of the normal range of noise signals recorded from the fetal scalp electrode is 17%. As the noise level contaminating the FECG increases, the ability of the monitors to reject the noise and determine the correct FHR decreases. At high noise levels there are marked differences in the accuracy of the FHR determined by different EFMs.

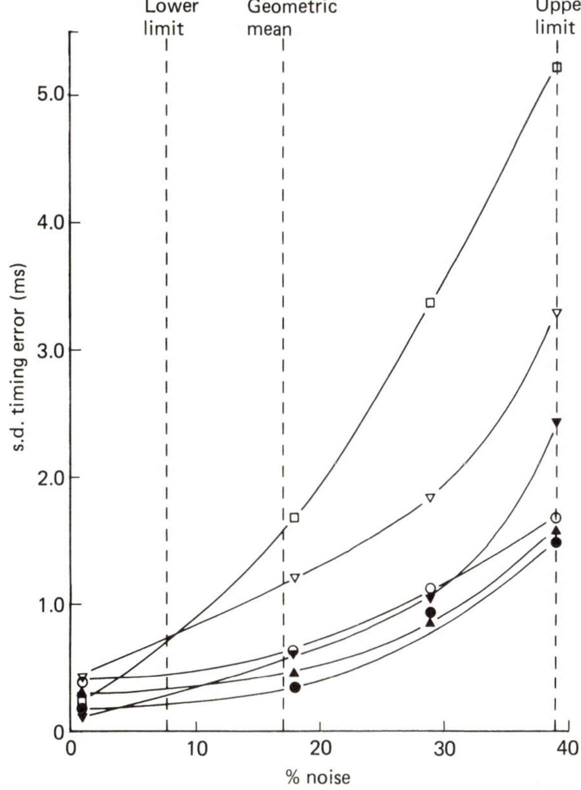


*Figure 4*. Standard deviation of the time-error distributions plotted against the signal-to-noise ratio of a simulated FECG for four EFMs. ▲—▲ 112; ●—● 8040A (120 b.p.m.); ○—○ 8040A (180 b.p.m.); □—□ 5005; ▼—▼ FM3R ECG; ▽—▽ FM3R AbdECG

The beat-to-beat variation of the human FHR is small. Wheeler *et al* (6) found that in the human fetus the standard deviation of the interval differences was 6.2 ms ± 1.9 (mean ± s.d.) and that of the interval differences between fetuses which were resting and those which were active was 1.7 ms ± 2.4 (mean ± s.d.). Wickham *et al* (7) quote a figure of mean 2.3 ms ± 0.3 s.e. for the beat-to-beat variation. The value given by Dawes *et al* (2) is about 2 ms and they concluded that this figure may be due to factors other than true physiological changes in the FHR. Dalton *et al* (1) showed that in the fetal sheep blockage of the sympathetic and parasympathetic system decreased the FHR variability dramatically although 35-40% of short-term and long-term FHR variability remained. The residue has a value of 0.6 ms ± 0.03 (mean ± s.e.) and was explained in terms of system noise, intrinsic variability of the heart, humoral agents other than catecholamines, and changes in the cardiac axis. Although the values of beat-to-beat variation reported in the literature were measured using research equipment designed for the precise measurement of FHR, it is unlikely that the precision of measurement of FHR exceeds that of the best EFM investigated in this study. The standard deviation of the time-error measured in this study refers to a single QRS-wave timing-error. If the FHR interval is considered, then the timing-errors due to two QRS-wave detections must be taken into account, in which case the time-error is likely to be up to 50% greater than the values shown in Figure 4.

The timing-error due to noise is likely to account for the major part of the beat-to-beat variability.

When the FHR or QRS-wave trigger-pulses from commercially available EFMs are used to calculate indices of FHR variability (3, 4, 5) it is important to define the levels of noise so that the indices measure a physiological change and not changes in the noise level of the FECG signal.

Care should be taken to maximize the signal-to-noise ratio of the FECG by careful electrode preparation. Reduction of electromyographic activity and electrode movement artefact may be obtained by sedation of the woman in labour, if this is considered appropriate.

Great importance has been attached by many obstetricians to the need for EFMs to measure the FHR with a beat-to-beat interval accuracy. However, the slow speed of the EFM chart-recorder (1 cm/min) and the scale sensitivity (30 b.p.m/cm) make it impossible to detect changes in the order of 1 ms. It has been shown that the noise will cause errors in the determination of FHR of the same order as those having physiological significance and that there is large variation in the ability of different commercially available EFMs to reject noise signal and calculate a precise FHR. Commercially available EFMs are therefore only useful to measure baseline FHR variation.

## Acknowledgements

The study described above is part of a larger project on the evaluation of fetal monitors and is funded by the Department of Health and Social Security, Scientific and Technical Branch. The author thanks I A Sutherland and P J Steer for their advice in the preparation of this paper.

## References

1. Dalton K J, Dawes G S and Patrick J E. The autonomic nervous system and fetal heart rate variability. *American Journal of Obstetrics and Gynecology,* 146, 456-462 (1983).

2. Dawes G S, Visser G H A, Goodman J D S and Levine D H. Numerical analysis of the human fetal heart rate: modulation by breathing and movement. *American Journal of Obstetrics and Gynecology,* 140, 535-544 (1981).

3. Nageotte M P, Freeman R K, Freeman A G and Dorchester W. Short-term variability assessment from abdominal electrocardiogram during the antenatal period. *American Journal of Obstetrics and Gynecology,* 145, 566-569 (1983).

4. Saini V D and Maulik D. Computation of short-term fetal heart-rate variability from heart-rate waveforms. *Computers in Biology and Medicine,* 12, 81-86 (1982).

5. Tromans P M, Sheen M A and Beazley M. Feto-maternal surveillance in labour: a new approach with an on-line microcomputer. *British Journal of Obstetrics and Gynaecology,* 89, 1021-1030 (1982).

6. Wheeler T, Cooke E and Murrills A. Computer analysis of fetal heart rate variation during normal pregnancy. *British Journal of Obstetrics and Gynaecology,* 86, 186-197 (1979).

7. Wickham P J D, Dawes G S and Belcher R. Development of methods for the quantitative analysis of the fetal heart rate. *Journal of Biomedical Engineering,* 5, 302-308 (1983).

Chapter 19

# The fetal phonocardiogram

**J Morgenstern, T Abels, R Leblanc, U Naumann, H Schettler, P Wolf**

## Introduction

This paper describes one part of a 'stand-alone' fetal monitoring system, consisting of special multi-element transducers, a nine-channel telemetry system and a special purpose microcomputer.

The data presented here were derived from chronically instrumented fetal lambs.

## The three-part study

The purpose of this study may be summarized by three questions, which are used as guidelines.

### Is it possible to set up a beat-to-beat FHR-monitor based on the phonocardiogram?

The original heart sounds (HS) were digital bandpass filtered (30-100 Hz) and analysed (HP 900-Computer) in parallel with the ECG, the arterial blood pressure and the electromagnetically measured stroke volume (SV). The HS were analysed by four different algorithms:

(a) Computing the envelope curve (EV) (Process mainly to overcome the difficulties in correctly determining the beginning of each HS) and evaluating
  (i) the parameter describing the EV
  (ii) the HS-parameter defined by the EV
(b) Discrete Fourier transformation (DFT)
(c) Linear Prediction (LP)
(d) Autocorrelation.

Since the DFT is a time consuming process even for very fast computers, its real time application is possible only with several restrictions. The LP has also been used with only a few predictors.

Figure 1 shows an example of these methods. At the top several original HS are displayed. Two first HS and two second HS are marked by brackets 1 1, 3 3 and 2

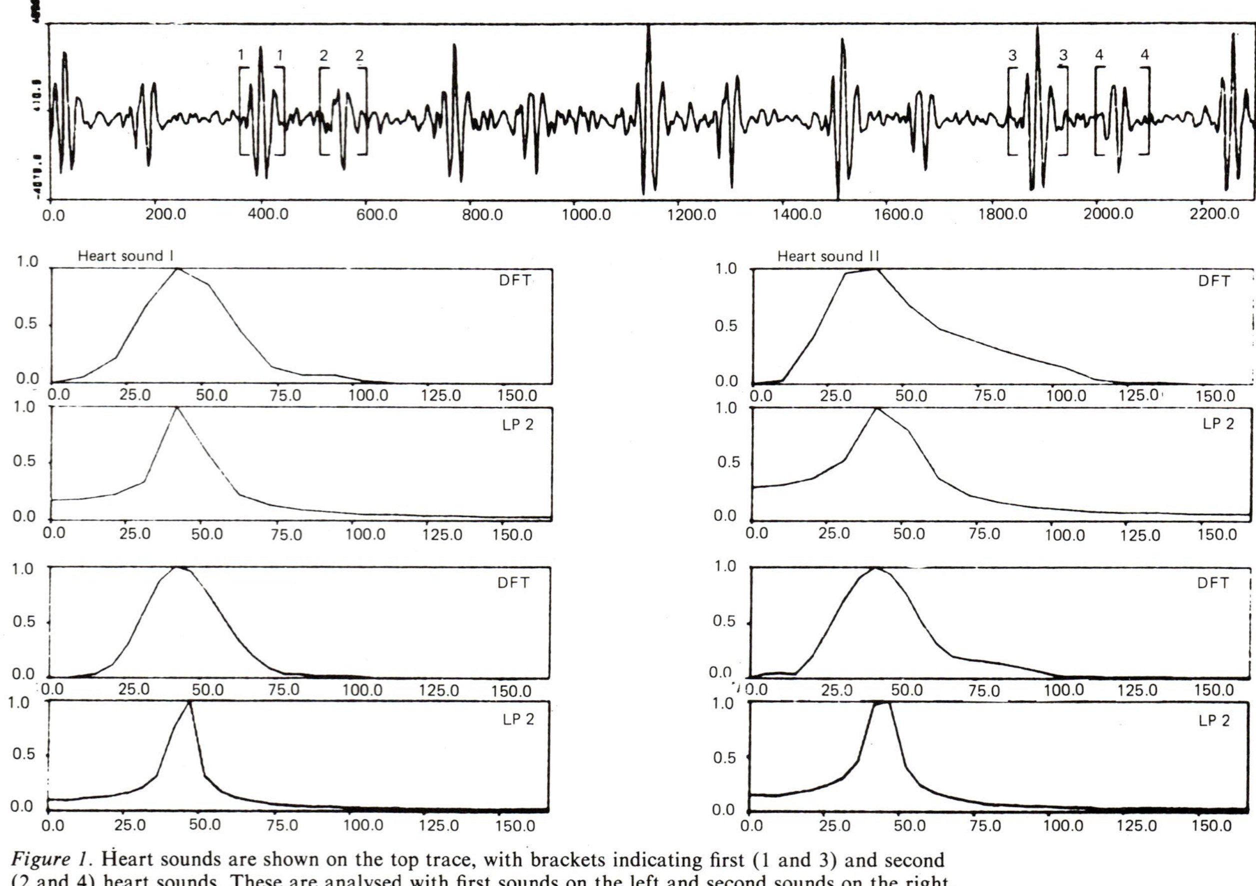


*Figure 1*. Heart sounds are shown on the top trace, with brackets indicating first (1 and 3) and second (2 and 4) heart sounds. These are analysed with first sounds on the left and second sounds on the right, showing (top to bottom): frequency-amplitude spectra after discrete fourier transformation (DFT), and after linear prediction (LP)

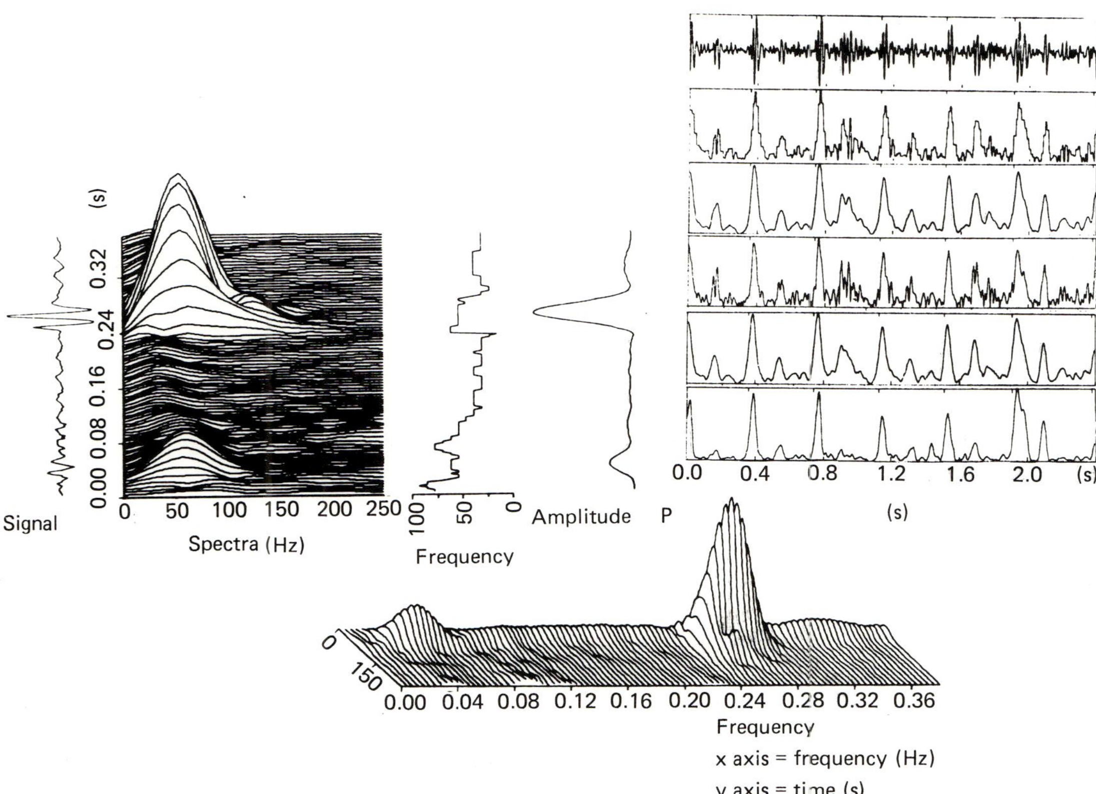


*Figure 2.* Left (signal): Original heart sound (one heart cycle); half left (spectra): DFT-spectra in successive order; right (amplitude): Max. amplitude for each DFT-spectrum; half right (frequency): Frequency at max. amplitude; bottom right (frequency): DFT-spectra rotated by 90°; top right: ST for five different algorithms together with original recording

2, 4 4, respectively. The contents of these brackets are analysed by DFT and LP and the results are shown below. The first field on the top left shows the frequency distribution after DFT while the LP-results are depicted underneath. The results of the two first HS are on the left hand side while the two second HS are on the right. It is obvious that the results concerning DFT and LP are comparable. The dominating frequencies are around 50 Hz for both HS. The distributions of the second HS seem to be more skewed to higher frequencies.

A continuous on-line assessment could be performed by examining the data in the above mentioned way for each new digitized data point. For off-line evaluation a 40 ms window was shifted in 2 ms (digitizing rate) steps over the signal. The results of such a procedure are shown in Figure 2. In this Figure, on the left, in the vertical axis, an original recording of one complete heart cycle is shown. The first window-result after DFT, is shown as the first amplitude/frequency spectrum parallel to the horizontal axis, expressed in Hz. The next spectrum in parallel gives the result derived from the window shifted by 2 ms. Corresponding to the first and second heart sounds, the frequency distributions are increasing and showing peaks where the original HS occur. From each spectrum the maximum amplitude and the frequency at maximum amplitude were computed. These two spectra are plotted on the right of the figure in the vertical axis. The spectrum of the amplitudes clearly points with its two extreme values to the first and second HS, respectively. The course of this spectrum could be easily redrawn from the 3D-spectrum (Figure 2, bottom right) by connecting the extreme value from each spectrum. The continous application of this process, the so-called spectral tracking (ST), is shown in Figure 2, top right, for several HS calculated by DFT, LP and three more algorithms. Since the methods are slightly different, and show different senstivity and specifity, a simultaneous application of at least three of

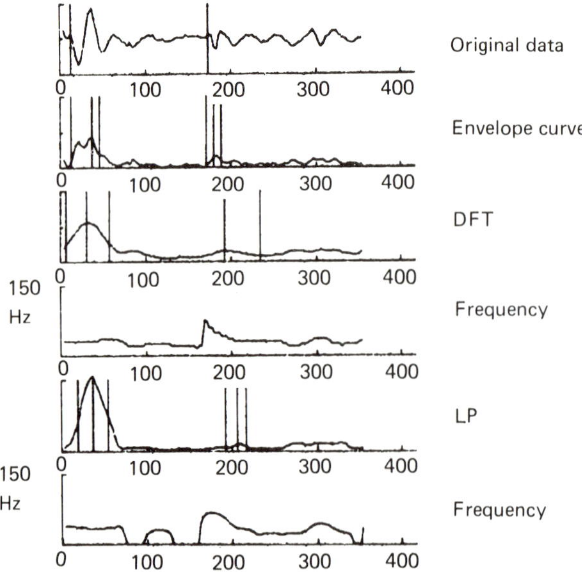


*Figure 3.* Control picture during evaluation (from top to bottom): Original but filtered HS (one heart cycle) with vertical bars at max. R-wave (from ECG) and diacrotic notch (from arterial blood pressure); envelope curve; DFT-amplitudes; DFT-frequencies; LP-amplitudes; LP-frequencies. The x-axis is scaled in ms

them seems reasonable and effective. The ST findings are fed into a logic tree to evaluate the most probable heart rate.

**Are there any specific beat-to-beat parameters available from each first or second heart sound that reflect FHR changes?**

From each peak in the spectral tracking display, the widths at half amplitude were detected and the corresponding original HS signal analysed for frequency, duration and amplitude . During the course of evaluation a control picture - Figure 3 - could be displayed. This Figure shows in relation to the HS (top trace) where, for example, DFT and LP have detected the HS - two vertical bars at half width - which define the areas of evaluation for that specific cardiac cycle. The corresponding frequencies are depicted in the traces 4 and 6, respectively.

With this second question we are looking for characteristic HS parameter changes. Thus we have chosen a FHR-trace with a severe pattern. In order to give an impression of the cardiovascular situation in Figure 4 besides the HR-trace, the left (L) and

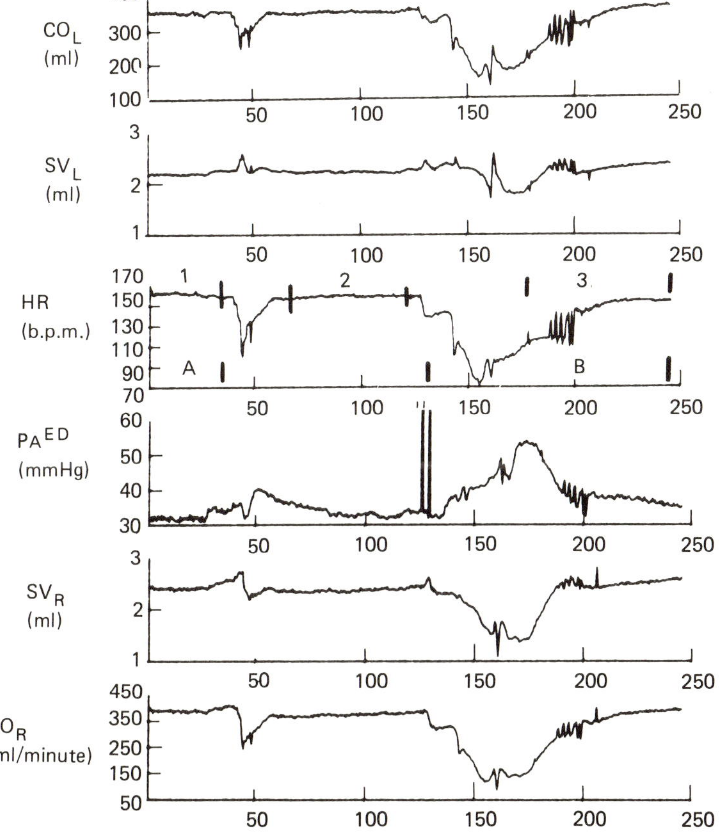


*Figure 4.* Six traces during severe cardiovascular changes. The abbreviations are: CO cardiac output, SV stroke volume, HR heart rate, $P_A$ arterial blood pressure, ED end diastolic, L left, R right. The x-axis is scaled in s

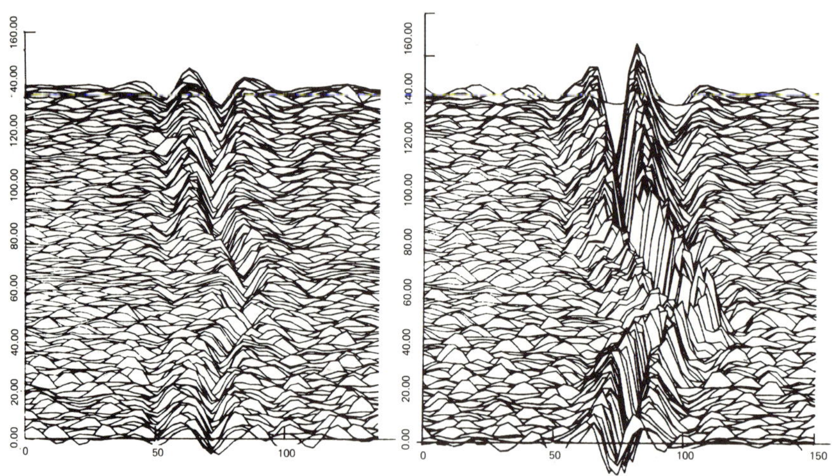


*Figure 5.* For the severe HR deceleration (*see Figure 4*) the filtered first HS (left) and second HS in successive order triggered by the ECG R-wave

right (R) SV, the after-load ($P_A$) and both cardiac outputs (CO) are shown. Although both SV are decreasing, they do not seem to be completely synchronized. In Figure 5 the first (left) and second HS are plotted in successive order. This plot starts well before the beginning of the severe deceleration. Each HS was triggered by the maximum of the R-wave. For further explanation how such figures are built up see (1).

Besides the somewhat lower or even diminished first upstroke of the first HS in the deceleration - which would trigger uncertainties and result in so-called jitter - and the increased amplitude of the second HS, there are no changes clear enough to be distinguished. These results are supported by the beat-to-beat computed numerical values, which are shown in Figure 6 (left for the first and right for the second HS). The three traces following the RR interval trace are the amplitude a, the duration d and the frequency f. The only pronounced change occurs in the course of the amplitude of the second HS. All the other parameters do not change simultaneously with the FHR-changes. The mean values with s.d. for the total trace and the two marked subtraces A and B (see Figure 4) are shown in Table 1.

**TABLE 1. Mean values for the total trace and two subtraces.**

| *HS* | *Total* (n=627) | | *A* (n=174) | | *B* (n=124) | |
|---|---|---|---|---|---|---|
| | *First* | *Second* | *First* | *Second* | *First* | *Second* |
| a (aU) | 11.1 | 19.7 | 11.9 | 17.0 | 10.2 | 27.6 |
| | 1.6 | 4.7 | 1.0 | 1.3 | 2.0 | 4.2 |
| d (ms) | 52.1 | 47.0 | 50.2 | 47.4 | 55.7 | 45.4 |
| | 8.2 | 3.3 | 3.0 | 2.4 | 12.8 | 3.3 |
| f (Hz) | 42.0 | 53.0 | 41.6 | 54.6 | 43.7 | 50.0 |
| | 2.3 | 9.1 | 0.7 | 7.9 | 3.8 | 8.9 |

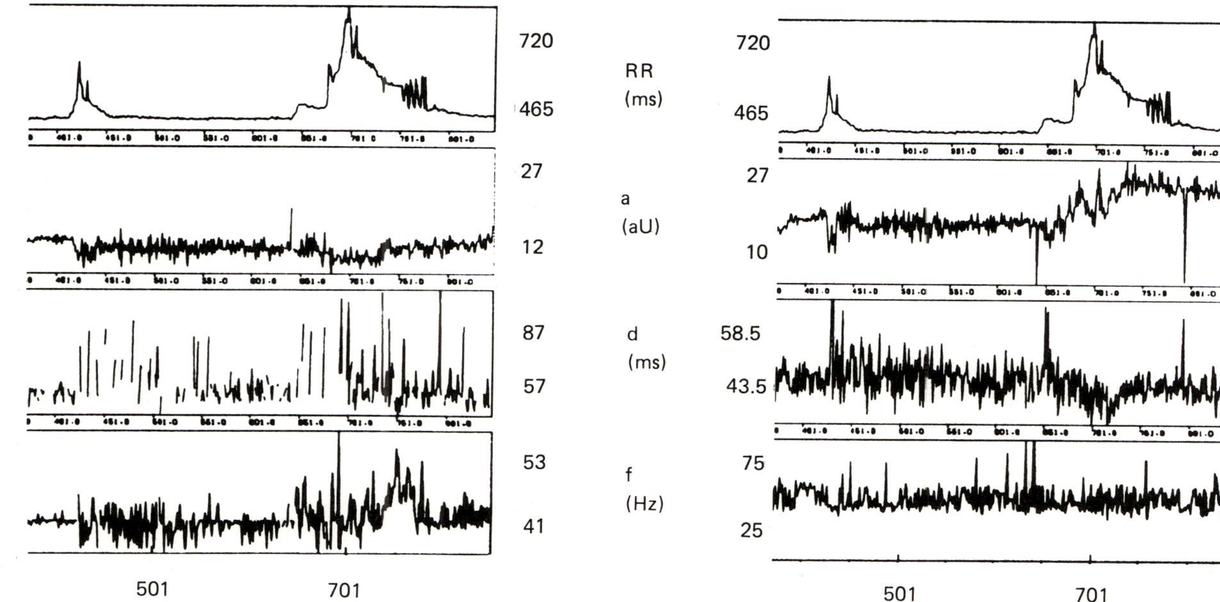


*Figure 6*. HS parameters (left first HS) calculated beat-to-beat from DFT. Top to bottom: RR-interval (inverse HR); a = amplitude (aU); d = HS duration in ms i.e. width at half amplitude (*see* vertical bars in Figure 3); f = frequency in Hz

Although there are statistically highly significant differences between the first and second HS, especially in the amplitude, a, and in the frequency, f, none of these parameters reflects FHR-changes. Since the origins of the HS is still a controversial subject, we do not want to enter this discussion. But, on the other hand, the fact that the severe FHR deceleration is neither reflected in a change of this HS duration nor in the HS frequency, but only in the HS amplitude, supports the hypothesis that the first HS is due to the contraction of the heart muscle without much contribution from the dynamics of the mitral valve or the left ventricle. In answering the second question, these findings could be summarized by the fact that due to these parameters and the described methods there is no way to discriminate the two HS beat-to-beat.

In conclusion, it therefore seems that the chief source of the HS is based on muscle contraction.

The results so far are not very satisfying. Especially the fact that the severe haemodynamic changes are in no way reflected in any HS-parameters and there is no difference in the parameters, although we had the impression that the overall spectrum (Figure 2) seems to show characteristic differences in the first and second HS. These disappointing results implicitly answer the third question:

### Do any of the HS-parameters offer the possibility to calculate the fetal SV indirectly?

This research idea was based on the assumption that the heart is a pump which generates the HS. Therefore SV changes might be reflected in HS alterations.

Thus we started another method of evaluation, without any filtering of the data. From each amplitude/frequency spectrum we detected all extreme values. Each first and second HS was represented by several amplitude and corresponding frequency values. By connecting points with nearly the same amplitude we constructed loops with changing frequencies.

The mean values with s.d. for the three subtraces 1,2 and 3 (see Figure 4) are shown in Table 2. For the first HS we found three main frequencies. While the frequency around 25 Hz appears only in 40 of 201 beats within the first subtrace and the frequency 34.5 Hz only in 68 of 132 beats within the second subtrace, the frequency around 25 Hz does not appear in the third part.

While the amplitudes (aU) of the low frequencies are increasing from 16.8 to 22.1,

**TABLE 2. Mean values with s.d. for the three subtraces.**

| *Sub-trace* | | *First HS* | | | *Second HS* | |
|---|---|---|---|---|---|---|
| 1 | N | 201 | 40 | 193 | | 201 |
| | f | 12.1(0.8) | 25.0(1.6) | 34.8(2.4) | | 30.1(1.6) |
| | a | 16.8(1.7) | 17.0(1.7) | 21.3(3.4) | | 40.2(4.1) |
| 2 | N | 132 | 112 | 68 | | 150 |
| | f | 12.6(1.0) | 24.4(1.6) | 34.5(4.0) | | 30.9(1.9) |
| | a | 18.4(2.5) | 24.1(4.1) | 24.1(5.7) | | 43.3(6.0) |
| 3 | N | 106 | | 101 | 107 | 65 |
| | f | 15.2(1.0) | | 37.4(2.3) | 15.2(1.5) | 36.2(2.0) |
| | a | 22.1(4.8) | | 16.1(5.4) | 20-7(4.8) | 56.9(12.0) |

N=No. of beats, f=frequency (Hz), a=amplitude (aU).

the higher components only increase from 21.3 to 24.1 and decrease to below starting level to 16.1.

For the second HS we mainly found only one frequency starting with 30.1 Hz and ending up with 36.2 Hz for the third subtrace. In the third subtrace an additional frequency of 15.2 Hz appears for all 107 cases, while the high frequency of 36.2 Hz is only present in 65 beats. These new findings offer a completely alternative way of differentiation between the two HS, and since the briefly described method of HS-mapping reflects some haemodynamic changes, we hope to answer the third question positively.

## Conclusion

In conclusion, the evaluation of the fetal phonocardiograms during haemodynamic changes cannot be done by simply picking up the frequency with the highest amplitude. It is rather a dynamic process with changing frequencies and amplitudes.

## Reference

1. Morgenstern J H, Czerny H, Schmidt H, Schulz J and Wernicke K. Systolic time intervals (STI) as a measure of myocardial contractility. In *Fetal and Neonatal Physiological Measurements,* edited by P Rolfe. Tunbridge Wells, Pitman Medical (1980).

Chapter 20

# Observations on the evolution of human fetal acidosis

**N C Smith, W P Soutter, F Sharp**

## Introduction

When human fetal hypoxia occurs, acidosis develops as a result of carbon dioxide retention and lactate accumulation, although it has never been clearly established if hypercapnia and lacticacidaemia occur simultaneously or separately. It has been postulated that the acidosis due to hypercapnia is more acute, transitory and of earlier onset than that due to lacticacidaemia which results from a more severe hypoxic insult, develops more slowly, lasts longer and is therefore more harmful to the fetus (1,4,6).

In the normal steady state the fetal acid-base status is determined by that of the mother. When placental gaseous exchange is impaired, carbon dioxide accumulates in the fetus and is converted to carbonic acid which dissociates into hydrogen and bicarbonate ions. The hydrogen ions are buffered by non-bicarbonate buffers, the most important being haemoglobin. Once these buffers become saturated, a fall in pH occurs. Lactic acid also accumulates in the fetal blood and tissues as a consequence of hypoxia. Glycogen, glucose and other minor sugars, under normal conditions are broken down anaerobically to pyruvate and then aerobically, via the tricarboxylic acid cycle, to form carbon dioxide and water with the release of energy in the form of adenosine triphosphate (ATP). When hypoxia occurs aerobic metabolism is halted and pyruvate is converted to lactate which accumulates in the tissues and blood. Under anaerobic conditions, sixteen times as many glucose molecules have to be broken down to produce the same energy as would be obtained under aerobic conditions. The lactic acid produced is buffered by both bicarbonate and non-bicarbonate buffers but once these are saturated a fall in pH occurs. The fetal kidneys are capable of excreting hydrogen ions although acidosis may compromise this function (2). The fetal lungs probably have no acid-base regulatory function.

The lack of understanding of the evolution of fetal acidosis has been compounded by difficulty in measuring lactate in the small samples obtained from the fetal scalp. Indirect measures of the lactate concentration have been made using the base excess (1,4), the base excess calculated at a haemoglobin concentration of 5g/100 ml (3), or the pH after equilibration of the blood sample with carbon dioxide at a tension of 40 mmHg (6). The conventional spectrophotometric method of lactate assay takes about 60 minutes and requires at least 1.0 ml of blood, to which strong acid has to be added after the sample has been placed on ice. A much faster electrochemical enzymatic method of lactate assay was developed (5), taking only 90 seconds, and a commercially available Lactate Analyser was subsequently developed. Soutter and co-workers (1978) evaluated this instrument, and they recommended its use for fetal scalp blood lactate assay by a technique which involved minimal handling of the sample and which had clinical applicability for the detection of intrapartum hypoxia (9).

## Patients and methods

Fetal scalp blood (FSB) samples were obtained on 306 occasions from 215 fetuses. An AVL 937C microanalyser (8) was used to measure the FSB gases, pH and derived values, and a Roche Lactate Analyser 640 (9) to measure the FSB lactate concentrations.

The normal ranges of values were derived from FSB sampled from fetuses in whom, during the preceding hour, the baseline heart rate had been between 120-160 beats/minute with no decelerations, who were born in good condition with 1 and 5 minute Apgar scores greater than six, and whose birth weights were greater than 2.5 kg. Cases were excluded if intravenous 10% glucose, fructose, haemacel, plasma or blood had been administered to the mother. Ninety-seven FSB samples, taken at different cervical dilations, fulfilled these criteria of normality, and the results were pooled to obtain the limits of the normal values which, for the purposes of this analysis, were derived from the 95% confidence limits (mean ± 2 s.d.) (7). Thus, $PCO_2$ values greater than 6.7 kPa (50.5 mmHg), pH values less than 7.26 and lactate values greater than 2.9 nmol/1 were considered abnormal (Table 1)

**TABLE 1. Limits of normal values.**

| *Parameter* | *Confidence limit (95%)* |
|---|---|
| $PCO_2$ | 6.7 kPa (50.5 mm Hg) |
| pH | 7.26 |
| Lactate | 2.9 nmol/1 |

## Results

In the 306 FSB samples there was a good correlation between the $PCO_2$ and pH values (r = -0.7) and between the lactate and pH values (r = -0.7). The correlation was poorer between the base deficit and pH values (r= -0.6) and between the base deficit and lactate values (r = -0.5) (Table 2). One hundred and five of the 306 FSB

**TABLE 2. Correlation coefficients between $PCO_2$, pH, lactate and base deficit in fetal scalp blood.**

| | *$PCO_2$* | *pH* | *Lactate* |
|---|---|---|---|
| pH | −0.7 | | |
| Lactate | 0.4 | −0.7 | |
| Base deficit | 0.1 | −0.6 | +0.5 |

**TABLE 3. Abnormal acid-base parameters found in 306 fetal scalp blood samples.**

| *Abnormal parameters* | *Number* |
|---|---|
| pH+$PCO_2$+lactate | 24 |
| pH+$PCO_2$ | 4 |
| pH+lactate | 3 |
| pH | 3 |
| $PCO_2$ | 41 |
| Lactate | 23 |
| $PCO_2$+lactate | 7 |
| Total with one or more abnormal values | 105 |

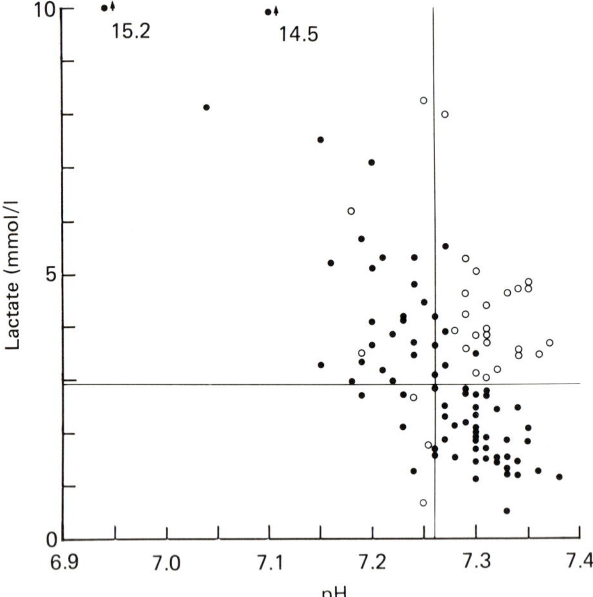


*Figure 1.* The relationship between fetal scalp blood lactate and pH values in samples with at least one abnormal parameter. O—O normal $PCO_2$; ●—● abnormal $PCO_2$

samples had one or more abnormal $PCO_2$ , pH or lactate values (Table 3, Figures 1 and 2). Thirty-four FSB samples had abnormal pH values: 24 of these had existing abnormal $PCO_2$ and lactate values; four had abnormal $PCO_2$ but normal lactate values; three had abnormal lactate but normal $PCO_2$ values; and three had normal $PCO_2$ and lactate values. Forty-one FSB samples had abnormal $PCO_2$ values only, and 23 FSB samples had abnormal lactate values only. In seven FSB samples there were abnormal $PCO_2$ and lactate values but normal pH values.

Hypercapnia and lacticacidosis were commonly found in association with a sudden profound fetal bradycardia as a result of uterine hypertonicity due to intravenous oxytocic overdosage (Table 4). Repeat measurements on the nine FSB samples

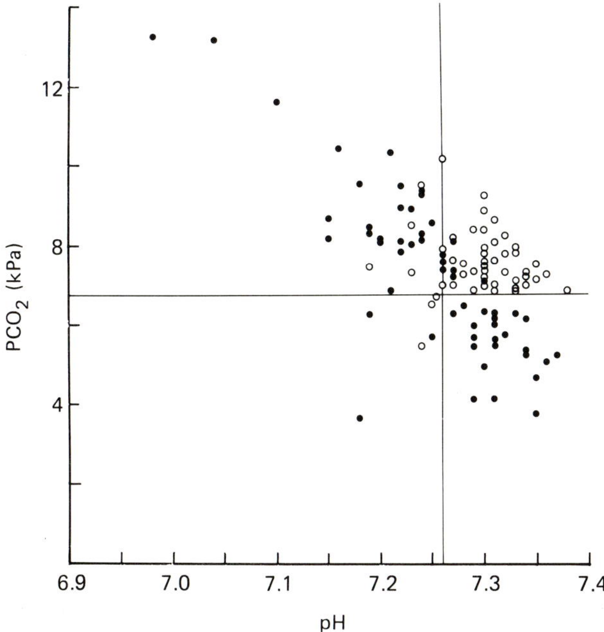


*Figure 2.* The relationship between fetal scalp blood $PCO_2$ and pH values in samples with at least one abnormal parameter. O—O normal lactate; ●—● abnormal lactate

**TABLE 4. Pairs of fetal scalp samples, the first taken during a prolonged bradycardia, the second after the fetal heart rate was normal.**

| *Time interval between samples (minutes)* | *$PCO_2$ (kPa)* | *pH* | *Lactate (nmol/l)* |
|---|---|---|---|
| 25 | — | 7.24 | 8.22 |
| | 4.8 | 7.40 | 2.72 |
| 90 | 6.3 | 7.27 | 8.00 |
| | 5.9 | 7.38 | 2.44 |
| 75 | — | 7.20 | 2.58 |
| | 4.9 | 7.39 | 1.25 |
| 30 | 11.6 | 7.10 | 14.5 |
| | 5.6 | 7.29 | *5.0* |
| 132 | 8.1 | 7.24 | 3.43 |
| | 5.6 | 7.27 | *3.30* |
| 95 | 7.5 | 7.23 | 4.11 |
| | *6.9* | 7.29 | 2.81 |
| 67 | 9.3 | 7.24 | 4.90 |
| | *7.1* | 7.35 | 2.02 |
| 120 | 9.5 | 7.22 | 3.91 |
| | *7.9* | 7.37 | 1.85 |
| 55 | 9.6 | 7.23 | 1.27 |
| | *8.2* | 7.27 | 1.83 |

Abnormal values in the second samples are shown in *italic*.

obtained after the hypertonicity had resolved and the fetal heart rate had returned to a normal rate revealed no significant acidosis in any of these samples. However, lacticacidaemia was still evident in two samples and hypercapnia in four.

## Discussion

The good correlation between rising $PCO_2$ values and falling pH values and between rising lactate values and falling pH values implies that hypercapnia and lacticacidaemia are principally responsible for causing a fall in pH. The poor correlation between the base deficit and lactate values suggests that the base deficit is a poor measure of lacticacidaemia.

The postulate that the acidosis due to hypercapnia is more acute, transitory and of earlier onset than that due to lacticacidaemia could not be substantiated by the results of the study, since 24 of the 34 (70%) FSB samples with abnormal pH values had associated abnormal $PCO_2$ and lactate values, four samples had evidence of acidosis as a consequence of hypercapnia only and three samples had acidosis due to lacticacidaemia only. In the human fetus it seems likely that hypoxia causes a fall in pH because of simultaneously elevated carbon dioxide and lactate levels. This suggests that the fetus resorts to anaerobic metabolism almost as soon as placental gaseous exchange is impaired to such an extent as to cause hypercapnia.

Of the 105 samples with abnormal $PCO_2$ , pH or lactate values, 41 had abnormal $PCO_2$ values only and 23 had abnormal lactate values only, although this interpretation depends on the chosen cut-off between normal and abnormal values (7). However, regardless of the exact cut-off values used, hypercapnia or lacticacidaemia may be present without necessarily causing a fall in pH, probably reflecting the action of fetal blood buffers until they become saturated when a fall in pH will result. The finding of co-existent hypercapnia and lacticacidaemia without an abnormal pH was unusual, occurring in only seven samples.

Recovery from fetal acidaemia following hypoxia due to uterine hypertonus was associated with an almost simultaneous return of lactate and $PCO_2$ values to normal (Table 4). This suggests that the acidosis due to lactate accumulation may be as rapid in onset and as transient as that due to hypercapnia.

In conclusion, in the human fetus acidosis due to hypoxia is probably caused by the simultaneous accumulation of carbon dioxide and lactate. This acidosis may be acute and short-lived and there may not be separate respiratory and metabolic components as there are in the human adult.

## Acknowledgements

This research was supported by a grant from the Scottish Hospital Endowments' Research Trust (HERT 544). We thank Professor Whitfield for checking the script.

## References

1. Beard R W, Morris E D and Clayton S G. Fetal blood sampling in clinical obstetrics. *Journal of Obstetrics and Gynaecology of the British Commonwealth*, 73, 562-570 (1966).

2. Daniel S S, Baratz R A, Bowe E T *et al.* Elimination of hydrogen ion by the lamb fetus and newborn. *Paediatric Research*, 6, 584 (1972).

3. Jacobson L and Rooth G. Interpretative aspects of the acid-base composition and its variation in fetal scalp blood and maternal blood during labour. *Journal of Obstetrics and Gynaecology of the British Commonwealth,* 78, 971-980 (1971).
4. Khazin A F, Hon E H and Quilligan E J. Biochemical studies of the fetus 111. Fetal base and Apgar scores. *Obstetrics and Gynecology,* 34, 592-609 (1969).
5. Racine P, Klenk H O and Kochsiek K. Rapid Lactate determination with an electrochemical enzymatic sensor: clinical usability and comparative measurements. *Zeitschrift für Klinische Chemie und Klinische Biochemie,* 13, 533-539 (1975).
6. Saling E and Schneider D. Biochemical supervision of the fetus during labour. *Journal of Obstetrics and Gynaecology of the British Commonwealth,* 74, 799-811 (1967).
7. Smith N C, Soutter W P and Sharp F. Fetal scalp blood lactate as an indicator of intrapartum hypoxia. *British Journal of Obstetrics and Gynaecology,* 90, 821-831 (1983).
8. Soutter W P, Aithchison T C, Thorburn J and Sharp F. An evaluation of the AVL 937C blood-gas and pH microanalyser. *British Journal of Anaesthesia,* 48, 1211-1218 (1976).
9. Soutter W P, Sharp F and Clark D M. Bedside estimation of whole blood lactate. *British Journal of Anaesthesia,* 50, 445-450 (1978).

Chapter 21

# Reservations about the methods of assessing at birth the predictive value of intrapartum fetal monitoring including premature interruption of the feto-placental circulation

**Peter M Dunn**

## Introduction

Modern methods of monitoring the status of the fetus using electronic heart rate recordings and intermittent fetal scalp pH measurements represent a great advance (13). However, they are by no means free from very real hazards of application, interpretation and management (5,12,15,21). Therefore, judgement must be exercised before using them in the 'low risk' labour.

In this paper I wish to draw attention to the fallibility, and even danger, that may be associated with some of the methods commonly used at birth to assess the success or failure of intrapartum monitoring in predicting fetal distress and birth asphyxia.

In 1982-1983 Sykes and his colleagues (23,24) in Oxford drew attention to the frequent mismatch between the assessment of the intrapartum condition of the fetus using the methods just mentioned, and the assessment of the condition of the infant at birth as determined by the Apgar score and umbilical artery pH. I welcomed their paper as I have long been worried by what seemed to me to be the unjustified faith placed by many workers on these methods of assessing at birth the correctness of the prediction of intrapartum status (3).

## Limitations of the Apgar score

Let us first consider the Apgar score. This provides a simple but very crude clinical summary of an infant's condition following delivery. What is often forgotten or ignored is that the score may itself be influenced by management including resuscitation technique. For instance, resuscitation in the head-down position and pharyngeal aspiration with a mucus catheter may both depress the Apgar score. The score may also be influenced by the timing of cord clamping. Thus, Figure 1 demonstrates the Apgar scores of two groups of infants that I studied in 1964, recorded immediately after delivery (0-5 seconds), at 1 minute and at 5 minutes in relation to whether the umbilical cord was clamped at the moment of birth (0-1 second), or after a delay of at least 3 minutes but before delivery of the placenta. Observe the 'cross-over' in the Apgar scores of the two groups between 1 and 5 minutes. Thus, the age at which the score is recorded may be critical. Likewise the accuracy of timing is clearly most important too. Furthermore, it also became apparent in this study that there were

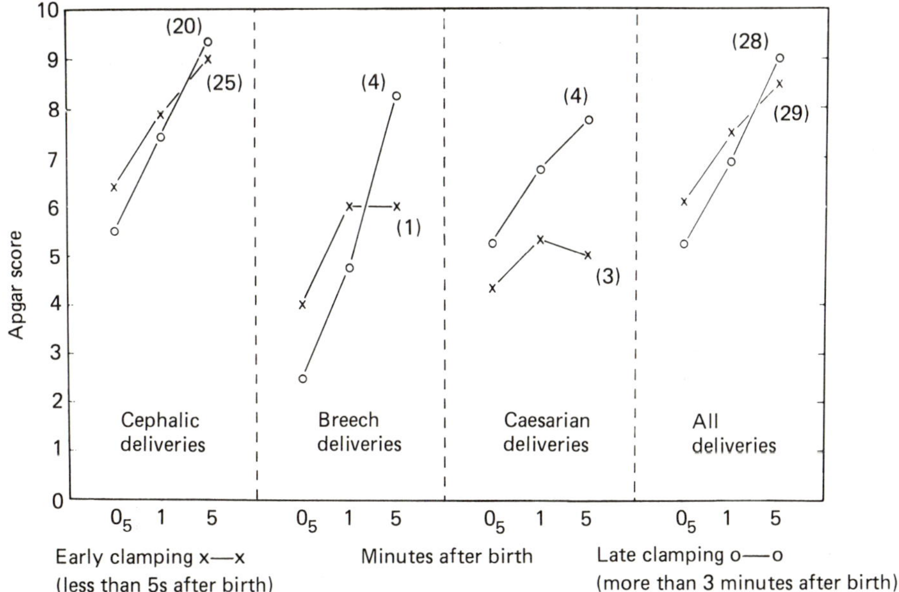


*Figure 1.* Apgar scores of infants 37–43 weeks' gestation at 0–5 seconds, 1 minute and 5 minutes after delivery in relation to whether the cord was clamped at the moment of birth (1 second) or after at least 3 minutes but before delivery of the placenta (P.M. Dunn, unpublished observations)

in this study that there were considerable differences in the observer errors between experienced and relatively inexperienced clinical staff.

Some of the difficulties can be illustrated in relation to an infant who was born by the breech at term. Although his Apgar score was only 1 immediately after delivery, it had risen to 9 by 1 minute and to 10 by 5 minutes. The umbilical vein pH was 7.19 at birth which was similar to the maternal venous pH of 7.20. However, the pH of blood taken from the infant's heel at the age of 6 minutes was only 6.88. This big difference was likely to be due to the fact that the umbilical cord has been compressed and pulseless for some 12 minutes during the second stage of labour. Undoubtedly, the heel blood sample reflected the infant's status at birth more accurately than the cord blood.

Another factor which may have a profound effect on the Apgar score without necessarily being related to fetal distress, is the administration of drugs to the mother

**TABLE 1. Factors that may modify the effect of fetal distress (hypoxia) on the status of the infant after delivery.**

| |
|---|
| Severity and length of hypoxia |
| Gestational age |
| Nutritional status—glycogen reserves |
| Drugs given to mother |
| Birth trauma |
| Method of delivery |
| Management at birth |
| Other postnatal events |

during labour. Drugs such as the opiates or diazepam will often influence the establishment of respiration, the tone of the infant, and indeed all the clinical signs included in the score.

Drugs are only one of the factors that may modify the status of the infant at delivery and also possibly modify the effect that hypoxia may have on the baby (Table 1). These include the severity and duration of the hypoxia, the gestational age of the baby, the nutritional status of the infant (including glycogen reserves), the occurrence of birth trauma, the method of delivery, management at birth, and other postnatal events.

It is also necessary to consider the degree to which events occurring *after* the diagnosis of fetal distress and before delivery may alter the status of the baby at birth (Table 2). These include the length of the interval between diagnosis and delivery (often 30 minutes or more), maternal stress, the posture adopted by the mother, any drugs which may be given to the mother including oxygen, and the management of delivery itself.

**TABLE 2. Events occurring between the diagnosis of fetal distress and delivery that may alter the status of the infant at birth.**

| |
|---|
| Length of the interval |
| Maternal stress |
| Posture of the woman |
| Drugs given to the mother (including oxygen) |
| Delivery technique |

The rapidity with which fetal status and pH may change is well recognized. Dawes and his colleagues (7), for example showed that the pH of an asphyxiated fetal lamb may fall from 7.5 to 7.0 in just 10 minutes. In particular, management of the second stage (1) may have a great influence on the degree of fetal acidosis at birth. Among the factors which must be taken into account and which may be influenced by management are: the degree of muscular effort made by the mother, breath-holding during pushing efforts, aortic or inferior vena caval compression due to maternal supine posture, and the use of drugs that cause the uterus to contract or relax (Table 3).

**TABLE 3. Factors causing fetal acidosis during the second stage.**

| |
|---|
| Maternal muscular effort |
| Breath holding during pushing |
| Aortic inferior vena caval compression—supine posture |
| Cord compression |
| Fetal skull compression |
| Reduced placental exchange |
| Fetal hypoxia |

## Clamping the cord

I would like to return to the common practice of immediately clamping the umbilical cord at birth in order to obtain samples of umbilical arterial and venous blood. The

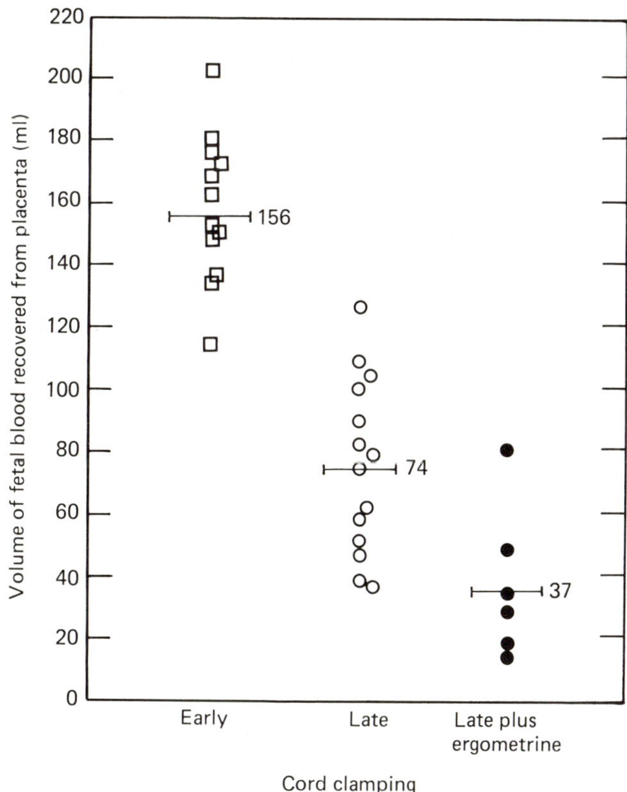


*Figure 2.* Volume of residual blood in the placentae of 32 normal term infants delivered per vaginam in relation to whether the cord was clamped at the moment of birth (within 1 second) or after at least 3 minutes but before delivery of the placenta. Some of the mothers of the late clamped cases had received ergometrine 0.5 mg at delivery (P.M. Dunn, unpublished observations)

fact that this practice may have a profound effect on the baby appears to be ignored. These effects may be haemodynamic or volumetric in character. Thus, Figure 2 shows the impact that cord clamping had on the residual placental blood volume of 32 normal term infants delivered (per vaginam) according to whether the cord was clamped at the moment of birth ('early') or after an interval of 3 or more minutes but before placental delivery ('late') (P M Dunn, unpublished observations). The latter group has been subdivided according to whether egometrine (0.5 mg) was given to the mother with the delivery of the shoulders. The mean residual volumes were 156, 74 and 37 ml, respectively. These differences, equivalent to more than a litre of blood in an adult, were reflected in the status of the infant. Indeed a great variety of animal and human studies (including those of the author) over the last two to three decades have repeatedly demonstrated the effect that cord clamping has, not only on the blood volume and haematocrit of the infant, but also on a whole range of other parameters including the onset of respiration, blood pressure, atrial pressure, the plasma proteins, pulmonary lymph flow and indeed the way the infant adapts or fails to adapt to extra-uterine life (2,9,18,19,20,25,27, P M Dunn, unpublished observations).

Adaptation to extra-uterine life depends on the achievement of adequate alveolar ventilation, accompanied by a fall in pulmonary vascular resistance, a greatly increased pulmonary blood flow and other secondary changes in the circulation. The key to successful adaptation appears to be the replacement of the lung fluid, which fills the alveolus prior to delivery, by air. Evacuation of this fluid is partially achieved during vaginal delivery by thoracic compression during the second stage of labour and, after birth, by pulmonary lymphatic drainage aided by the 'milking' action of respiratory movements and a low central venous pressure.

Clearance of lung fluid is often inadequate when the preterm infant is delivered by Caesarean section, particularly when the latter is elective. The baby has been deprived of the vaginal squeeze to the thorax and respiratory movements may be weak or absent because of such factors as maternal anaesthesia, a compliant rib cage, and increased airway resistance as well as lack of surfactant. In addition, cord clamping at delivery of vigorously pulsating umbilical vessels will cut off the low resistance placental circulation and might be expected to cause a sharp rise in systemic blood pressure. In the presence of a continuing high pulmonary vascular resistance, the heart may exhibit transitory 'failure' with raised pulmonary and central venous pressures. Raised pulmonary venous pressure might then be expected to lead to pulmonary oedema with the extravasation of plasma proteins causing inactivation or displacement of surfactant and hyaline membrane formation. Meanwhile, a raised central venous pressure would impede pulmonary lymphatic drainage, a situation which would be exacerbated if the infant were then resuscitated in the head-down position.

## Proposed optimum delivery and resuscitation techniques for preterm infants and Caesarean section

This hypothesis was founded on a range of clinical observations made while I was working at the Birmingham Maternity Hospital in 1960-1961. As a result, a delivery technique was devised to try to bypass the above problems at preterm Caesarean delivery (11). The technique was as follows:

(1) Two members of the paediatric staff attend all preterm Caesarean deliveries. One 'scrubs up' and armed with sterile mucus catheter and warmed sterile towel, stands next to the obstetrician.

(2) The obstetrician delivers the baby's head and then passes while the anaesthetist injects an oxytocic agent into the mother's arm vein. The uterus will contract in response to this injection after a delay of 45-50 seconds.

(3) 30 seconds after the injection the obstetrician completes the delivery of the baby who is then wrapped in the warm towel and laid on his side on the mother's legs. The paediatrician then gently clears the mouth and nose.

(4) As the uterus contracts the obstetrican eases the placenta out through the incision with minimal handling or traction of the cord. (If the placenta has been damaged and the cord has to be clamped, this should be done as near to the placenta as possible.)

(5) The placenta is then placed inside the warmed towel alongside the baby and the whole unit is transferred to the resuscitation platform where the infant is placed on a head-up slope with the placenta lying alongside the body.

(6) The status of the infant is then assessed, the time being usually 1-2 minutes after delivery.

(7) If the infant is breathing vigorously, is pink, has a good peripheral circulation, has no evidence of inspiratory retraction, has a good alveolar air entry and umbilical pulsation has ceased at the umbilicus, then the cord may be clamped and divided, and the infant transferred to the special care nursery or ward.

(8) If these conditions are not satisfied and especially if the infant's gestational age is less than 32 weeks, the infant should be intubated and intermittent positive pressure ventilation (IPPV) maintained for 10-15 minutes. *It is vital to use the minimum positive pressure* sufficient to bring about a steady improvement since the lung fluid is incompressible and the use of higher pressure may cause alveolar duct rupture. The main purpose of the IPPV is to milk alveolar fluid steadily into and along the pulmonary lymphatics towards the central venous pool.

(9) Meanwhile, the placenta remains alongside the infant so that if for any reason the central venous pressure rises, blood may flow retrogradely down the umbilical vein (in which there are no valves) to the placenta. If, on the other hand, the infant is thought to be hypovolaemic and hypotensive, the placenta may be raised above the levels of the baby to encourage placental transfusion.

(10) When the conditions described in section 7 have been achieved, the cord will be found to be white and non-pulsatile and may then be divided in the usual way. It is, of course, vital to keep the infant warm during the whole period.

Independent of this work, Landau and his colleagues (16) had reported delivering a few infants by Caesarean section with their placentae raised high with a view to encouraging a placenta transfusion, a technique subsequently reported also by Secher and Karlberg (1962) (22) and Vardi (1965) (26). Unfortunately, such a practice may also lead to hypervolaemia and polycythaemia.

The success that followed the introduction of the technique described above, first in Birmingham in 1961, then in Warwick 1962-1963 and in Bristol in 1970-1971, has been briefly described elsewhere (11). Neonatal mortality from respiratory distress syndrome among preterm Caesarean infants was almost eliminated and, following the 1970-1971 study, the technique came into routine use in the University of Bristol Department of Obstetrics and Gynaecology. During 1972 and 1973 all the 36 preterm infants delivered by Caesarean section in the Department survived, except for two with lethal malformations. This was in sharp contrast to the 25% mortality among such infants that had been our experience up till that time, with the umbilical cords having been divided at once in the conventional way.

Although the hypothesis on which this delivery technique was based rested on clinical observation, experimental evidence in support has accumulated over the years, including observations on the effect that cord clamping has on the heart rate (4), the systemic blood pressure, the pulmonary vascular resistance (6) and the volume and characteristics of pulmonary lymph (17). The clinical observations on neonatal 'foaming' following Caesarean delivery (and cord clamping) by Klein (1972) (13) are also of interest. Studies made in Bristol in 1964 (P M Dunn, unpublished observations) also provided support for the hypothesis that the infant's blood volume, blood pressure and haematocrit were least disturbed when the cord was not clamped and the placenta delivered and laid at the same level as the baby. Indeed, this practice was widely followed throughout most of the word until the recent spread of Western obstetrics. Even today the majority of babies delivered vaginally in the rural areas of developing countries are not separated from their placentae until the latter has delivered, and has lain alongside the infant until all pulsation has ceased (10).

## Conclusions

By keeping the placental circulation intact and at the same level as the infant while pulmonary respiration is established, a premature rise in systemic blood pressure is avoided, a 'safety valve' is provided for raised central venous pressure, and the stage set for best acheiving vascular normovolaemia (Table 4). May I therefore end with

**TABLE 4. Intact umbilical circulation at delivery.**

| |
|---|
| Avoidance of premature rise in systemic blood pressure |
| Provision of safety valve for raised central venous pressure |
| Provides best opportunity for achieving normovolaemia |

a plea that we reconsider and hopefully discontinue the potentially harmful practice of immediate cord clamping in order to obtain samples of umbilical artery and vein blood, and use instead if necessary blood taken from the infant by heel-prick. It is true that the term infant is remarkably resilient especially when delivered (per vaginam). However, even term infants may be made seriously ill by this practice and preterm infants are put at great risk. I am particularly concerned at the possibility that immediate cord clamping, by causing a dramatic and abrupt rise in systemic blood pressure in an asphyxiated preterm infant whose lungs are still fluid-filled, may lead to a surge in cerebral blood flow and intraventricular haemorrhage. As Hippocrates reminded us: 'First, we must do no harm'.

May I end with a quotation from a book written by the English obstetrician Thomas Denman in 1801(8):

'...the common method of tying and cutting the umbilical cord in the instant the child is born, is likewise one of those errors in practice that has nothing to plead in its favour but custom ... is it possible that this wonderful alteration in the human machine should properly be brought about in one instant of time, and at the will of a bystander? Let us leave the affaire to nature, and watch her operations and it will soon appear that she stands not in need of our feeble assistance, but will do the work herself at a proper time, and in a better manner. In a few minutes the lungs will gradually be expanded and the great alterations in the heart and blood vessels will take place. As soon as this is perfectly done, the circulation in the umbilical cord will cease of itself ... By this rash, inconsiderate method of tying the umbilical cord before the circulation in it is stopped, I doubt not but many children have been lost, many of their prinicpal organs have been injured, and foundations laid for various disorders'.

## References

1. Adamson T M, Boyd R D H, Hill J R, Normand I C S, Reynolds E O r and Strang L B. Effect of asphyxia due to umbilical cord occlusion in the foetal lamb on leakage of liquid from the circulation and on permeability of lung capillaries to albumin. *Journal of Physiology*, 207, 493-505 (1970).

2. Arcilla R A, Oh W, Lind J and Blankenship W. Portal and atrial pressures in the newborn period. A comparative study in infants born with early and late clamping of the cord. *Acta Paediatrica Scandinavica*, 55, 615-625 (1966).

3. Bowe E T, Beard R W, Finsker M, Poppers P J, Adamsons K and James L S. Reliability of fetal blood sampling: maternal and fetal relationships. *American Journal of Obstetrics and Gynecology* , 107, 279-287 (1970).

4. Brady J P and James L S. Heart rate changes in the fetus and newborn infant during labour, delivery and the immediate neonatal period. *American Journal of Obstetrics and Gynecology* , 84, 1-12 (1962).
5. Chalmers I. Trials of intrapartum monitoring. *Perinatal Medicine, 6th European Congress, Vienna 1978* , edited by O Thalhammer, K Baumgarten and A Pollak, 260-265. Stuttgart, George Thieme Publications (1979).
6. Dawes G S, Jacobson H N, Mott J C, Shelley H J and Stafford A. The treatment of asphyxiated, mature foetal lambs and rhesus monkeys with intravenous glucose and sodium bicarbonate. *Journal of Physiology* , 169, 167-184 (1963).
7. Dawes G S, Mott J C, Shelley H J and Stafford A. The prolongation of survival time in asphyxiated mature foetal lambs. *Journal of Physiology* , 168, 43-64 (1963).
8. Denman T. *An introduction to the practice of midwifery*. 3rd Edition, Printed for J Johnson, St Paul's Churchyard, London, 253 (1801).
9. Dunn P M. Cord occlusion and the onset of respiration. *Proceedings of the Society of Pediatric Research,* Abstract 160 (1967).
10. Dunn P M. Comment in *Year Book of Paediatrics*. Edited by S S Gellis, 16-17. Chicago, Year Book Medical Publishers (1967-1968).
11. Dunn P M. Caesarean section and the prevention of respiratory distress syndrome of the newborn. *Perinatal Medicine,* 3rd European Congress, Lausanne 1972. Edited by H Bossart, J M Croz, A Huber, L S Prod'hom and J Sistek, 138-145. Bern, Hans Huber (1973).
12. Dunn P M. Problems associated with fetal monitoring during labour and conclusions on the benefits and hazards of fetal and neonatal monitoring. *Perinatal Medicine,* 6th European Congress, Vienna 1978. Edited by O Thalhammer, K Baumgarten and A Pollak, 270-273 and 297-299. Stuttgart, Georg Thieme Publications (1979).
13. Huch A and Huch R. The insights derived from perinatal monitoring. *Perinatal Medicine,* 6th European Congress, Vienna 1978. Edited by O Thalhammer, K Baumgarten and A Pollak, 284-293. Stuttgart, Georg Thieme Publications (1979).
14. Klein M. Asphyxia neonatorum caused by foaming. *Lancet,* 1, 1089-1091 (1972).
15. Kloosterman G J. Intrapartum benefits and hazards of monitoring. *Perinatal Medicine,* 6th European Congress, Vienna 1978. Edited by O Thalhammer, K Baumgarten and A Pollak, 279-283. Stuttgart, Georg Thieme Publications (1979).
16. Landau D B, Goodrich H B, Franka W F and Burns F R. Death of Cesarean infants: a theory as to its cause and a method of prevention. *Journal of Pediatrics,* 36, 421-426 (1950).
17. Modanlou H, Yeh S Y, Hou E H and Forsythe A. Fetal and neonatal biochemistry and Apgar scores. *American Journal of Obstetrics and Gynecology,* 117, 942-951 (1973).
18. Oh W, Lind J and Gessner I H. Circulatory and respiratory adaptation to early and late cord clamping in newborn infants. *Acta Paediatrica Scandinavica,* 55, 17-25 (1966).
19. Oh W, Oh M A and Lind J. Renal function and blood volume in newborn infants related to placental transfusion. *Acta Paediatrica Scandinavica,* 55, 197-210 (1966).
20. Oh W, Wallgren G, Hanson J S and Lind J. The effects of placental transfusion on the respiratory mechanics of normal term infants. *Pediatrics,* 40, 6-12 (1967).
21. Pillai M. Fetal monitoring during labour. *Lancet,* 1, 67 (1984).
22. Secher O and Karlberg P. Placental and blood transfusion for newborns delivered by Caesarean section. *Lancet,* 1,1203-1205 (1962).
23. Sykes G S, Johnson P, Ashworth F, Molloy P M, Gu W, Stirrat G M and Turnbull A C. Do Apgar scores indicate asphyxia? *Lancet,* 1, 494-496 (1982).
24. Sykes G S, Molloy P M, Johnson P, Stirrat G M and Turnbull A C. Fetal distress and the condition of newborn infants. *British Medical Journal,* 287, 943-945 (1983).
25. Usher R, Shephard M and Lind J. The blood volume of the newborn infant and placental transfusion. *Acta Paediatrica Scnadinavica,* 52, 497-512 (1963).
26. Vardi P. Placental transfusion. An attempt at physiological delivery. *Lancet,* 1, 12-13 (1965).
27. Yao A C and Lind J. *Placental transfusion.* 1-175. Springfield, Illinois, C C Thomas (1982).

Part 3

# Blood Gas

Chapter 22

# Skin surface gas partial pressures and transcutaneous blood gas analysis

D W Lübbers

## Introduction

Since $O_2$ and $CO_2$ can easily diffuse through the epidermis, the question arose whether the skin could be used as a 'window' through which internal processes concerning the $O_2$ and $CO_2$ metabolism and transport could be followed non-invasively. When a Clark-type $PO_2$ electrode (1) is put on the skin surface of an adult forearm, the results are disappointing. The $PO_2$ histogram (measured at a room temperature of 27°C, breathing air) shows mostly very low $PO_2$ values, the mean being close to zero (Figure 1). Breathing pure oxygen has only a very small affect on the skin surface $PO_2$, $P_sO_2$ (3, 14). This shows that under normal conditions, the 'window' is closed. To find out more about the internal processes with non-invasive methods, we must investigate how this 'window' can be opened, if at all.

An important finding is that the 'window' starts to open if skin blood flow increases. With drug-induced hyperaemia, skin surface $PO_2$ increases. Figure 2 shows the $PO_2$

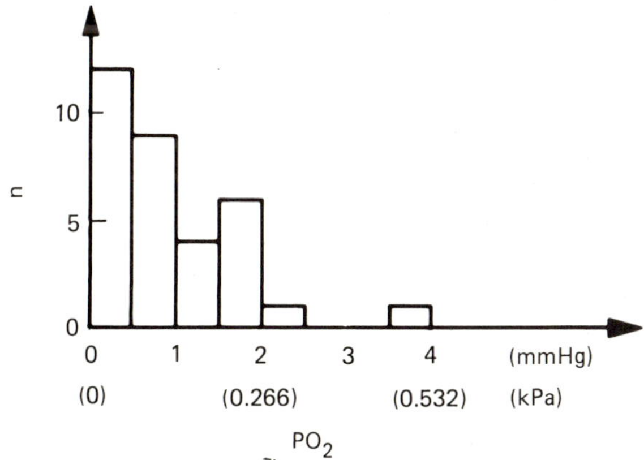


*Figure 1*. Histogram of the $PO_2$ on the surface of the non-hyperaemized adult skin. On normal skin, $PO_2$ is almost zero (mean $PO_2$ = 0.85 mmHg (0.11 kPa)); (breathing air, room temperature: 27°C; temperature of covered skin: 34.5°C; n = 33) (3)

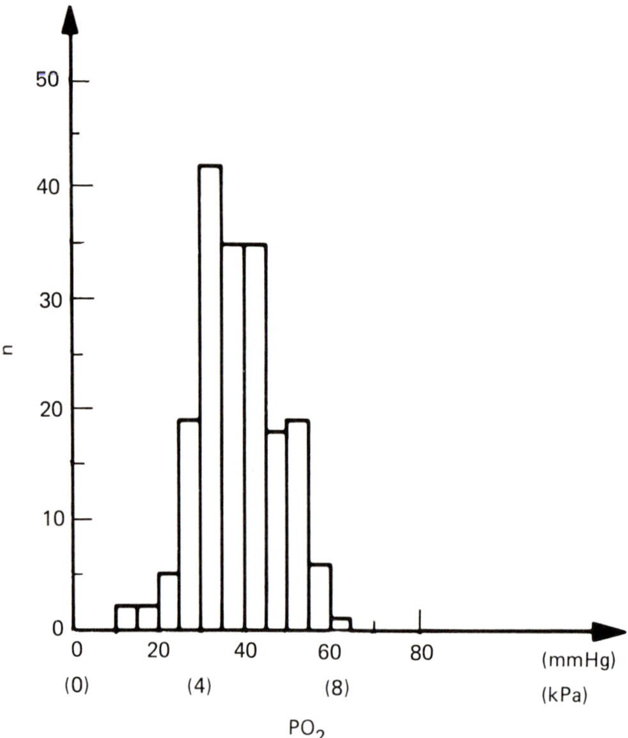


*Figure 2.* Histogram of the skin surface $PO_2$ of adults with drug-induced hyperaemia (Finalgon). Mean $PO_2$ = 36 mmHg, (4.8 kPa) n = 100; (breathing air, temperature of uncovered skin 35.5 – 36.5°C) (15)

histogram after application of Finalgon, a nicotinic acid compound. The very low $PO_2$ values have disappeared. All skin surface $PO_2$ values react to changes in arterial $PO_2$, but also to changes of local flow (for example brought about by inflating a cuff around the upper arm). Since these manoeuvres do not change tissue respiration, the $P_sO_2$ reflects changes in the availability of oxygen to the tissue.

## Oxygen balance equations - the importance of blood flow

The way in which the $O_2$ availability affects tissue oxygenation can be deduced from simple balance equations. In steady state the oxygen delivery to the tissue equals the $O_2$ consumption.

$$\underbrace{(C_{a,O2} - C_{v,O2})\dot{B}}_{O_2 \text{ delivery}} = \underbrace{AVD_{O2} \cdot \dot{B} = \dot{V}_{O2}}_{O_2 \text{ consumption}} \qquad \mathbf{1}$$

with $C_{a,O2}$= arterial $O_2$ concentration;
$C_{v,O2}$ = venous $O_2$ concentration;
$AVD_{o2}$ = arterial venous oxygen concentration difference;

$\dot{B}$ = blood flow;
$\dot{V}_{02}$ = rate of oxygen consumption.
From equation 1 the following equations are obtained:

$$C_{v,O2} = C_{a,O2} - \dot{V}_{O2}\frac{1}{\dot{B}} \qquad 2$$

$$\frac{C_{v,O2}}{C_{a,O2}} = 1 - \frac{\dot{V}_{O2}}{C_{a,O2} \cdot \dot{B}} = 1 - R_{O2} = f_{O2} \qquad 3$$

$$R_{o2} = \frac{C_{a,O2} - C_{v,O2}}{C_{a,O2}} \qquad 4$$

Equation 3 shows that the venous oxygen concentration, $C_{v,o2}$, changes with the flow, $\dot{B}$, in a hyperbolic way (13, 15, 17, 18, 19). In Figure 3 such a hyperbola is calculated using a skin $O_2$ consumption of $\dot{V}_{o2}$ = 0.3 ml $O_2$/(100 g.min) and an arterial oxygen concentration of 2.1 ml $O_2$/l. At a flow of 1.42 ml/(100 g.min), the available oxygen is used up so that $C_{v,o2}$ is zero.

In a homogeneous tissue supplied by a straight capillary this would result in a linear decrease of blood $O_2$ concentration from the arterial to the venous end (Figure 3, left side, lowest trace). Because of the hyperbolic nature of the relationship $C_{v,o2}$ vs $\dot{B}$, at first, with increasing flow, $C_{v,o2}$ increases steeply. At a flow of 5 ml/(100

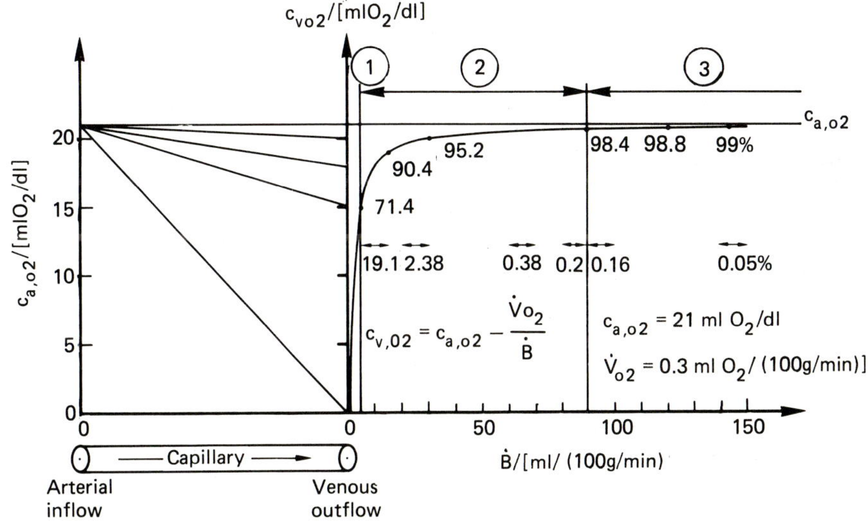


*Figure 3.* Circulatory hyperbola for the overall $O_2$ supply of the skin. With a constant $C_{a,o2}$ = 21 ml/dl and an $O_2$ consumption $\dot{V}$ = 0.3 ml/(100 g.min) the flow $\dot{B}$ is calculated according to equation 2. The numbers at the dots of the curve describe $C_{v,o2}$ as a percentage of $C_{a,o2}$. There are three different regions: (1) $C_{v,o2}$ changes with flow, (2) distinct changes of $C_{v,o2}$ with flow changes, (3) $C_{v,o2}$ is almost independent of flow. The horizontal lines with two arrows correspond to a flow change of 10 ml/(100g.min), and the adjacent numbers to the concomitant percentage change of $C_{v,o2}$ (18)

g.min), $C_{v,o2}$ has already reached 71.4% of the arterial $O_2$ concentration ($f_{o2} = 0.714$ or $R_{o2} = 0.286$). Then the increase becomes smaller, it reaches 98% of $C_{a,o2}$ with $\dot{B}$ = 90 ml/(100 g.min) and then levels off. Skin blood flow values of 100 ml/(100 g.min) and higher have been reported in heat induced hyperaemia (13).

It is interesting to note that the change in $C_{v,o2}$ caused, for example, by a flow change of 10 ml/(100 g.min) depends very much on the absolute flow value. At 5 ml/(100 g.min) the change of the $C_{v,o2}$ is 19.1% of $C_{a,o2}$. At 90 ml/(100 g.min) it decreases to 0.2% and then becomes gradually smaller. This different sensitivity to flow changes distinguishes three different regions in the circulatory hyperbola (Figure 3). In region 1, changes of flow have drastic effects on $C_{v,o2}$, whereas larger changes of $C_{a,o2}$ are needed to produce changes in $C_{v,o2}$. In region 2, the middle part of the hyperbola, flow changes as well as changes of $C_{a,o2}$ affect $C_{v,o2}$ and, in region 3, flow changes have practically no effect on $C_{v,o2}$, but $C_{v,o2}$ values mirror $C_{a,o2}$. Equations 3 and 4 show that the quotient $\dot{V}_{o2}/(C_{a,o2}.\dot{B})$ determines the slope of the hyperbola: the numerator tells us how much oxygen is needed, the denominator how much oxygen is offered. The ratio of both values is decisive for tissue oxyenation.

## Venous and skin surface $O_2$ values

How is the venous oxygen concentration $C_{v,o2}$ of the balance equation related to the skin surface $PO_2$? To reach the skin surface, oxygen has to be transported from the capillary blood through the epidermis. Since, within the tissue, $O_2$ is transported by diffusion, there is an oxygen pressure gradient across the epidermis. The epidermis receives its oxygen from the upper part of the capillary loop, the capillary dome. The loop-shaped capillaries obtain their blood from arterioles and small arteries which come from the subpapillary arterial plexus. The epidermis consists of a viable layer (approximately 20 - 30 μm thick) which is covered by a dead layer (approximately 10 - 20 μm thick). The skin surface $PO_2$ measures that of $PO_2$ in the capillary dome but is reduced by the $PO_2$ gradient across the epidermis. The capillary dome corresponds to the middle of the capillary; therefore,

$$C_{a,o2} - C_{d,o2} = 0.5\ AVD_{o2}$$

where $C_{d,o2}$ is the capillary dome oxygen concentration.

The oxygen pressure is obtained from the oxygen concentration according to Henry's law: $C_{o2} = s \cdot PO_2$ (s = solubility coefficient). In blood, most of the oxygen is chemically bound to haemoglobin: $C_{o2} = 1.34.C_{hb} \cdot S_{o2}$ (where $C_{hb}$ = haemoglobin concentration; $S_{o2}$ = oxygen saturation).

## Circulatory hyperbola for $CO_2$

In a similar way, a circulatory hyperbola can be calculated for $CO_2$ (19). In Figure 4 $C_{co2}$ increases linearly from the arterial to the venous end; trace 'a' corresponds to a flow of 1.42 ml/(100 g.min) (see Figure 3). $C_{v,co2}$ approaches $C_{a,co2}$ at lower flow values than those corresponding in Figure 3. The $CO_2$ concentration in the middle of the capillary corresponds to the capillary dome ($C_{d,co2}$). In the physiological range the $CO_2$ dissociation curve can be taken as being linear.

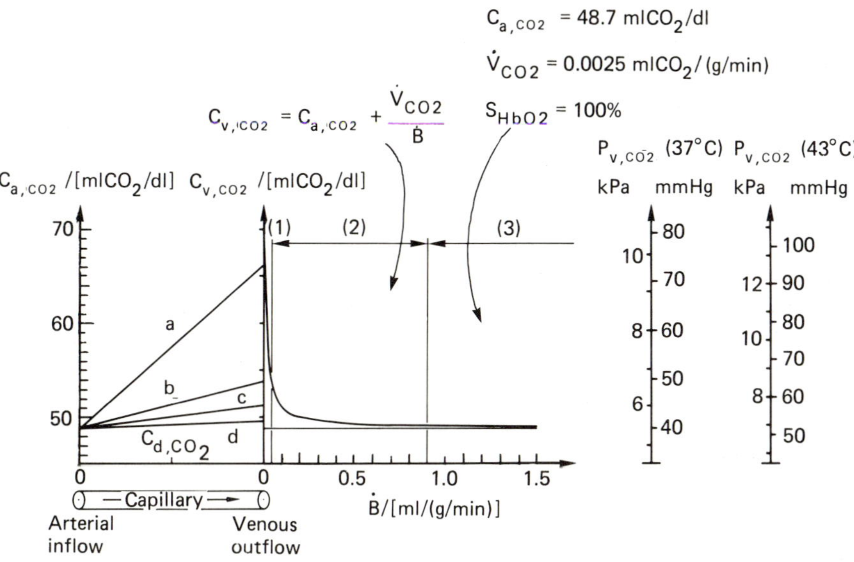


*Figure 4.* The circulatory hyperbola for the overall $CO_2$ exchange of the skin. $S_{HbO2}$: $O_2$ saturation of haemoglobin. For further explanation *see Figure 3* (20)

## The capillary loop model

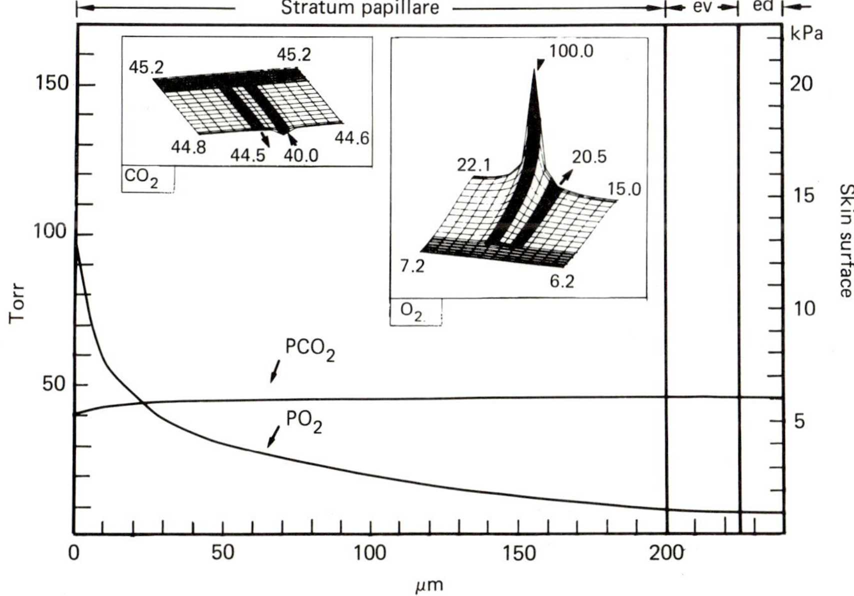


*Figure 5.* $PO_2$ and $PCO_2$ profiles along the arterial limb and across the epidermis (insets $PO_2$ and $PCO_2$ fields over a cross-section of the epidermis and the capillary loop); blood flow 1 ml/(100g.min), temperature 37°C, skin surface covered with an impermeable layer (7)

For a general understanding, the balance equations are sufficient. However, for a more quantitative description other model assumptions have been tried (16, 20). We have developed the capillary loop model by which the gas exchange processes between the skin and the surroundings as well as during the measurements, can be simulated (4, 5, 7). Figure 5 shows the calculated $PO_2$ and $PCO_2$ fields around the capillary loop and across the epidermis at low blood flow (1 ml/(100 g.min)) at 37°C. The z-axis gives the values of $PO_2$ and $PCO_2$ . One can see the enormous difference between the $PO_2$ and the $PCO_2$ field is apparent. This occurs because of the difference in solubility coefficients and the chemical binding of $O_2$ and $CO_2$ (the relation between the diffusional conductivity of $O_2$ and $CO_2$ is 1:16). To transport the same amount of $O_2$ and $CO_2$ , oxygen needs a much larger gradient.

The lower part of Figure 5 shows $PO_2$ and $PCO_2$ profiles along the arterial limb of the capillary and across the epidermis: with a $P_aO_2$ of 100 mmHg (13.33 kPa), $P_sO_2$ amounts to around 7 mmHg (0.93 kPa). The $PO_2$ profile shows that there is a gradient from the tissue to the venous capillary. Therefore, $O_2$ shunt diffusion occurs. At high flow values it amounts to 5%, but at low flow values it increases to 20%. In the $PCO_2$ field the $P_aCO_2$ of 40 mmHg (5.33 kPa) increases to only 45.2 mmHg (6.03 kPa) on the skin surface. The $CO_2$ shunt amounts to 10 - 15% at low and to 3 - 5% at high flow values. It is interesting to note that $PO_2$ and $PCO_2$ do not vary much on the skin surface.

In Figure 6 the circulatory hyperbola for the capillary dome $PO_2$ is calculated for the straight capillary model (squares) and the capillary loop model (circles) (13). At low flow values there is a distinct difference between both curves, and the reason for this is the $O_2$ shunt diffusion. The lowest curve shows the skin surface $PO_2$ . Comparing the circulatory hyperbola for $PO_2$ with the circulatory hyperbola for $O_2$ concentration shows that the $P_{d,o2}$ values do not approach the $P_aO_2$ as close as $C_{v,o2}$ approaches $C_{a,o2}$. The reason being that at a blood $PO_2$ of 100 mmHg (13.3 kPa) a small change in $CO_2$ corresponds a large change in $PO_2$ . The figure demonstrates that the general

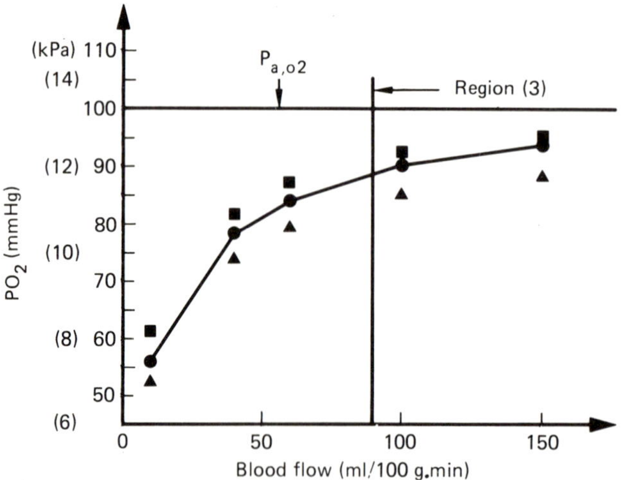


*Figure 6.* Transcutaneous $PO_2$ and $PO_2$ of the capillary dome vs flow (capillary loop model). With low flow values, the $P_{d,o2}$ without shunt (■) equation 2 is always higher than the $P_{d,o2}$ with diffusion shunt (●) (capillary loop model). At high flow values, the influence of $O_2$ shunt diffusion on the $P_{d,o2}$ is very much reduced. ▲ corresponds to the skin surface $PO_2$ (13)

conclusions drawn for the simple balance model also hold for the more complicated capillary loop model, at least at high flow values.

The analysis demonstrates that skin surface $PO_2$ gives mainly information about the local regulation of oxygen supply to the epidermis (see equation 2). The arterial $O_2$ concentration and the $O_2$ pressure of the arterial blood ($C_{a,o2}$) are determined by lung respiration and blood haemoglobin.

## Peripheral vascular resistance

Local blood flow, $\dot{B}$, is determined by the peripheral perfusion pressure, pp (11) and is regulated by changes of the local vascular resistance, r. At a given difference between arterial and venous peripheral perfusion pressure ($pp_a$- $pp_v$), the $O_2$ offer amounts to:

$$\dot{B} \cdot C_{a\,O2} = \frac{pp_a - pp_v}{r} \cdot C_{a,O2} \qquad 5$$

However, if we are interested in looking through the skin, in opening the window further to see how much oxygen is offered to the epidermis, then we must abolish local vascular reactions. In systematic studies we have found that this can be achieved by heating the skin surface to 43 - 45°C (10, for review see 13). Arterioles and small arteries are completely dilated by heat, so that the vascular resistance becomes constant and a minimum. Equation 5 shows that under this condition, $\dot{B}$ depends only on the peripheral perfusion pressure which is determined by central blood pressure and the state of the circulatory system. Therefore, the skin surface $PO_2$ with abolished regulation of local blood flow monitors the balance between the available and consumed oxygen. If the $O_2$ consumption remains constant, the balance depends on the state of circulation as well as the arterial oxygen partial pressure and concentration. If the aterial oxygen partial pressure is known, the ratio $tcPO_2/P_aO_2$ gives information about the state of the circulation and, if it is known that circulation is at its maximum (region 3 of the circulatory hyperbola), $tcPO_2$ reflects the arterial $PO_2$.

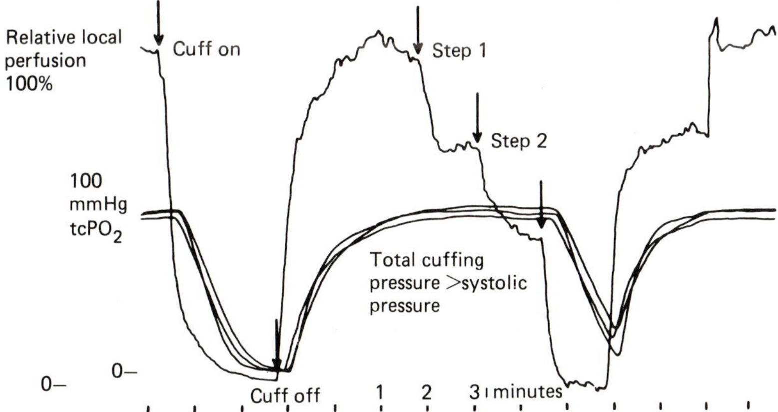


*Figure 7.* Recording of 'relative local perfusion' and $tcPO_2$ (3 channels) from an electrode affixed to the forearm. Partial cuff occlusion (step 1, step 2) had an obvious effect on relative local perfusion but no influence on $tcPO_2$ (15)

The latter situation is shown in Figure 7. $TcPO_2$ was measured by a $PO_2$ electrode with 3 Pt wires (15 $\mu$m diameter) heated to 45°C and fixed on the forearm of an adult (15). The electrical power needed to maintain the tissue temperature was used as an indicator of the relative local perfusion. Blood flow was reduced by inflating a cuff around the upper arm. With a certain delay, all 3 $tcPO_2$ traces went to zero. After pressure release there was no reactive hyperaemia because of the maximum dilation. The cuff was then inflated in two steps which both reduced blood flow but did not change $tcPO_2$. Only the third decrease of flow changed the $tcPO_2$. With such a high flow the $O_2$ available to the tissue was so large that $tcPO_2$ reflected changes in arterial $PO_2$ and not in blood flow.

## Factors affecting $tcPO_2$–$P_aO_2$ relationship

### Temperature

Several factors influence the relationship between $tcPO_2$ and $P_aO_2$ (5,13,23). There is a non-linear relationship between blood oxygen concentration and oxygen partial pressure, the $O_2$ dissociation curve which is caused by the chemical binding of oxygen to haemoglobin. The gradient of the $O_2$ dissociation curve $\Delta CO_2 / \Delta PO_2$, depends on the absolute $PO_2$. It is large in the range 20 - 80% oxygen saturation of haemoglobin and then decreases. Above a $PO_2$ of 200 mmHg haemoglobin is completely saturated with $O_2$. The $O_2$ dissociation curve is influenced by $CO_2$ and pH, but also by temperature. Therefore, the local heating of blood in capillaries and arterioles increases the blood $PO_2$. The $PO_2$ increase is obtained by multiplying by the temperature coefficient for blood, $g_{O_2} = \exp(\Delta T \times 0.056)$. Similarly, the blood $PCO_2$

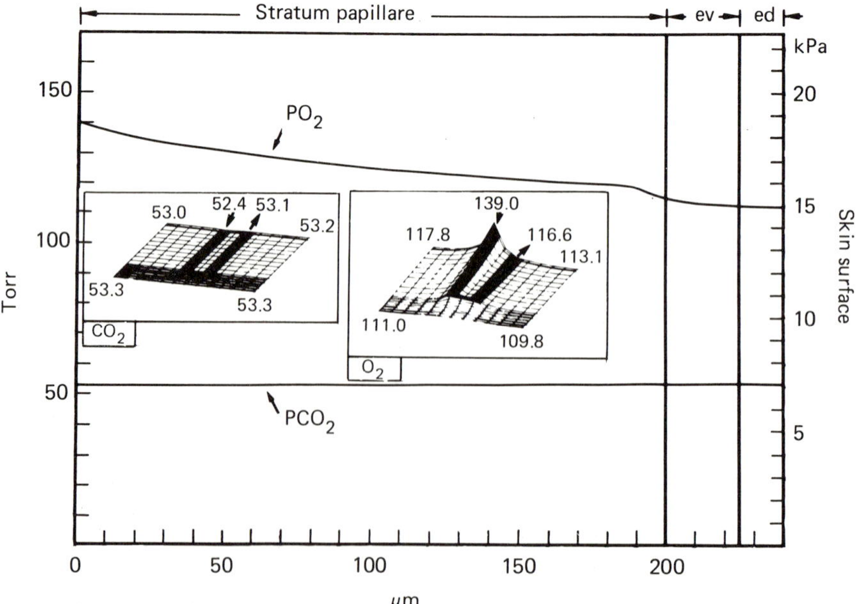


*Figure 8.* $PO_2$ and $PCO_2$ profiles along the arterial limb and across the epidermis (insets $PO_2$ and $PCO_2$ fields of the epidermis and the capillary loop); blood flow = 100 ml/(100g.min), temperature 43°C, skin surface covered with an impermeable layer (7)

increases with increase of temperature, the temperature coefficient being $g_{CO2} = \exp(\Delta T \times 0.045)$ (13,22).

Figure 8 shows $PO_2$ and $PCO_2$ fields as well as $PO_2$ and $PCO_2$ profiles for skin heated up to 43°C ($g_{O2}$ (43°C) = 1.399;$g_{CO2}$ (43°) = 1.310) (7). With increasing temperature the $P_aO_2$ increased from 100 mmHg (13.33 kPa) to 139.9 mmHg, the $P_aCO_2$ from 40 mmHg (5.33 kPa) to 52.4 mmHg (6.99 kPa). It is assumed that flow increased to 100 ml/(100g.min) and that $\dot{V}_{O2}$ was 0.4 ml/(100 g.min) at a respiratory quotient of 0.8. The $tcPO_2$ amounted to 111 mmHg (14.80 kPa) and the $tcPCO_2$ to 53.5 mmHg (7.11 kPa).

## Haemoglobin content and blood flow

The capillary loop model can be used to calculate the relationship between $tcPO_2$ vs $P_aO_2$ (8). Figure 9 shows the influence of a variation of the haemoglobin content

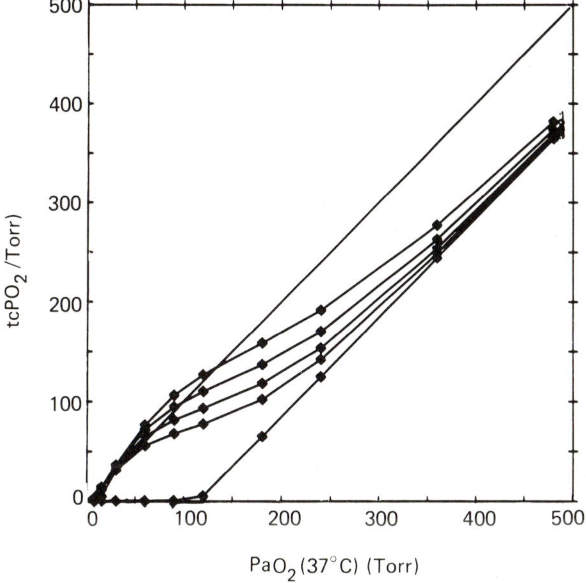


*Figure 9*. Transcutaneous $PO_2$ calibration curves, $tcPO_2$ (43°C) vs $P_aO_2$ (37°C) for blood with five different haemoglobin contents. (For further explanations *see text*) (8)

($\dot{V}_{O2}$ = 0.4 ml $O_2$ /100 g.min), B = 100 ml/(100 g.min). At a $P_aO_2$ of 90 mmHg without haemoglobin (lower curve), skin completely consumes the arterial oxygen and $tcPO_2$ is zero. Above this $P_aO_2$ , the $tcPO_2$ just starts to increase, but only at a $P_aO_2$ of around 120 mmHg does it increase almost in parallel with the line of identity, at a distance of about 115 mmHg below. The other curves describe the effect of haemoglobin 2, 4, 8 and 16 g/dl blood (0.31, 0.62, 1.2 and 2.5 mmol/l) on the $tcPO_2$. The $O_2$ dissociation curve produced non-linear curves and they cross the line of identity at low $PO_2$ values, become larger, but then cross the line again.

Similar curves are obtained with variations of flow as shown in Figure 10. They

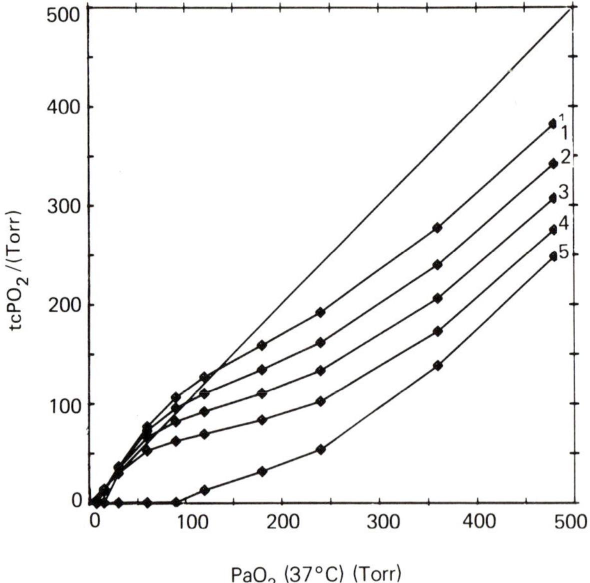


*Figure 10.* Transcutaneous calibration curves, $tcPO_2$ (43°C) vs $P_aO_2$ (37°C) for different blood flow values (1 = 100 ml/(100g.min), 2 = 50 ml/(100g.min), 3 = 25 ml/(100g.min), 4 = 10 ml/(100g.min), 5 = 1 ml/(100g.min)) (8)

are calculated for a haemoglobin concentration of 16 g/dl (2.5 mmol/l). Since the $CO_2$ dissociation curve is linear, the $tcPCO_2$ vs $P_aCO_2$ curves are linear.

## Electrode $O_2$ consumption

The polarographic measurement of $tcPO_2$ consumes oxygen which must diffuse from the capillary dome through the epidermis. The effect of this additional $O_2$ transport on the $tcPO_2$ is shown in Figure 11 (13). A Pt wire was first covered by a cellophane membrane (thickness 12 μm) and a Teflon membrane (thickness 12 μm), (Figure 11a). The $PO_2$ at the platinum surface was zero so that a $PO_2$ profile between zero and $P_{d,O2}$ was produced. From the capillary dome there was a small $PO_2$ decrease within the viable part of the epidermis but then a larger one in the stratum corneum because of the high diffusional resistance of this layer. The $PO_2$ difference between $P_{d,O2}$ and the $tcPO_2$ is marked by a heavy line; it amounted to 13 mmHg (1.73 kPa). Figure 11b shows measurements with a Teflon membrane of 50 μm thickness. In this case, the $O_2$ consumption of the electrode became smaller and the diffusional resistance between the capillary dome and Pt surface was mainly determined by the Teflon membrane. The difference $P_{d,O2}$ - $tcPCO_2$ was 4 mmHg (0.53 kPa).

A small $O_2$ consumption of the electrode also has another advantage, as is shown in Figure 12 (6). Here, at first in contact with air, a Teflon membrane was placed on the epidermis and then covered by a gas impermeable electrode, so that $PO_2$ decreased. The skin was then immediately heated up to 43°C (second arrow) so that blood flow increased to 100 ml/(100 g min). The upper one of the three traces corresponds to an electrode without $O_2$ consumption (D = 0), the middle one to an electrode with a Pt wire of 40 μm diameter (D = 40), and the lowest one to a diameter of about 140

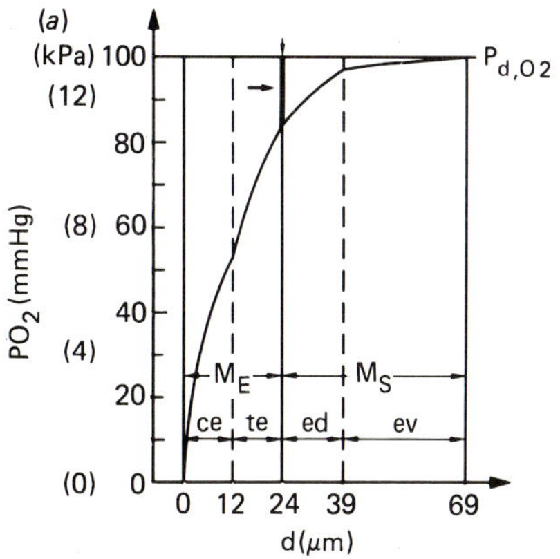


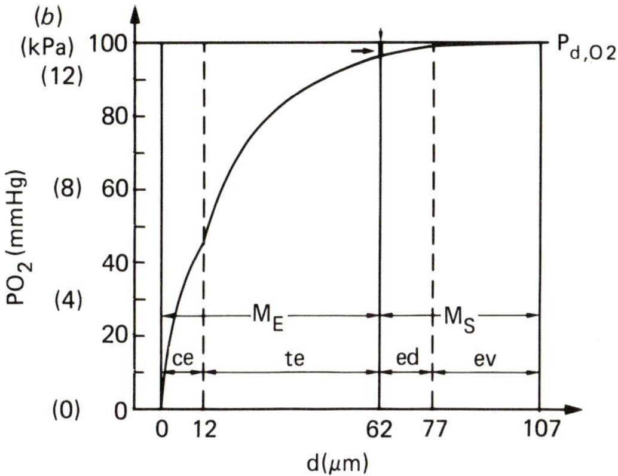


*Figure 11.* Polarographic measurement of skin surface $PO_2$: $PO_2$ profile in the electrode membrane and the epidermis (small diameter of platinum wire). (arrow: total $\Delta PO_2$ across the epidermis (heavy line); $M_E$ = electrode membrane; ce = cellophane; te = Teflon; $M_S$ = epidermis; ed = dead part of the epidermis; ev = viable part of the epidermis) (13)

μm (D = ∞) which completely covers the tissue around a capillary loop. When respiring 100% oxygen the arterial $PO_2$ increases from 90 mmHg (12 kPa) to 600 mmHg (80 kPa). During this manoeuvre the $tcPO_2$ of the electrode (D = 0) increases from 104 mmHg (13.87 kPa) to 504 mmHg (67.20 kPa), that of electrode (D = 40) from 80 mmHg (10.67 kPa), to 344 mmHg (45.87 kPa) and the $tcPO_2$ (D = ∞) measures first 40 mmHg (5.33 kPa) and then 88 mmHg (11.73 kPa). This demonstrates clearly that the actual signal measured by the $tcPO_2$ electrode depends very much on its properties. After occlusion of blood flow, the $PO_2$ decreases correspondingly to the $O_2$ consumption of tissue and the electrode. This can be clearly seen by comparing the gradients of the three traces: the lowest trace is the steepest one. A $tcPO_2$ electrode with a large cathode and a Mylar membrane was introduced by Eberhard et al (2).

For practical application we have proposed a compromise for the electrode construction, so that $P_aO_2$ increase by heat is approximately cancelled by the $O_2$ consumption

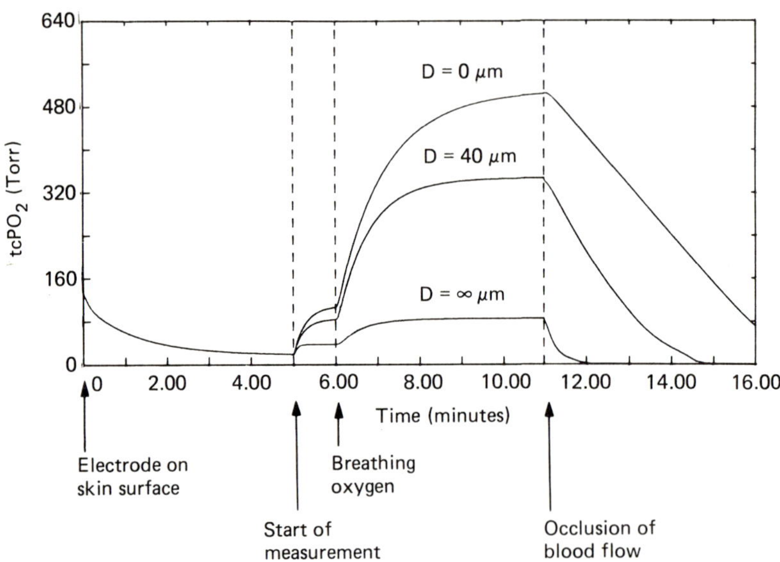


*Figure 12.* Calculated transients of $tcPO_2$ at different measuring conditions. The skin surface is covered by a 12 μm Teflon membrane, so that $PO_2$ diffusion can only occur at the area where the electrode consumes oxygen. D = diameter of this area (electrode diameter). For further explanations *see text* (6)

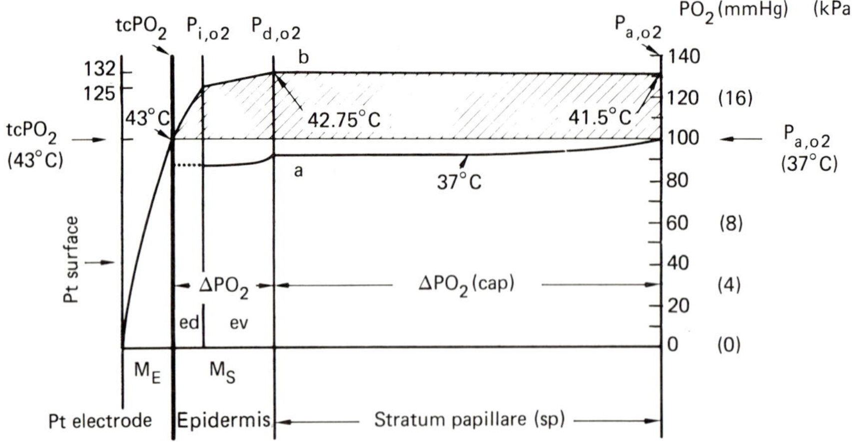


*Figure 13.* $PO_2$ profile in the epidermis and in the membrane in front of a platinum wire with heat induced hyperaemia and polarographic $PO_2$ measurements. It is assumed that the temperature decreases from 43°C at the skin surface to 41.5°C at the arterial inflow. For further explanations *see text* and *Figure 12* (13)

of the electrode (10). This is achieved by careful selection of the diameter of the platinum wire and the thickness of the membrane. The procedure is schematically shown in Figure 13. Here, $P_aO_2$ at 37°C equals $tcPO_2$ at 43°C. Figure 14 shows the correlation between $tcPO_2$ and arterial $PO_2$ (for more details see 9, 12, 13, 21). $TcPO_2$ measurements in newborns with intact circulation show a surprisingly good correlation

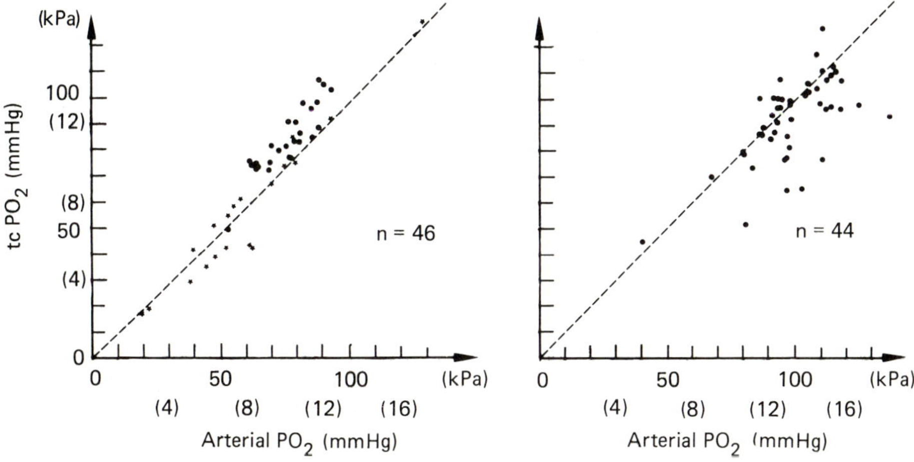


*Figure 14.* Comparison of the arterial $PO_2$ (37°C) and corresponding transcutaneous $PO_2$ values (43°C; 12 μm cellophane and 12 μm Teflon). Left: 46 blood samples from 25 healthy (●) and 9 sick infants (*), Right: 44 blood samples from 28 women during labour (15)

curve (region 3 of the circulatory hyperbola) (15). As expected from the analysis, the middle range $tcPO_2$ values tend to lie above the line of identity. With adults the scattering is much larger. The reason for this scattering is a greater variation in skin capillarization and thickness of epidermal layers. Also blood flow regulation is more pronounced, so that even in normal persons variations of $tcPO_2$ values are found.

## Linear relation between $tcPCO_2$ and $P_aCO_2$

In the physiological range the $tcPCO_2$ vs $P_aCO_2$ relationship is linear. During $PCO_2$ measurements tissue $PCO_2$ equilibrates with the electrode and $P_aCO_2$ must be temperature corrected. Measurements have shown that the difference between $tcPO_2$ and the temperature corrected $P_aCO_2$ value of the blood was rather variable (9, 12) but mostly larger than that expected from model calculations (7). The reason for this discrepancy has to be investigated; it may be that the $CO_2$ production of the skin is higher than that assumed or that at high flow values, carboanhydrase limits the $CO_2$ reaction.

## The value of $tcPO_2$ and $tcPCO_2$ in shock

The first applications of $tcPO_2$ and $tcPCO_2$ measurements were to monitor arterial blood gases. Most of these measurements were performed under the tacit understanding that 'excess' hyperaemia (region 3 of the circulatory hyperbola) was always present. Later it was found that also in circulatory disturbances, as in shock, $tcPO_2$ and $tcPCO_2$ measurements were valuable if the transcutaneous values were compared with arterial blood gases. Under conditions in which the blood supply to the periphery, especially to the skin, is reduced and peripheral perfusion pressure decreases, $tcPO_2$ decreases and $tcPCO_2$ increases (9, 12, 13, 24, 25, 26, 27).

## Conclusion

In conclusion, the practicc of thc transcutaneous measurement of $PO_2$ and $PCO_2$ can be well explained from the theory. The weak point of the currently available electrodes is their inability to measure local blood flow. If this could be improved then it would be much easier to interpret the transcutaneous $PO_2$ and $PCO_2$ values. I hope for further improvements in the future.

## References

1. Clark L C Jr. Monitor and control of blood tissue oxygen tensions. *Transactions of the American Society for Artificial Internal Organs,* 2, 41-48 (1956).
2. Eberhard P, Hammacher K and Mindt W. Perkutane Messung des Sauerstoffpartialdruckes. *Methodik und Anwendungen,* Stuttgart Proc Medizin-Technik, p.26 (1972).
3. Evans N T S and Naylor P F D. The systemic oxygen supply to the surface of human skin. *Respiratory Physiology,* 3, 21-27 (1967).
4. Grossmann U. Smmulation of combined transfer of oxygen and heat through the skin using a capillary loop model. *Mathematics and Biological Sciences,* 61, 205-236 (1982).
5. Grossmann U and Lübbers D W. Analysis of epidermal oxygen supply by simulation of oxygen partial pressure fields under varying conditions. *Critical Care Medicine,* 9, 734-735 (1981).
6. Grossmann U and Winkler P. Transients of gas exchange processes in the upper skin calculated by the capillary loop model. In *Oxygen Transport to Tissue VI,* edited by D F Burley et al. New York, Plenum Press, in press (1984).
7. Grossmann U, Winkler P and Lübbers D W. Coupled transport of $O_2$ and $CO_2$ within the upper skin simulated by the capillary loop model. In *Oxygen Transport to Tissue V,* edited by D W Lubbers, H Acker, T K Goldstick, E Leniger-Follert, New York, Plenum Press, in press (1984).
8. Grossmann U, Winkler P and Lubbers D W. The effect of different parameters (temperature, $O_2$ consumption, blood flow, haemoglobin content) on the $tcPO_2$ calibration curves calculated by the capillary loop model. In *Oxygen Transport to Tissue VI,* edited by D F Bruley et al. New York, Plenum Press, in press (1984).
9. Huch A, Huch R and Lucey J F (eds). *Continuous transcutaneous blood gas monitoring,* The National Foundation - March of Dimes. Birth Defects: Original Article Series, vol XV, 4, New York, A R Liss, 1979.
10. Huch A, Huch R, Meinzer K et al. Eine schnelle, beheizte Pt-Oberflaechenelektrode zur kontinuierlichen Uberwachung des $PO_2$ beim Menschen. *Elektrodenaufbau und -eigenschaften,* Stuttgart, Proc Medizin-Technik, p.26, (1972).
11. Huch A, Lubbers D W and Huch R. Der periphere Perfusions-druck: eine neue nicht-invasive Messgroesse zur Kreislaufueberwachung von Patienten. *Anaesthesist,* 24, 39 (1974).
12. Huch R and Huch A. *Continuous transcutaneous blood gas monitoring,* New York, Basel, Marcell Dekker (1983).
13. Huch R, Huch A and Lübbers D W. *Transcutaneous $PO_2$* , New York, Thieme, Stuttgart, Thieme-Stratton Inc. (1981).
14. Huch R, Lubbers D W and Huch A. Quantitative continuous measurement of partial oxygen pressure on the skin of adults and newborn babies. *Pfluegers Archivs,* 337, 185-198 (1972).
15. Huch R, Lubbers D W and Huch A. The transcutaneous measurement of oxygen-carbon dioxide tensions for the determination of arterial blood gas values with control of local perfusion and peripheral perfusion pressure: theoretical analysis and practical application. In *Oxygen Measurement in Biology and Medicine,* edited by J P Payne and D W Hill. pp.121-138, Butterworth, London (1975).
16. Kimmich H P and Kreuzer F. Model of oxygen transport through the skin as basis for absolute transcutaneous measurement of $PaO_2$ . *Acta Anaesthiologica Scandinavica,* 68, 16 (1978).
17. Lubbers D W. Theoretical basis of transcutaneous blood gas measurements. *Critical Care Medicine,* 9, 721-733 (1981).
18. Lubbers D W. Cutaneous and transcutaneous $PO_2$ and $PCO_2$ and their measuring conditions. In *Continuous Transcutaneous Blood Gas Monitoring,* edited by A Huch, R Huch and J F Lucey. The National Foundation - March of Dimes. Birth Defects: Original Article Series, Vol XV, pp.13-32, New York, A R Liss, 1979.

19. Lubbers D W and Grossmann U. Gas exchange through the human epidermis as a basis of $tcPO_2$ and $tcPO_2$ measurments. In *Continuous Transcutaneous Blood Gas Monitoring,* edited by R Huch and A Huch; New York, M Dekker Inc, in press (1982).
20. Quinn J A. Gas transfer through the skin: a two layer model relating transcutaneous flux to arterial tension. In *Oxygen Transport to Tissue III,* edited by I A Silver, M Erecinska and H I Bicher. New York, Plenum Press, pp.175-181.(1978).
21. Severinghaus J W. Workshop on methodological aspects of transcutaneous blood gas monitoring. *Acta Anaesthesiologica Scandinavica,* 68 (1978).
22. Severinghaus J W. A combined transcutaneous $PO_2$ -$PCO_2$ electrode with electrochemical $HCO_3$ stabilization. *Journal of Applied Physiology,* 51, 1027-1032 (1981).
23. Severinghaus J W, Stafford M and Thunstrom A M. Estimation of skin metabolism and blood flow with $tcPO_2$ and $tcPCO_2$ electrodes by cuff occlusion of the circulation. *Acta Anaesthesiologica Scandinavica,* 68, 9-15 (1978).
24. Shoemaker W C and Vidyasagar R. Physiological and clinical significance of $PtcO_2$ and $PtcO_2$ . *Critical Care Medicine,* 10, 689 (1981).
25. Tremper K K, Shoemaker W C and Shippy C R. Transcutaneous oxygen monitoring of critically ill adults, with and without low flow shock. *Critical Care Medicine,* 9, 706-709 (1981).
26. Versmold H T et al. Limits to $tcPO_2$ monitoring in sick neonates: relation to blood pressure, blood volume, peripheral blood flow and acid base status. *Acta Anaesthesiologica Scandinavica,* 68, 88-90 (1978).
27. Waxman K, Sadler R, Eisner M E, Applebaum R, Tremper K K and Mason E R. Transcutaneous oxygen monitoring of emergency department patients. *American Journal of Surgery,* 146, 35-38 (1983).

Chapter 23

# Blood gas analysis in the unstressed human fetus at 17-22 weeks' gestation

**I Z Mackenzie, B Castle, P Johnson**

## Introduction

Current assessment of fetal well-being during the antenatal period in the human has relied upon observations of fetal heart rate (FHR) patterns, fetal limb and chest wall movements, ultrasound measurements of the fetal anatomy and liquor volume, and the quantitation of various hormones and biochemical constituents in maternal blood and urine. Access to the fetal circulation might provide a direct, precise assessment of the fetal state, relating both to its acute condition and chronic compromise in the way that scalp blood sampling has been utilized during the intrapartum period.

With the development of fibre-optic fetoscopy equipment, fetal blood sampling has become a recognized investigation for prenatal diagnosis of disorders only detectable by fetal blood analysis (5,6) and with attention to technique, methods of obtaining pure samples of fetal blood have been perfected (7,10). With experience, samples can be reliably obtained from the umbilical cord where identification of the vessels can be determined by the colour of the blood contained, whether oxygenated in the umbilical vein or de-oxygenated in the umbilical arteries. By using this technique, samples of whole blood have been collected from the fetus during mid-gestation and blood gas analysis performed to determine normal values in the human fetus under near physiological conditions.

## Patients and Methods

Sixty-eight patients at 17-22 weeks gestation, admitted for induction of abortion by intra-amniotic injection of prostaglandins, have been studied. Each gave informed signed consent to be investigated and prior approval of the principle of fetoscopic research using fetal blood sampling techniques had been given by the Local Hospital Ethics Committee. Fetoscopy using a Storz fetoscope, No 26300C, was performed by the technique previously described (7). Pre-medication with papavaretum 20 mg i.m. was given 1-2 hours pre-operatively and diazepam 5 mg i.v. 5-10 minutes prior to fetal blood sampling in each case; local anaesthetic infiltration into the anterior abdominal wall was performed immediately prior to instrumentation.

All patients were investigated in a resting, non-agitated state in a supine position breathing air. A maternal venous blood sample was collected from the antecubital fossa at the start of the procedure and samples were collected under continuous direct vision from the umbilical vein and/or one of the umbilical arteries in either order, preventing contamination by amniotic fluid. In 10 cases, a sample of the intervillous blood was aspirated from the placenta avoiding the major surface vessels. All samples were collected into pre-heparinized syringes and blood gas analyses were performed within 30 minutes of collection. pH, $PO_2$, $PCO_2$, ABE and percentage oxygen saturation were measured using an ABL automatic blood gas analyser (Radiometer, Copenhagen). Kleihauer tests were performed on all the fetal and placental samples.

In six cases following the initial sampling from the umbilical vein, the patient breathed 100% oxygen via a face mask for 2-4 minutes and a further sample was collected from the vein for blood gas analysis: in all but two cases, the second sample was collected using the same needle siting for asiration without interval removal.

Following the collection of samples, a therapeutic dose of $PGE_2$ was instilled intra-amniotically to induce abortion.

## Results

The Kleihauer test confirmed that all the samples collected from the umbilical cord were pure fetal blood and those from the placenta were predominantly maternal (0-less than 5 fetal RBC per 50 LPF).

Table 1 lists the mean (± s.d.) and range of blood gas results obtained in the 68 patients studied: in 42 cases, matched umbilical arterial (FA) and umbilical venous (FV) samples were obtained. The base excess values did not differ significantly in the blood obtained from maternal vein from that in the fetal artery and vein, while the only significant difference observed between maternal vein and fetal vein was the degree of oxygen saturation (p less than 0.02: Student's *t*-test). By comparison, significant differences (p less than 0.0001) were noted in the other indices measured between fetal vein and fetal artery and maternal vein and fetal artery.

There was a positive correlation for pH between maternal vein and fetal artery (r = 0.326, 48 degrees of freedom, p less than 0.025) and fetal vein (r = 0.352, 55

**TABLE 1. Blood gas values at fetoscopy at 17–22 weeks' gestation (values given are mean ±1 s.d.) with range of values in parentheses.**

| | *IVS* | *FV* | *FA* | *MV* |
|---|---|---|---|---|
| n | 10 | 59 | 52 | 65 |
| pH | 7.41±0.03 | 7.36±0.03 | 7.32±0.03 | 7.36±0.03 |
| | (7.36−7.48) | (7.26−7.41) | (7.25−7.38) | 7.30−7.41) |
| $PCO_2$ | 28±6 | 37±3 | 42±4 | 38±4 |
| (mmHg) | (19.3−38.6) | (28.1−46.6) | (35.3−50.1) | 26.3−47.0) |
| $PO_2$ | 83±24 | 43±9 | 23±6 | 40±12 |
| (mmHg) | (60.2−129.1) | (19.5−69.7) | (12.0+37.9 | (20.8−81.7) |
| ABE | 6±3 | 4±2 | 4±2 | 4±2 |
| | (2.1−12.2) | (0.3−8.9) | (0.9+9.7) | (0.6−10.8) |
| % O | 295±3 | 74±11 | 35±13 | 68±16 |
| saturation | (91.0−98.8) | (23.7−92.1) | (11.0−64.5) | (31.1−95.1) |

IVS=intervillous space; FV=fetal umbilical vein; FA=fetal umbilical artery; MV=maternal vein

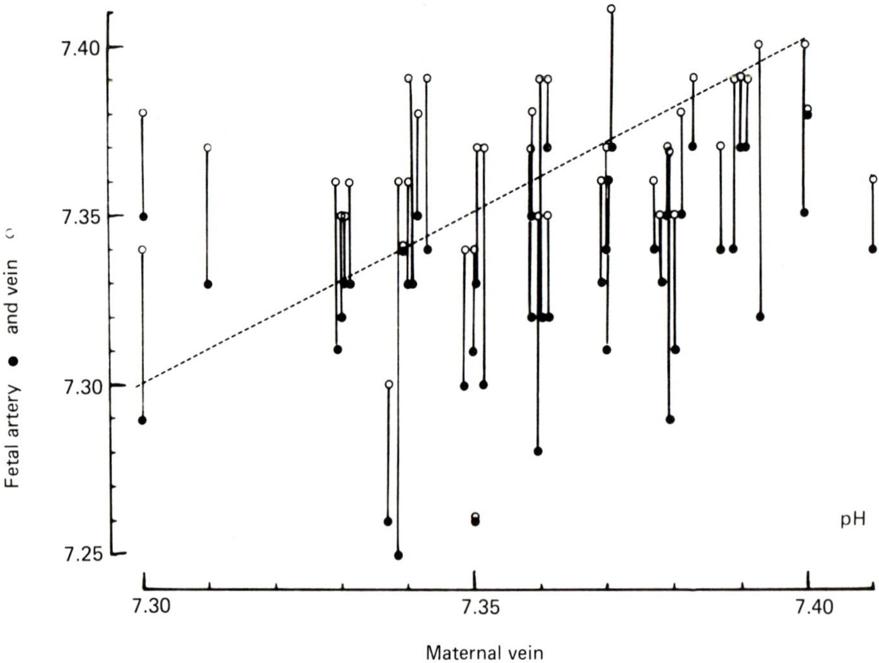


*Figure 1.* Relationship between maternal vein and fetal umbilical artery and vein pH, in 42 matched samples. The dotted line is the line of identity

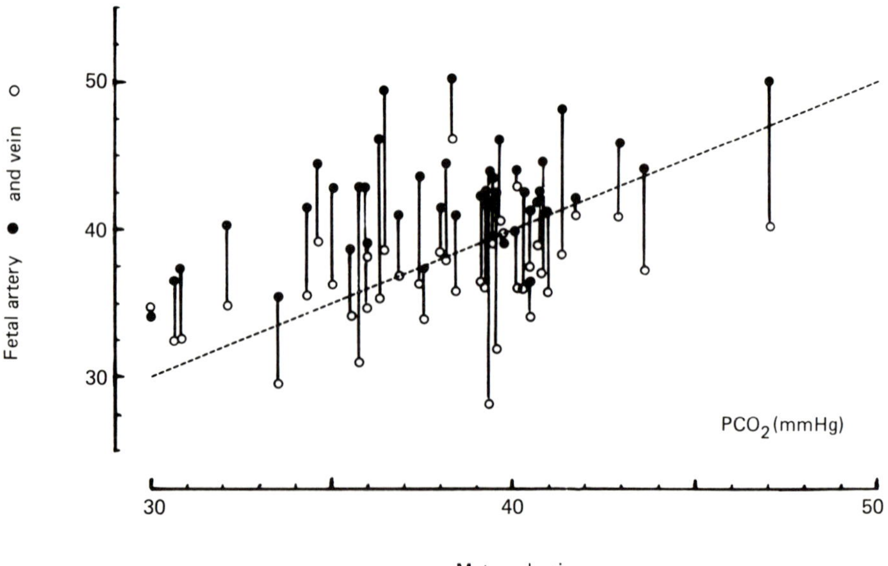


*Figure 2.* Relationship between maternal vein and fetal umbilical artery and vein $PCO_2$ in 42 matched samples

d.f., p less than 0.01) (Figure 1). With the exception of four cases, the pH in the fetal artery was always lower than in the maternal vein; no similar association existed between fetal vein and maternal vein. In no case was the fetal vein pH lower than the fetal arterial pH. There was no correlation between maternal vein and fetal vein for $PO_2$. However, in no patient was the fetal $P_aO_2$ higher than in the maternal vein, while in almost half the cases the fetal $P_vO_2$ was lower than in the maternal vein; the mean gradient between fetal and maternal vein was 3 mmHg. In no case was the fetal $P_aO_2$ greater than 35 mmHg and in only three instances was the $P_vO_2$ less than 35 mmHg.

The fetal $P_aCO_2$ was lower than the maternal value in only two cases. However, in contrast to $P0_2$, there was a positive correlation between maternal vein and fetal artery (r = 0.4868, 48 d.f., p less than 0.001) and fetal vein (r = 0.3149, 55 d.f., p less than 0.02) (Figure 2). In two patients, the fetal $P_vCO_2$ was marginally higher than the $P_aCO_2$: the other indices measured in these two cases confirmed that the correct vessel assignment had been made.

Figure 3 illustrates the relationship between blood gas values in the seven cases in whom all four blood samples (maternal vein, fetal vein and artery, and intervillous blood) were obtained. Gradients in the expected direction for $PO_2$, $PCO_2$ and pH were found between intervillous blood and the fetal vein values with significant

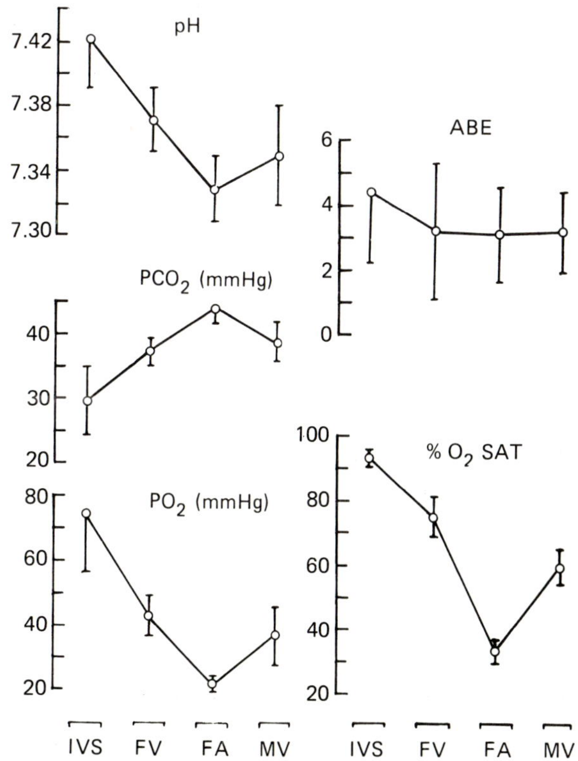


*Figure 3.* Blood gas analyses of samples of blood from peripheral maternal vein (MV), intervillous blood (FVS), fetal umbilical artery (FA) and fetal umbilical vein (FV) obtained in seven patients (values illustrated are mean ± 1 s.d.)

differences existing for each of these values (p less than 0.05); there was no significant difference in base excess.

The effect of breathing 100% oxygen for 2-4 minutes on fetal $P_vO_2$, $P_vCO_2$, and percentage oxygen saturation is shown for individual cases in Figure 4. There were no significant differences between the pre-oxygenation and post-oxygenation pH, $PCO_2$ and base excess. The mean pH was unchanged at 7.38 ml. However, although the initial pH range was small at 7.37 - 7.39 for the six patients studied the post-oxygenation range was widened to 7.32 - 7.45. The change in $PCO_2$ with oxygenation was variable: in three cases there was a fall in $PCO_2$ associated with a marked increase in $PO_2$, while in the other three cases there was a slight fall in $PCO_2$ with a small increase in $PO_2$. pH in these cases tended to change in the reverse direction to $PCO_2$. The increase in $PO_2$ from 39 ± 4 to 82 ± 31 was significant (p less than 0.05: Wilcoxon's signed ranks test) and percentage oxygen saturation from 73 ± 6 to 95 ± 4 was also significant (p less than 0.05: Wilcoxon signed ranks test). The base excess increased in five of the six patients.

In no instance did pregnancy gestation over the range studied appear to influence the results obtained for fetal blood gas values.

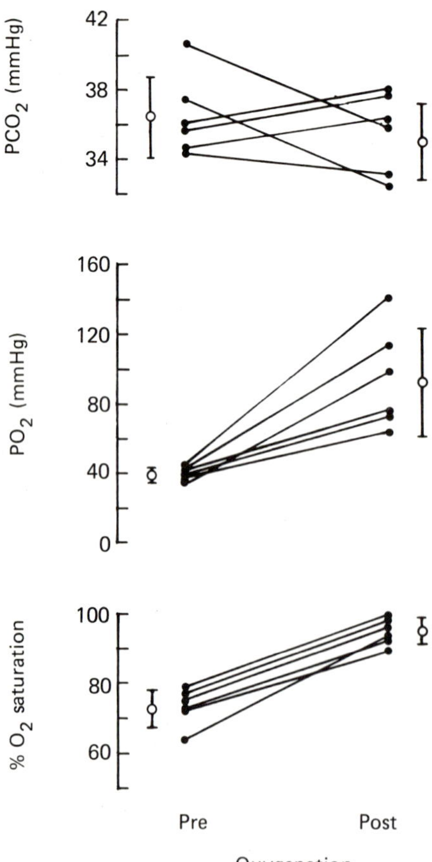


*Figure 4.* The effect upon fetal vein $PCO_2$, $PO_2$ and percentage oxygen saturation of the mother breathing 100% oxygen for 2–4 minutes in six patients. (Mean ± 1 s.d. values are also shown)

## Discussion

The observations reported of fetal blood gas status during mid-gestation in the human fetus are probably unique. While some maternal stress may have been provoked at the prospect of the study procedure and impending therapeutic abortion and some fetal sedation inevitably resulted from the administration of medication to the patient, the conditions for the study were considered to be as near physiological as possible to permit sampling of the intact fetal circulation. Various reported series of diagnostic fetoscopic fetal blood sampling from the umbilical cord (7,11) indicate that the technique probably causes little or no significant disturbance to fetal cardiovascular dynamics. Umbilical vein samples collected at full term pregnancy during delivery by elective Caesarean section in the unit in Oxford have produced mean values for pH 7.31 ± 0.04, $PCO_2$ 42 ± 5, $PO_2$ 28 ± 9 and base excess -4 ± 2; the respective arterial values were pH 7.23 ± 0.05, $PCO_2$ 54 ± 6, $PO_2$ 14 ± 6, and base excess -5 ± 3 (P Johnson, unpublished data). Comparison of these data with the present results supports the view that the samples collected at fetoscopy were from unstressed fetuses.

Comparison of the results in the present series with those previously published for human and animal models is difficult since the former have generally been obtained using general anaesthesia (12) while the latter have generally been performed at a later gestational stage and using chronic preparations. Observations in the sheep (2), goat (8), cow (4) and pig (4) indicate that there is a $PO_2$ difference between maternal vein and fetal vein varying between 17-24 mmHg. For the mare (3) the difference is only 1.5 - 3.0 mmHg. We cannot provide comparative data because we did not measure uterine venous values. Although a maternal vein (40 ± 12) to fetal vein (43 ± 9) difference of 3 mmHg existed, the ranges were wide suggesting a variable difference between uterine efferent and peripheral vein measurements.

As shown in Figure 1, there was no consistent gradient between maternal and fetal vein $PCO_2$ with mean values of 38 mmHg and 37 mmHg, respectively; in the sheep, goat, cow and pig, a consistent downward gradient of 3 - 5 mmHg from fetal vein to maternal vein has been found with no obvious gradient in the mare. This is also reflected in the vein-to-vein pH differences; in the present study and in the mare (4) the fetal and maternal venous pH values were similar whereas a pH difference of 0.04 - 0.05 is found in other species (12).

The positive direct correlation found in the present study for pH and $PCO_2$ between both fetal vessels and the maternal vein, suggests that the fetal state is influenced by the maternal respiratory status at the time of sampling. In those patients with a mild respiratory acidosis, both fetal vessels tended to have lower pH values and higher $PCO_2$ values.

Maternal arterial blood would have provided more information but it was not considered ethically acceptable to approach patients to assist in this way. As an alternative, samples of blood were aspirated from the placenta from the intervillous space. Compared with the other samples collected, the ranges of values for pH, $PCO_2$, $PO_2$ and base excess were greater in intervillous blood. The probable explanation for this is the blind nature by which the sampling was performed. The tip of the aspiration needle could either be in an efferent or afferent limb of the intervillous space. However, the gradient for these indices compared with both fetal vein and artery were all in the expected direction. Worthwhile interpretation of these results must await the collection of a larger number of samples.

Breathing 100% oxygen for a few minutes produced a large increase in oxygenation of fetal umbilical vein blood. A similar observation was made by Quilligan et al (9) in women undergoing Caesarean section using regional block anaesthesia. These workers noted an increase in mean $PO_2$ from 16.8 mmHg before oxygenation to 26.1 mmHg in four patients studied These increases occurred after the patient had been breathing 100% oxygen by mask for 5 minutes and are less than those observed in the present study. These differences could be explained by the differences in gestational period, the technique of sampling and the anaesthesia used. Since the basal $O_2$ values in that study were well below those measured at elective section at term (18 vs 28) it is likely that uteroplacental blood supply was compromised. Fetal skin surface measurements ($FP_sO_2$ ) in labour have shown that maternal $O_2$ administration causes a rise in $FP_sO_2$.

Whether the early second trimester fetus has higher $O_2$ and lower $CO_2$ levels than at term is not certain. Nonetheless, some of the high venous levels of $O_2$ found, especially after $O_2$ administration raise questions as to the physiological mechanisms involved as well as the possible effects of fetal hyperoxia. There are many factors involved in oxygen delivery to, and $CO_2$ removal from, the fetus. For example, early in gestation the distance between maternal and fetal circulation is much greater than at term, whereas oxygen consumption of the placenta is much less. Chronic catheterization of the very young fetus in experimental animals has been unsuccessful to date and thus it is likely that measurements such as the ones reported here, coupled with other physiological variables such as blood pressure, ECG and blood flow may provide unique data on early fetal development. The general similarity of results, however, supports the view that the administration of oxygen to the maternal organism can produce a significant and rapid increase in fetal oxygenation. The observation of $PCO_2$ rising in three cases and falling in three cases with pH moving in the reverse direction can probably be explained in terms of the maternal respiratory response to the administration of oxygen-rich air to breathe: in three, a marked increase in $PO_2$ occurred with a fall in $PCO_2$ due to increased respiratory effort while in the other three the responses were hypoventilation with a smaller increase in $PO_2$ , a rise in $PCO_2$ with a fall in pH. This observation further supports the view that the maternal respiratory status rapidly influenced the fetal status during these studies.

The question remains as to whether the higher $O_2$ and lower $CO_2$ values in both fetal vein and artery found at fetoscopy at 17 - 22 weeks reflect a genuine physiological difference between early and late gestation or simply a more normal physiological state than is found at term elective Caesarean section. The latter is suggested by the fact that the values above for elective Caesarean section were perhaps surprisingly only marginally better than those found after labour. Comparison of our data with those published from other animal species is not entirely appropriate since the latter are generally from chronically catheterized fetuses and made comparatively late in gestation.

Furthermore, species differences in materno-placental vascular anatomy have been considered important in determining fetal blood gas levels.

Having established values for blood gases in the venous and arterial circulation in the unstressed human fetus during mid-pregnancy, further avenues of research are now possible. A direct assessment of fetal well-being in at-risk pregnancies could now be possible, allowing a more precise antenatal management of such cases (I Z Mackenzie and B M Castle - unpublished data). By using blood gas analyses of samples collected from the umbilical cord it has been possible to differentiate from which vessel the sample has been collected, allowing further observations on fetal physiology including protein and hormone synthesis and placental transfer (1,13) and with the application of techniques of measuring umbilical blood flow, more precise kinetic studies will now become available during mid-gestation in human pregnancy.

## Acknowledgements

The authors wish to acknowledge the technical assistance and expert nursing care provided by Sister Jane Ferguson.

## References

1. Aynsley-Green A, Soltesz G, Jenkins P A and Mackenzie I Z. The metabolic and endocrine milieu of the human fetus and mother at 18-21 weeks of gestation. II. Blood glucose, lactate, pyruvate and ketone body concentrations. In: *Biology of the Neonate,* (in press).
2. Comline R S and Silver M. Daily changes in fetal and maternal blood of conscious pregnant ewes with catheter in umbilical and uterine vessels. *Journal of Physiology (London),* 209; 567-586 (1970).
3. Comline R S and Silver M. $PO_2$, $PCO_2$ and pH levels in the umbilical and uterine blood of the mare and ewe. *Journal of Physiology (London),* 209; 587-608 (1970).
4. Comline R S and Silver M. A comparative study of the blood gas tensions, oxygen affinity and red cells 2, 3. DPG concentrations in fetal and maternal blood in the mare, cow and sow. *Journal of Physiology (London),* 242, 805-826 (1974).
5. Cordesius E, Gustavii B and Mitelman F. Prenatal chromosomal analysis of fetal blood obtained at fetoscopy. *British Medical Journal,* 280, 1107 (1980).
6. Kan Y W, Golbus M S, Trecartin R F and R A Filly. Prenatal diagnosis of beta thalassaemia and sickle cell anaemia. *Lancet,* 1, 269-271 (1977).
7. I Z Mackenzie and D A Maclean. Pure fetal blood from the umbilical cord obtained at fetoscopy; experience with 125 consecutive cases. *American Journal of Obstetrics and Gynecology,* 138, 1213-1218 (1980).
8. Prystowsky H, Meschia G and Barron D H. The oxygen tension in the placental bloods of goats. *Yale Journal of Biological Medicine,* 32, 441-448 (1960).
9. Quilligan E J, Vasicka A, Aznar R, Lipsitz P J, Moore D and Bloor B M. Partial pressure of oxygen in the intervillous space and the umbilical vessels. *American Journal of Obstetrics and Gynecology,* 79, 1048-152 (1960).
10. Rodeck C H and Campbell S. Sampling pure fetal blood by fetoscopy in second trimester of pregnancy. *British Medical Journal,* 2; 728-730 (1978).
11. Rudolph A M, Heyman M A, Teramo K A W et al. Studies on the circulation of the previable human fetus. *Paediatric Research,* 5, 452-460 (1971).
12. Silver M, Steven DH, Comline RS. In: *Fetal and Neonatal Physiology.* Barcroft Centenary Symposium. Ed: R S Comline, K W Cross, G S Dawes, P W Nathanielsz, pp. 245-271. Cambridge University Press, London (1973).
13. Soltesz G, Harris D, MacKenzie I Z and Aynsley-Green A. The metabolic and endocrine milieu of the human fetus and mothers at 18-21 weeks of gestation. I. Plasma amino-acid concentrations. *Paediatric Research,* (in press).

Chapter 24

# Continuous simultaneous tissue-pH and transcutaneous carbon dioxide monitoring during labour

**C Nickelsen, S G Thomsen, T Weber**

## Introduction

Monitoring of the fetal heart rate has been the best available method of assessing fetal well-being during labour for more than a century. Until a few years ago, this monitoring was accomplished either by discontinuous use of a stethoscope or by continuous cardiotocography using ultrasound or fetal electrocardiography. Fetal heart rate monitoring often reveals heart rate abnormalities necessitating further investigation and for this purpose fetal blood sampling (FBS), with measurement of both pH and $PCO_2$, has been the best tool. Unfortunately, FBS often has to be carried out several times in order to avoid erroneous measurements (6) and to determine the progression or regression of an acidosis. The blood collection is difficult as it involves repeated amnioscopies and skin incisions, and it causes discomfort and anxiety to the mother.

In order to solve these problems the Kontron-Roche electrode for continuous tissue-pH (t-pH) measurement was introduced 7 years ago. Previous studies (5,11) have established the close correlation of t-pH to capillary as well as umbilical artery blood pH, and the combination of t-pH and cardiotocographic monitoring has proven its value (14). However, in contrast to FBS, the t-pH cannot give any information regarding the exact nature of an acidosis as the $PCO_2$ is unknown. During the last few years transcutaneous carbon dioxide (tc-$PCO_2$ ) monitoring has been practicable, and studies (4,10) have shown a close correlation of tc-$PCO_2$ to capillary and umbilical artery blood $PCO_2$. The next logical step in fetal monitoring would be to establish a continuous simultaneous monitoring of fetal heart rate, uterine contractions, t-pH and tc-$PCO_2$. This is a presentation of our preliminary results obtained by monitoring 22 deliveries.

## Materials and methods

Twenty-two parturients at term were included in this study after informed consent. The pregnancy was uncomplicated in 16 cases, while three patients suffered from pre-eclampsia, two from rhesus immunization and one from diabetes mellitus. Eighteen patients went into spontaneous labour and four had labour induced by prostaglandin $E_2$ pessaries.

The pH electrode and the $PCO_2$ transducer were applied when the cervical os was dilated more than 4 cm and the membranes had ruptured. The t-pH electrode used was a combined glass-reference electrode (Kontron-Roche), designed according to the concept described by Stamm *et al* (9). The active part of the electrode is the pH sensitive tip, measuring 1.3 mm in diameter and 1 mm in length. The reference electrode with a liquid/liquid junction placed around the glass electrode is an integral part of the electrode. The electrode was sterilized in three steps:

(1) the inner electrode with trioxane gas for 24 hours
(2) the invasive part of the electrode with fluid aldehydes for 30 minutes, and
(3) the rest of the electrode and electrical connections with trioxane gas for 24 hours.

The electrode was calibrated at pH 7.38 and pH 6.84 by sterile phosphate buffers (Radiometer) at 37°C. The buffer containers were mounted with sterile cylinders of 30 cm length to avoid contamination of the proximal part of the cable during calibration. A clinical pH-meter (PHM 75, Radiometer) was used for monitoring and t-pH values between 7.50 and 7.00 were recorded every tenth second in the lower trace of the cardiotocogram. Prior to the application of the t-pH electrode with Henners tool (1), a catheter was inserted to monitor intrauterine pressure. The fetal ECG was recorded by the spiral electrode attached to the pH electrode.

The tc-$PCO_2$ transducer (E5230, Radiometer) used was a specially designed, thermostated Severinghaus carbon dioxide electrode (7) with heating element, temperature sensor, glass pH electrode and reference electrode integrated in the transducer housing, measuring 15 mm in diameter and 11 mm in height. The generated heat is transferred from the heating element to the skin, producing vasodilatation and increasing the permability of the skin to $CO_2$. The tc-$PCO_2$ measurement is in fact a pH measurement in an electrolyte solution placed with the glass pH and reference electrode on the one side and a $CO_2$ permeable membrane on the other. The $CO_2$ released from the skin diffuses through the membrane causing pH of the electrolyte solution to change. As this pH change correlates with the $CO_2$ diffusion, $PCO_2$ can be calculated and recorded by the monitor (TCM20, Radiometer). The membrane was renewed before each study in order to avoid bacterial contamination. The transducer, connected to the monitor, was calibrated with 5% and 1O+ carbon dioxide/nitrogen gas (approximately 5.1 kPa and 10.1 kPa at normal ambient pressure). Following calibration, the transducer was sterilized in fluid aldehydes for 30 minutes and attached to the fetal head by a suction ring by means of a negative pressure of 20 kPa (12). No shaving or other preparations were performed prior to the application of the transducer, which was heated to a temperature of 44°C during monitoring. Application was carried out with two fingers without the use of any tool. If the monitoring time exceeded 4 hours, the transducer was removed and attached to another place in order to avoid heat damage to the skin. The tc-$PCO_2$ was recorded intermittently every tenth second on the FHR trace of the cardiotocograph (8030A, Hewlett Packard) as well as continuously on the carbon dioxide monitor. Furthermore, the energy used to heat the transducer ('heat consumption') was continuously recorded on the carbon dioxide monitor.

Immediately after delivery, blood samples were collected anaerobically from the umbilical artery and vein and analysed on a blood gas analyser (ABL3, Radiometer). Following each monitoring, both devices were recalibrated to evaluate their drift. The cardiotocogram and the t-pH, but not the tc-$PCO_2$, were used to decide whether interference was indicated during labour. A t-pH value between 7.20 and 7.15 was considered pathological and indicated delivery within the next 15 minutes. A t-pH of less than 7.15 indicated immediate delivery. A pathological cardiotocogram did not result in intervention, if t-pH was normal.

## Results

Four neonates were delivered by vacuum extraction, three because of suspected asphyxia and one because of a prolonged second stage of labour. Eighteen women delivered spontaneously.

In five cases the t-pH monitoring had to be discarded as unsuccessful for the following reasons. Usually, a low t-pH was only accepted as an indication for intervention if the reading was verified by reapplication, but in one case this procedure was not carried out, and the neonate was delivered by vacuum extraction because of bradycardia and a t-pH of 7.14 (not double checked). The child had an umbilical artery blood pH of 7.28 and Apgar scores of 10 both 1 and 5 minutes after delivery. One patient objected to continuous monitoring just after application of the t-pH electrode, and the monitoring was stopped. In two cases no acceptable pH-signals were obtained after two attempted applications. One recording was considered too short as the patient delivered only 5 minutes after application. Consequently, 17 t-pH recordings (77%) were successful even during the second stage of labour and until delivery.

Five of the tc-$PCO_2$ recordings also had to be discarded as unsuccessful. The two cases in which there was first objection and second monitoring of only 5 minutes duration were the same as those described above. Three measurements were unsuccessful because of technical problems with the monitor or loss of transducer membrane during sterilization. Consequently, 17 tc-$PCO_2$ recordings (77%) were successful. In some cases the tc-$PCO_2$ transducer slipped out of the suction ring during the second stage of labour, but reapplication was easy and a reliable tc-$PCO_2$ was available within 2 minutes.

The drift of the t-pH electrode was less than 0.12 pH-units in all cases (mean 0.035). Three recordings revealed drifts of 0.9-0.12 pH-units, while the drift in all other cases was less than 0.04. The tc-$PCO_2$ transducer drifted from 0-25% (mean 5.5%). In three cases the drift was 10, 12 and 25%, respectively, while it was less than 8% in the remaining cases.

At delivery the t-pH correlated linearly with the umbilical artery blood pH ($r= 0.72$, p less than 0.01). If the three cases with excessive drift were omitted, the correlation coefficient was 0.76 (p less than 0.001). As the tc-$PCO_2$ was measured at 44°C, the arterial $PCO_2$ was corrected according to the anaerobic temperature coefficient of $CO_2$ in blood (8) before correlation and regression were studied. The arterial $PCO_2$ at 37°C was multiplied by 1.402 to compensate for the temperature difference. A linear correlation between tc-$PCO_2$ and arterial blood $PCO_2$ was found ($r=0.51$, p less than 0.05), but omitting the three cases with excessive drift, the correlation coefficient was 0.78 (p less than 0.001). The blood gas analyser calculated the standard base excess of umbilical artery blood ($A_{umb}$ SBE) at delivery). From the t-pH and the tc-$PCO_2$ corrected 37°C a 'tissue/transcutaneous standard base excess' (t-SBE) was calculated using either the Siggaard-Andersen nomogram or the formula

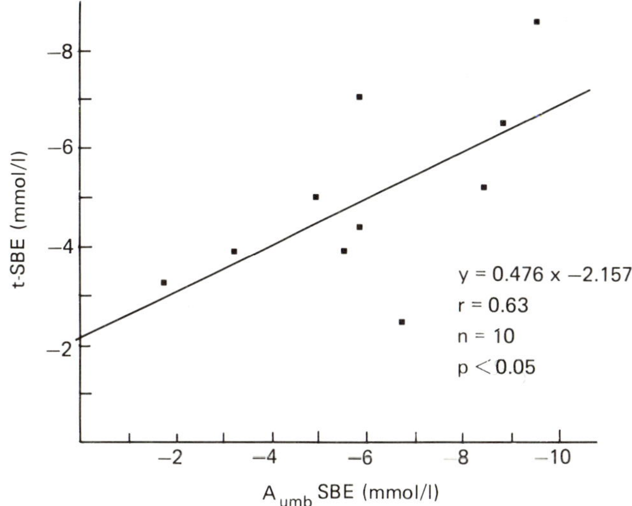


*Figure 1.* Correlation between standard base excess of umbilical artery blood ($A_{umb}$SBE) and 'tissue/transcutaneous standard base excess' (t-SBE) at delivery

describing the nomogram (8). Excluding the unsuccessful recordings and those with excessive drift, 1O tracings were left. The t-SBE correlated linearly to $A_{umb}$ SBE (r= 0.63, p less than 0.05) (Figure 1).

The following cases illustrate the additional use of t-pH and tc-$PCO_2$ in cardiotocographic monitoring.

Figure 2 illustrates the monitoring of a 31-year-old primipara with a normal pregnancy. The cardiotocogram represents the seventh hour of the first stage of labour. The deep deceleration in fetal heart rate was followed by an immediate tc-$PCO_2$ increase from 10 to 13 kPa, reaching its maximum within 6 minutes and returning to the starting level within 25 minutes. The t-pH at the onset of the deceleration was 7.29, decreasing slowly to a minimum of 7.20 in 25 minutes. During the next 20 minutes the t-pH increased to 7.25, and this value remained unchanged until delivery 2 hours later. The neonate was delivered by vacuum extraction because of a prolonged second stage of labour. Apgar scores were 9 and 10, 1 and 5 minutes after delivery, respectively. The umbilical artery blood pH was 7.21 and the $A_{umb}$ SBE -4.9 mmol/l.

Figure 3 shows the cardiotocogram during the second stage of labour in a 29-year-old primipara with an uncomplicated pregnancy and a first stage of labour lasting 9 hours, in which monitoring showed normal values. Variable decelerations were accompanied by a gradual t-pH decrease from a value of 7.28 to below 7.20. The pH electrode was consequently reapplied, and as the new t-pH value also decreased below 7.20, vacuum extraction was indicated. The t-pH/FHR electrode was removed to allow space for the vacuum extractor, and the infant was delivered 5 minutes later. The tc-$PCO_2$ level was constant at 7.5 kPa during the first 30 minutes of the t-pH decrease, but during the last 15 minutes until delivery tc-$PCO_2$ increased to approximately 11.5 kPa. Apgar scores were 7 and 10, 1 and 3 minutes, respectively, after delivery, but since the baby suffered from amniotic fluid aspiration, the Apgar score at 5 minutes was only 3. Umbilical artery blood pH was 7.11, $PCO_2$ (corrected to 44°C) was 11.8 and the $A_{umb}$ SBE was -9.5 mmol/l. The baby quickly recovered.

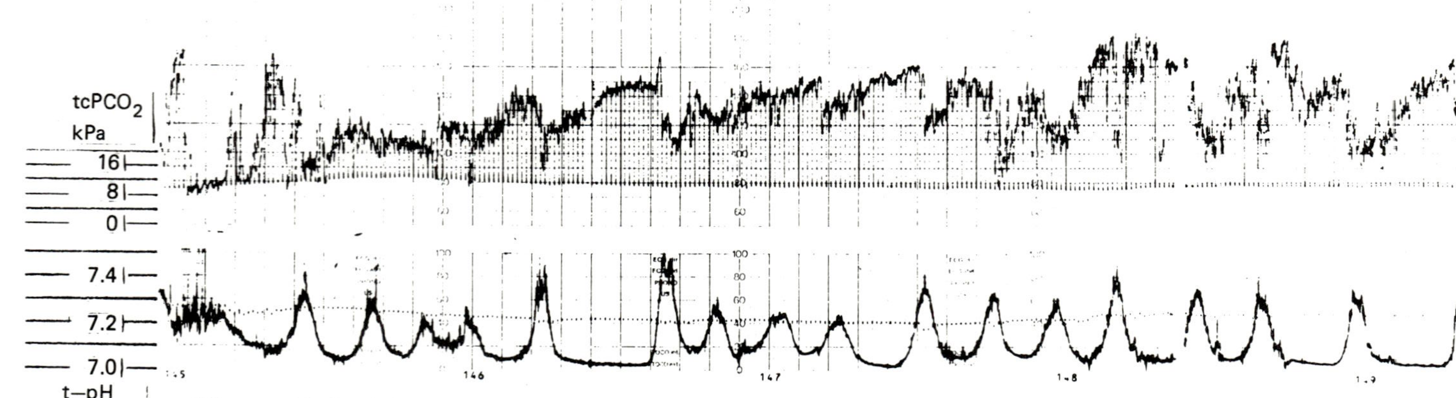


*Figure 2*. The cardiotocogram during 50 minutes of the first stage of labour illustrating a fetus suffering from respiratory acidosis. Fetal heart rate and transcutaneous carbon dioxide tension (tc-$PCO_2$) (end of vertical bars) is registered in the upper trace, tissue pH (t-pH) (dotted line) and intrauterine pressure in the lower trace. Paper speed 1 cm/minute

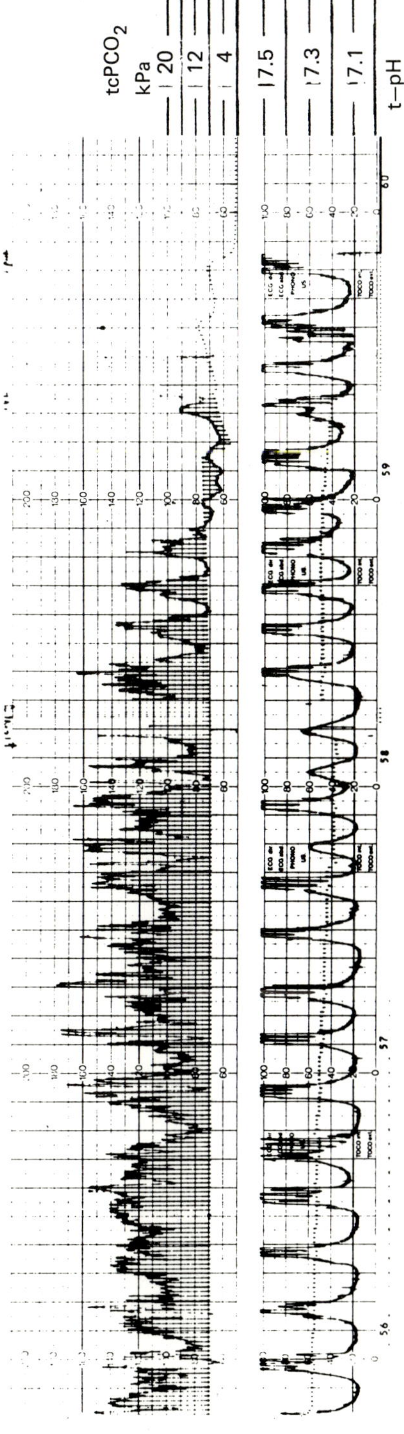


*Figure 3*. The cardiotocogram of the second stage of labour showing a fetus developing metabolic acidosis

## Discussion

In previous studies (13), continuous t-pH measurements with the Kontron-Roche electrode have been carried out with the same failure rate as in our study. The main reason for these problems is dislocation of the electrode tip from the skin incision, caused by tangential forces on the electrode during rotation and descent of the fetal head. This causes spuriously low values, and to avoid such 'false positives' we requested reapplication of the electrode before accepting a decreased pH value as true. On the other hand 'false negatives' (i.e. false normal values) have never been described. The cervix was sometimes located posteriorly and correct application of the electrode at a right angle to the head, without pressure from the edge of the cervical os, was impossible. The excessive drift of the electrode in three cases was probably caused by inadequate calibration.

The suction application of the tc-$PCO_2$ transducer is quick and simple. Usually, the tc-$PCO_2$ transducer was applied after the t-pH electrode and positioned under the edge of the cervical os on the side of the fetal head. The suction method for transcutaneous oxygen monitoring (tc-$PO_2$) has previously been reported; the results are comparable to those obtained by the glue fixation technique (12). These results are probably also valid in tc-$PCO_2$ monitoring, since exact contact and heating are less essential than in tc-$PO_2$ monitoring (2). As the $PCO_2$ monitor is constructed for neonatal monitoring, it switches off if the electrode is cooled below 30°C for more than 2 minutes. This happened during sterilization in two cases and was the major contributing factor to the failure rate of 23%. If the volume of sterilization fluid was small and the temperature not too low, the built-in heating element was able to maintain the temperature above the critical level. In the cases with excessive drift of the tc-$PCO_2$ transducer the same 1-year-old device was used, while the drift of newer transducers was acceptable.

Both t-pH and tc-$PCO_2$ correlated linearly to the respective values in the umbilical artery blood in this study. Carbon dioxide diffuses easily through human tissue (capillaries, intercellular and intracellular compartments), which is in accordance with the fact that the tc-$PCO_2$ in our study was very close to the $PCO_2$ of umbilical artery blood. The tissue-pH is measured in the intercellular fluid, and the values found by simultaneous t-pH and tc-$PCO_2$ monitoring must represent the values of intercellular fluid. The buffering capacity of intercellular fluid is mainly due to the bicarbonate content and because of the absence of haemoglobin and the low concentration of proteins, it has a lower buffering capacity than the blood. If, however, the peripheral circulation is normal, the blood is in equilibrium with the intercellular fluid. This was confirmed by the intimate correlation between t-pH and the umbilical artery blood pH in our study. According to these considerations, the buffering capacity of the extracellular compartment, including blood and intercellular fluid, must be taken into account when the amount of non-volatile acid is calculated. The calculation of the standard base excess does this, and in our study a linear correlation between t-SBE and SBE of the umbilical artery was demonstrated.

In the first example (Figure 2) the tc-$PCO_2$ increase seen immediately after the deceleration in fetal heart rate indicates a respiratory acidosis, as the t-pH decrease during the first 6 minutes is fully explained by the $CO_2$ accumulation. The continued decrease in t-pH, in spite of restoration of the tc-$PCO_2$ level, is explained by a complicating metabolic acidosis, since the calculated t-SBE decreased from an initial level of -1 mmol/l to -6 mmol/l during the first 25 minutes. During the last 20 minute period the fetus recovered, resulting in a t-SBE of -4 mmol/l, which is close to the umbilical artery value at delivery.

The second example illustrates the development of a metabolic acidosis with normal tc-$PCO_2$ values during the first part of the t-pH decrease. The calculated t-SBE was −7 mmol/l at the start and -10 mmol/l at delivery. Fetal acidosis is probably always accompanied by an elevation of $PCO_2$ (3), and the increase in tc-$PCO_2$ during the last minutes before delivery can be explained as secondary to the metabolic acidosis.

This preliminary study of simultaneous monitoring of t-pH and tc-$PCO_2$ seems to indicate that it is possible, by continuous monitoring, not only to detect an acidosis, but even to evaluate its precise nature.

Further development of the electrode and more extensive clinical testing must be awaited before this new technique can become clinically applicable.

## Acknowledgements

Tc-$PCO_2$ electrodes (E5230), tc-$PCO_2$ monitor (TCM 220) and pH-meter (PHM 75) were kindly placed at our disposal by Radiometer, Copenhagen.

## References

1. Flynn A M, Kelly J. The continuous measurement of tissue pH in the human fetus during labour using a new application technique. *British Journal of Obstetrics and Gynaecology,* 87, 666-668 (1980).
2. Frederiksen P S, Wimberley P D, Melberg S G, Witt-Hansen J and Friis-Hansen B. *Transcutaneous blood gas monitoring,* edited by R Huch and A Huch. London/New York, Marcel Dekker, (1983).
3. Goodlin R C and Kaiser I H. The effect of ammonium chloride induced maternal acidosis on the human fetus at term: I. pH, hemoglobin, blood gases. *American Journal of Medical Science,* 233, 662-675, (1957).
4. Hansen P K, Thomsen S G, Secher N J and Weber T. Transcutaneous carbon dioxide measurements in fetus during labour. *American Journal of Obstetrics and Gynecology,* in press.
5. Lauersen N H, Miller F C and Paul R H. Continuous intrapartum monitoring of fetal scalp pH. *American Journal of Obstetrics and Gynecology,* 133, 44-50 (1979)
6. Lumley J, Potter M, Newman W, Talbot J M, Wakefield E and Wood C. The unreliability of a single estimation of fetal scalp blood pH. *Journal of Laboratory and Clinical Medicine,* 77, 535-542 (1971).
7. Severinghaus J W, Stafford M and Bradley A F. Tc-$PCO_2$ electrode design, calibration and temperature gradient problems *Acta Anaesthesiologica Scandinavica Suppl,* 68, 118-122 (1978).
8. Siggaard-Andersen O. *The acid-base status of the blood,* 4th edition, Copenhagen, Munksgaard (1974).
9. Stamm O, Latscha U, Janecek P and Campara A. Development of a special electrode for continuous subcutaneous pH measurement in the fetal scalp. *American Journal of Obstetrics and Gynecology,* 124, 193-195 (1976).
10. Thomsen S G and Weber T. Fetal transcutaneous carbon dioxide tension during the second stage of labour. *British Journal of Obstetrics and Gynaecology,* in press.
11. Weber T, Hahn-Petersen S and Bock J E. Continuous fetal tissue pH recordings during labour. A preliminary report. *British Journal of Obstetrics and Gynaecology,* 85, 770-772 (1978).
12. Weber T and Secher N J. Continuous measurement of transcutaneous fetal oxygen tension during labour. *British Journal of Obstetrics and Gynaecology,* 86, 954-958 (1979).
13. Weber T. Continuous fetal scalp tissue pH monitoring during labour. *Acta Obstetrica et Gynaecologica Scandinavica,* 59, 217-223, (1980).
14. Weber T. Cardiotocography supplemented with continuous fetal pH monitoring during labour. *Acta Obstetrica et Gynaecologica Scandinavica,* 61, 351-355 (1982).

Chapter 25

# Transcutaneous $PCO_2$ monitoring of the fetus during labour

**Stephan Schmidt**

## Introduction

Transcutaneous monitoring of oxygen and carbon dioxide partial pressure ($tcPO_2$ and $tcPCO_2$) is a potentially important new method for the investigation of fetal physiology during labour, as well as a tool for fetal surveillance (1, 2, 3, 5, 12).

We have performed a clinical study in which $tcPCO_2$ was recorded in 224 fetuses during labour when suspect, prepathological or pathological heart rate patterns occurred. In 13 fetuses the pH of blood samples from the umbilical artery was less than 7.19. All infants were born in a vigorous condition with Apgar scores of more than 7.

## Methods and materials

A modified Severinghaus transducer was used for all the measurements. This device incorporates a heating element, a temperature sensor, a glass pH electrode and a reference electrode (12). By modification of a commercially available $tcPCO_2$ electrode (Radiometer E 5230), we have succeeded both in improving the application to the fetal head and also integrating an ECG electrode into the measuring chamber of the transcutaneous system, so that penetration of the fetal scalp becomes superfluous (11) (Figure 1). The measuring chamber in this combined transducer is filled with an electrolyte solution. This is achieved by means of a tube system situated within the fixing ring, which allows filling and overflow directly after the application of the transducer onto the fetal skin. This fluid serves as the conductor for the fetal heart action potential to the metal ring of the ECG electrode integrated in the $tcPCO_2$ device (Figure 1). Direct fetal heart rate recording can be performed with a commercial cardiotocograph. Another advantage achieved with the modification of the transducer is the provision of precisely defined conditions for the transcutaneous measurement when the measuring chamber is filled with a solution of known specification (7). Additionally, it is possible to detect a leakage directly after application when the adhesion of the fixing ring on the fetal skin may be only very slightly incomplete. In this case the contact solution would return either slowly or not at all via the outlet tube, and a re-application can be performed immediately.

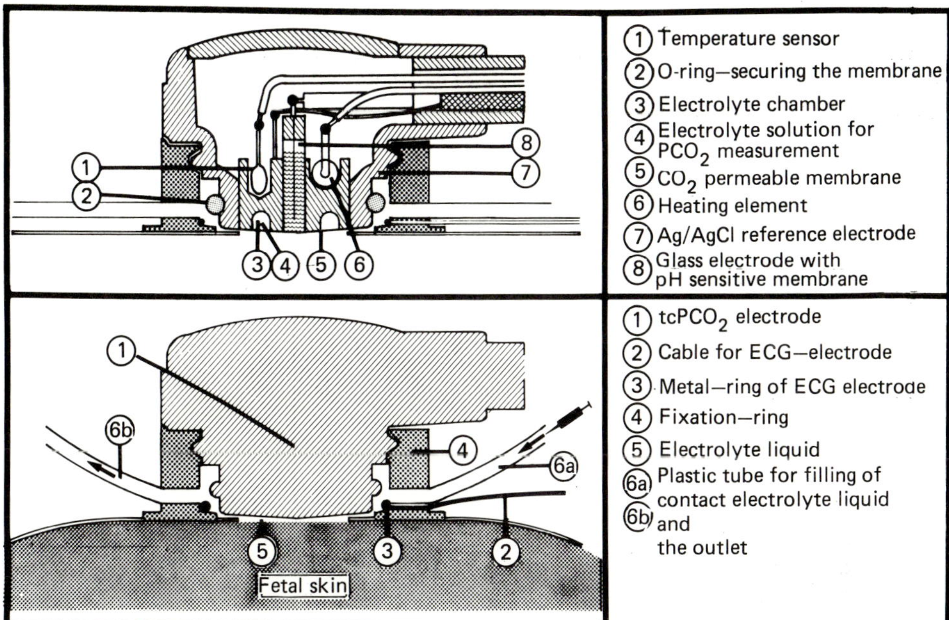


*Figure 1.* Schematic cross-section of the combined non-invasive electrode for the $tcPCO_2$ measurement and fetal heart rate recording (11)

A two-point calibration of the $tcPCO_2$ electrode with 5% and 10% carbon dioxide gas was performed at temperatures of 39°C and 44°C. The temperature of the skin surface rose by approximately 0.8°C for each 1°C above original tissue level, as indicated by the transducers. To elicit the electrode drift during the measuring procedure, controls were performed at the end of the measurements using 10% carbon dioxide gas (6). With the procedure chosen for measuring transcutaneous $PCO_2$ there was normally negligible drift.

The cervical dilatation at the time of application was more than 3 cm, while the lower pole had reached at least the interspinal plane. The application was performed by means of a fetal blood sampling tube. The fetal skin onto which the combined transducer was applied was swabbed and cleansed of blood, mucus, amniotic fluid and vernix, while hair was cut using scissors. The transducer was then fixed into an application forceps and a tissue adhesive (2-butylcyanoacrylate) was poured onto the contacting surface of the electrode. The device was then glued onto the prepared area of the fetal skin.

## Results

Of 242 attempts made, application was not successful in 18 cases. The transducer was dislodged eight times and a compression between the fetal head and the pelvic wall made re-application necessary in 10 cases.

For synoptical coverage of the results, the fetal heart rate (FHR), the labour, the transcutaneous carbon dioxide partial pressure ($tcPCO_2$ ) and the relative heat

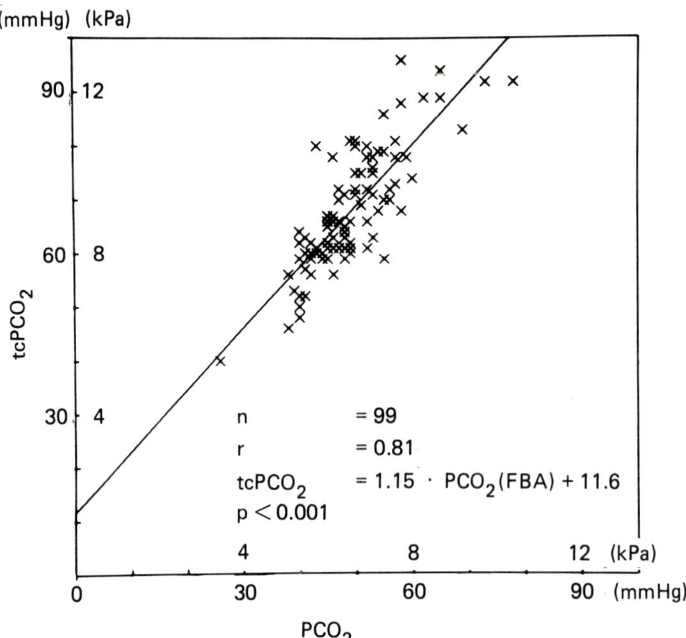


*Figure 2.* Correlation between transcutaneous carbon dioxide partial pressure ($tcPCO_2$) and the $PCO_2$ of fetal blood (FBA) at a measuring temperature of 44°C

variation of the electrode (mW) were traced polygraphically on a four-channel recorder. In order to describe the specific characteristics of the $tcPCO_2$ in the fetus we performed transcutaneous measurements at two different temperatures and correlated the $tcPCO_2$ values with the values of the fetal blood (8, 9). The comparisons of the transcutaneous $PCO_2$ measurement with the $PCO_2$ values of the fetal blood analysis showed a significant correlation at both measuring temperatures (p less than 0.001) (Figure 2). The correlation coefficient was higher at 44°C ($r = 0.81$) compared with the results at 39°C ($r = 0.74$).

## Discussion

When not corrected for the production of $CO_2$ in the skin (tissue factor) and for the effect of raised temperature (temperature factor), the transcutaneous values clearly exceeded the values of the fetal blood (Figure 2), (2, 7, 12).

It has previously been shown for $tcPO_2$ that the patterns of transcutaneous measurements are considerably influenced by the progress of labour (3). In order to investigate this influence on transcutaneous $PCO_2$ measurements, we tested their reliability at different stages of labour. We found that at identical measuring temperatures (44°C), the correlation coefficient (r) was higher during the first stage of labour ($r = 0.81$), compared with the data of the second stage of labour ($r = 0.76$). Also in the case of the development of a *caput succedaneum* the correlation coefficient was lowered, especially when the transducer temperature was 39°C. Local skin changes, on the other hand, seem to occur to a great extent at a measuring temperature

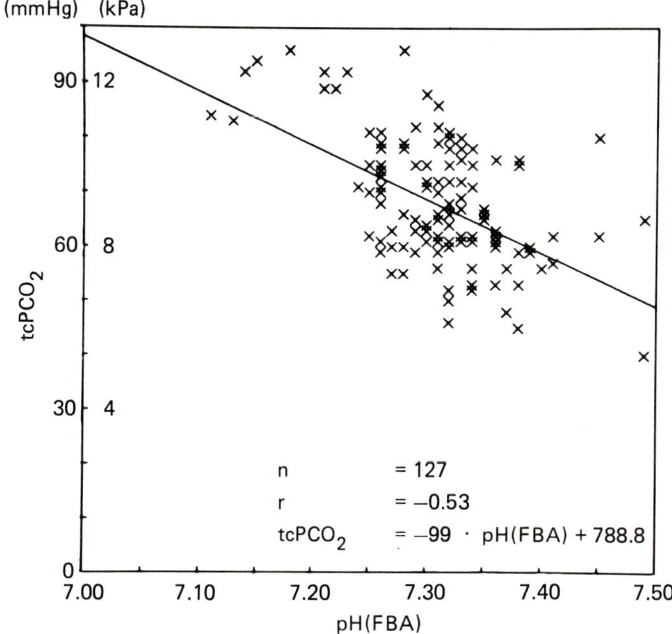


*Figure 3.* Correlation of $tcPCO_2$ and pH of fetal blood (FBA) at a measuring temperature of 44°C

of 44°C and can lead to less consistent values after a monitoring period of more than 150 minutes. Nevertheless, our analysis has proved that in spite of the influences of the progress of labour and the duration of measurement, there still remains a statistically significant conformity between carbon dioxide levels measured transcutaneously and the $PCO_2$ levels in the fetal blood (p less than 0.001).

Since pH measurements are one basis of fetal surveillance during labour we also investigated the correlation between $tcPCO_2$ and pH. An inverse and statistically significant correlation between $tcPCO_2$ and pH levels was found (Figure 3). The correlation coefficient (-0.53) was lower than that found for $tcPCO_2$ and $PCO_2$. This might be caused by the fact that the pH level is not only dependent on the blood $CO_2$ content, but is additionally determined by the degree of metabolic acidity, in particular by the lactic acid concentration (4, 10). When we compared the $PCO_2$ levels obtained transcutaneously with the actual pH level from fetal blood analysis, we found the $tcPCO_2$ levels increased when pH decreased. In the pH range 7.25-7.50 we found a considerable scattering of the $PCO_2$ levels measured transcutaneously (Figure 3). On the other hand, all the $tcPCO_2$ levels measured at 44°C and not corrected when a pre-acidosis occurred during labour, were above 9.33 kPa. This finding, which needs to be confirmed by a larger number of cases, suggests that the additional use of $tcPCO_2$ monitoring could reduce the number of fetal blood analyses that have to be performed. An incision for fetal blood sampling would be necessary only when pathological heart rate patterns emerge and additionally the $tcPCO_2$ recording exceeds the 9.33 kPa level.

Furthermore, the use of transcutaneous carbon dioxide monitoring is a helpful tool in the surveillance of the fetus during labour when the course of an acute complication is not clearly indicated by the fetal heart rate pattern (Figure 4). In this case the

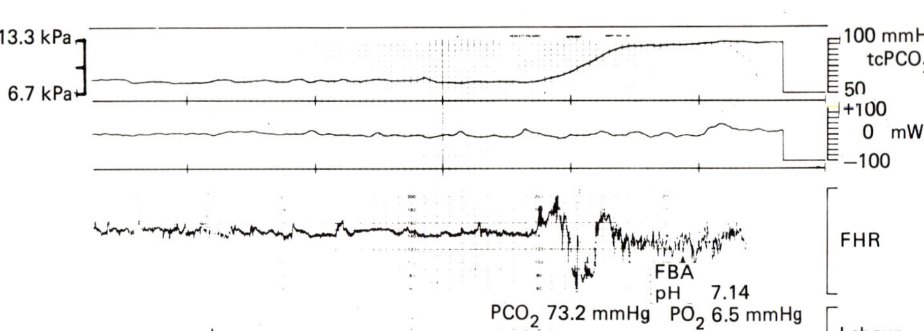


*Figure 4*. Polygraphic tracing of $tcPCO_2$, relative heat variation (mW), fetal heart rate (FHR) and labour during an acute intrauterine complication. The rise of the $tcPCO_2$ indicates clearly the development of fetal acidosis

development of a fetal acidosis is indicated by a rise of the $tcPCO_2$ from its original baseline to a level above 12.0 kPa. The baby was born after immediate Caesarean section before signs of clinical depression had developed.

## Conclusion

We conclude that $tcPCO_2$ monitoring proves to be a reliable method of detecting changes in $PCO_2$ levels during intrauterine complications. Its application to clinical medicine, especially when pathological fetal heart rate patterns are present, might diminish the frequency of fetal blood sampling and optimize the timing for operative delivery.

## References


1. Delpy D and Parker D. Transcutaneous measurement of arterial blood-gas tensions by mass spectrometry. *Lancet*, 1016-1017 (1975).
2. Huch A, Huch R, Arner B and Rooth G. Continuous transcutaneous oxygen tension measured with a heated electrode. *Scandinavian Journal of Clinical and Laboratory Investigations*, 31, 269-274 (1973).
3. Huch A and Huch R. Klinische und physiologische Aspekte der transkutanen Sauerstoffdruckmessung in der Perinatalmedizin. *Zeitschrift für Geburtshilfe und Perinatologie*, 179, 235-239 (1975).
4. Künzel W. Der Säure-Basen-Status im maternen und fetalen Blut während der Geburt und im Blut des Neugeborenen unmittelbar post partum. *Gynäkologie*, 7, 36-43 (1974).
5. Löfgren O. Continuous transcutaneous carbon dioxide monitoring of the fetus during labor. *Critical Care Medicine*, 9, 750-751 (1981).
6. Löfgren O. Drift of the $tcPCO_2$ measurement in vivo and in vitro. *Biotelemetry Patient Monitoring*, 9, 115-123 (1982).
7. Lübbers D W. Theoretical basis of the transcutaneous blood gas measurements. *Critical Care Medicine*, 9, 721-732 (1981).
8. Saling E. Neues Vorgehen zur Unteruchung des Kindes unter der Geburt (Einführung, Technik, Grundlagen). *Archiv für Gynäkologie*, 197, 108-115 (1962).
9. Saling E. Capillaries in the fetal scalp. *Lancet*, 1, 370-371 (1980).
10. Saling E. Fetal scalp blood analysis. *Journal of Perinatal Medicine*, 9, 165-177 (1981).
11. Schmidt S, Langner K, Rothe J and Saling E. A new combined non-invasive electrode for $tcPCO_2$ measurement and fetal heart rate recording. *Journal of Perinatal Medicine*, 10, 297-300 (1982).
12. Severinghaus J W, Stafford M and Bradley A F. $tcPCO_2$ electrode design, calibration and temperature gradient problems. *Acta Anaesthetica Scandinavica*, Supplement 68, 118-122 (1978).

Chapter 26

# Experimental head compression and transcutaneous oxygen tension in the fetal lamb

**A Verhoeff, T C Jansen, A R van der Wiel, H C S Wallenburg**

## Introduction

In several publications Huch and associates (1, 2) have advocated continuous transcutaneous measurement of oxygen tension on the fetal scalp as a reliable method of intrapartum surveillance of fetal oxygenation. There is good evidence that transcutaneously measured oxygen tension ($P_{tc}O_2$) in newborns (7) and adults (8) closely reflects central arterial oxygenation. However, doubts have been expressed with regard to the agreement between fetal scalp $P_{tc}O_2$ and systemic fetal oxygenation during labour (9, 10). Values of fetal scalp $P_{tc}O_2$ could be altered independently of fetal arterial $PO_2$ ($PaO_2$) due to compression of the fetal scalp capillary circulation by the pressure circle which develops between the fetal presenting part and the birth canal during uterine contractions (6). However, the importance of such a 'tonsure effect' (9) on fetal scalp $P_{tc}O_2$ cannot be examined in the human fetus during labour, since the oxygen tension in the fetal arterial circulation cannot be measured. For this reason we used the fetal lamb to assess the effect of experimental equatorial compression of the fetal head on scalp $P_{tc}O_2$ as related to systemic $PaO_2$.

## Materials and methods

Experiments were carried out in four pregnant Texel ewes at 135-140 days' gestation.

### Surgical preparation

Anaesthesia was induced with an intramuscular injection of ketamine hydrochloride 500 mg, atropine 0.5 mg, and sodium thiopental 300-500 mg intravenously. The animals were placed in a lateral position on the operating table, intubated and mechanically ventilated with 40% oxygen, 60% nitrous oxide and 0.5-4 volume per cent enflurane.

A polyvinyl catheter was inserted into the maternal aorta through a femoral artery. A lower midline laparotomy was performed and the pregnant uterine horn was exposed. A fetal hind limb was delivered through a small uterine incision in an area free of cotyledons and a polyvinyl catheter was placed in the fetal aorta via a femoral artery. The limb was returned into the amniotic cavity and the incision was closed.

A second window was made in an area over the fetal neck. The carotid arteries were located and a previously calibrated continuously recording intravascular $PO_2$ electrode (5) was inserted into the left carotid artery. An electromagnetic blood flow transducer (Skalar Medical Instruments) was fitted around the right carotid artery. The fetal head was then carefully delivered through the same window and the edges of the uterine incision were sutured to the skin to prevent loss of amniotic fluid.

A 65 mm wide inflatable rubber cuff contained within a perspex ring with an inner diameter of 94 mm was placed around the equator of the fetal skull just above the eyes (Figure 1). Care was taken not to compress the carotid arteries. A flat area of

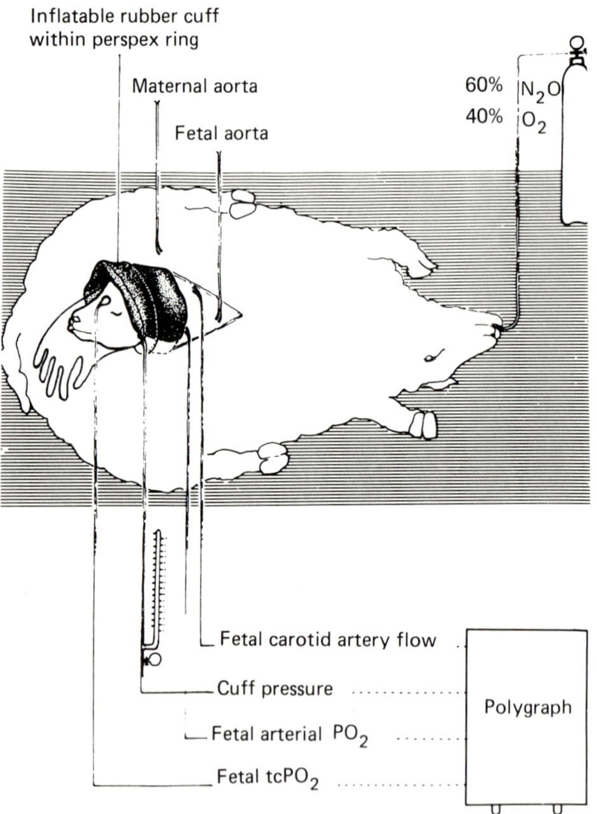


*Figure 1.* Schematic representation of the experimental animal preparation

the fetal scalp distal to the inflatable cuff and approximately between the eyes was shaved and a transcutaneous $PO_2$ transducer developed in our laboratory (14, 15) was attached to the fetal skin with a cyanoacrylate glue.

Figure 2 shows a schematic cross section of the transducer. It consists of a 50 $\mu$m diameter cathode and an Ag-AgCl reference electrode. The heating element has a resistance of 20 ohms. Two thermistors with a resistance of 10 000 ohms each at 20°C are used for measurement and control of the transducer temperature. The

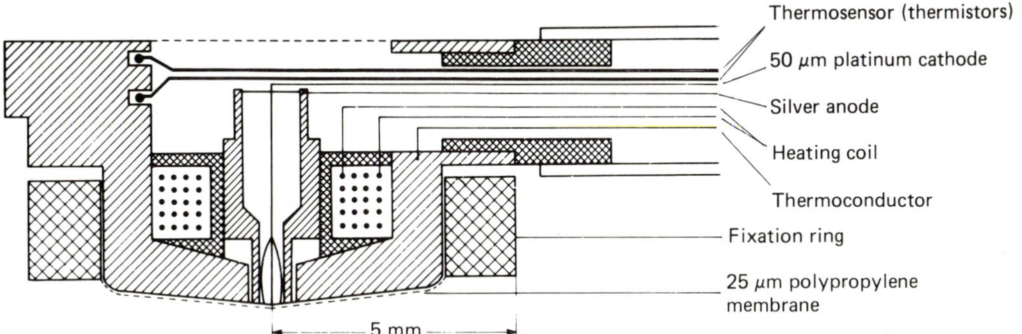


*Figure 2.* Schematic cross-section of the fetal transcutaneous $PO_2$ transducer

membrane consists of polypropylene of 12.5 μm thickness. The electrolyte is a buffered hygroscopic solution (pH 11.5). The transducer has thc following specifications:

a diffusion current, $I_d$ of 1.3 x $10^{-2}$ namp/mmHg $O_2$
a response time (t95%) of 6 seconds
a drift less than 5% over 48 hours
an oxygen consumption of 0.34 x $10^{-16}$ mole $O_2$ /s mmHg
a zero current $I_0$ less than 0.001 namp
a reproducibility of the measured diffusion current less than 5%
weight 1.8 g, external diameter 11.0 mm, height 5.25 mm.

The transducer is linked to an electronic instrument that gives a continuous indication of the $PO_2$ and regulates the temperature of the transducer to within 0.1°C of a preset level.

The device was heated to 45°C. The preparation was covered with warm saline-soaked towels.

### Measurements

Maternal and fetal arterial pressures were measured with pressure transducers (Gould Statham P23 ID) maintained at the level of the ewe's heart and continuously recorded.

Fetal heart rate was obtained from the arterial pressure signal. The signals from the fetal intravascular and transcutaneous $PO_2$ transducer were continuously recorded on a multichannel polygraph, together with the fetal carotid artery flow, fetal heart rate and the pressure in the inflatable cuff. Intracranial pressure was measured in one experiment through a needle inserted into the cisterna magna. The relative transducer heating energy required to keep the temperature of the $P_{tc}O_2$ transducer at a stable level of 45°C was not recorded.

### Experimental protocol

Experiments were begun 30-40 minutes after the placement of the $P_{tc}O_2$ transducer to allow stabilization. Two different experimental protocols were used in each sheep in a random order. According to the first protocol equatorial compression of the fetal head was induced stepwise by means of intermittent inflation of the cuff. Cuff pressure was increased from 0-70 mmHg and decreased to 0 mmHg in steps of 5-10 mmHg;

each pressure level was maintained for 1-2 minutes to allow the $PO_2$ transducers to stabilize.

The second protocol was designed to simulate fetal head compression during labour. The cuff pressure was gradually increased to 50-70 mmHg and decreased to 5-10 mmHg over a period of approximately 1 minute. This procedure was repeated every 2-3 minutes for 15-20 minutes.

Following these two experimental protocols, and after 15-20 minutes recovery period, fetal transcutaneous and arterial oxygen tensions were compared in the absence of fetal head compression over a wide range of normoxemic and hypoxemic values. Fetal hypoxemia was induced by slowly decreasing the oxygen content of the gas mixture inspired by the ewe. The time of exposure to hypoxia varied from 2 minutes for a 0% to 10 minutes for a 20% $O_2$ concentration.

The $PO_2$ transducers were removed at the end of the experiments and recalibration showed that virtually no drift had occurred.

## Results

### Comparison between fetal $P_{tc}O_2$ at various levels of oxygenation

The data points were obtained from the continuous oxygen tension tracings at 1-minute intervals after stabilization of the $P_{tc}O_2$ transducer output following a change in the composition of the gas mixture. At least 60 paired values of fetal $P_{tc}O_2$ and $PaO_2$ at various levels of normoxemia and hypoxemia in the absence of fetal head compression were obtained in each animal, yielding an r between 0.88 and 0.98 and a slope between 0.76 and 1.23. Good agreement was shown to exist over a wide range of low and normal oxygen tensions.

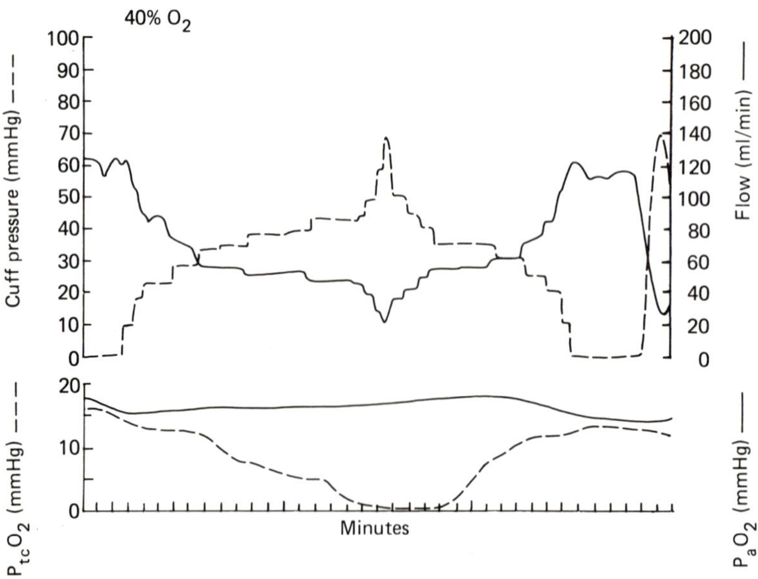


*Figure 3.* Fetal carotid artery flow, $P_{tc}O_2$ and $P_aO_2$ at stepwise altered cuff pressures

**Effect of fetal head compression on $P_{tc}O_2$ and $PaO_2$**

Fetal $P_{tc}O_2$ and $PaO_2$ remained stable at stepwise increased cuff pressures up to approximately 25 mmHg. At higher cuff pressures fetal $PaO_2$ remained unchanged, whereas $P_{tc}O_2$ showed a progressive fall to become zero at cuff pressures of 5-10 mmHg below the measured fetal systolic pressure, i.e. at 40-50 mmHg (Figure 3). At decreasing cuff pressures fetal $P_{tc}O_2$ returned to baseline values which were reached at the 20-25 mmHg level. Fetal $P_{tc}O_2$ continued to fall in the 1-2 minutes during which a cuff pressure of more than 25 mmHg was applied. There appeared to be a significant positive correlation in all cases between the time during which cuff pressures of more than 25 mmHg were maintained and the resulting progressive fall in fetal $P_{tc}O_2$ (Spearman test, p less than 0.001).

When labour-like fetal head compression with peak pressures of 50-70 mmHg and a duration of approximately 1 minute was simulated, fetal $PaO_2$ again remained stable, but $P_{tc}O_2$ showed a 30-60% fall (Figure 4). In these experiments $P_{tc}O_2$ started

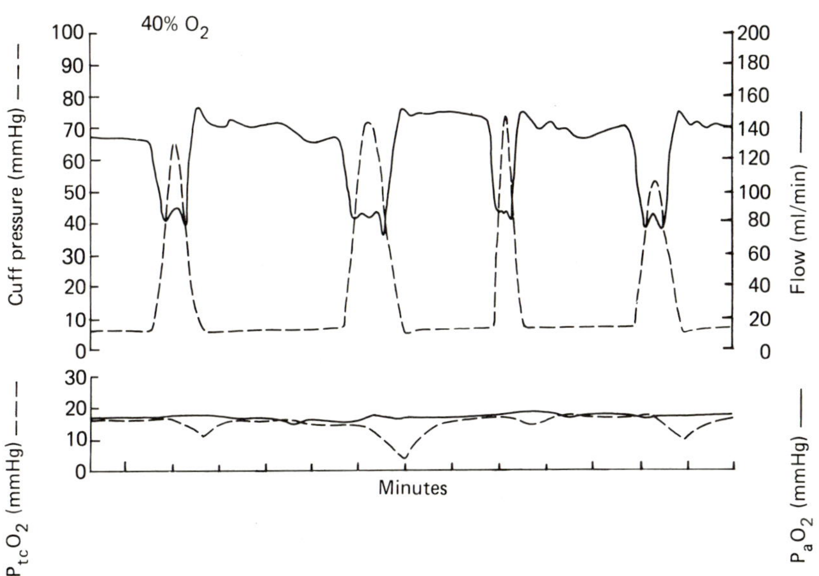


*Figure 4.* Fetal carotid artery flow, $P_{tc}O_2$ and $P_aO_2$ at 'labour-like' fetal head compression

to fall when peak compression values were obtained after 20-30 seconds, and the nadir of the $P_{tc}O_2$ curve occurred 40-50 seconds later.

**Effect of fetal head compression on fetal circulation**

Even a small increase in cuff pressure (10-25 mmHg) resulted in a simultaneous decrease in mean blood flow through the fetal carotid artery. A maximum fall in carotid artery flow to 25-40% of its original value was observed at cuff pressures of 50-60 mmHg (Figures 3 and 4); no further decrease in flow occurred at higher cuff pressures. On return of cuff pressures to 5-10 mmHg carotid artery flow appeared to increase briefly above its baseline value. The single experiment in which intracranial pressure was measured showed that the fall in carotid artery flow occurred in parallel with a rise in intracranial pressure from 12 to approximately 30 mmHg, reached at a cuff pressure of 50 mmHg. At higher cuff pressures no further rise in intracranial pressure or decrease in carotid artery flow was observed. Mean fetal arterial pressure remained constant at all cuff pressures. Fetal heart rate also remained constant in most experiments; in a few cases a fall of 10-20 beats per minute was observed in association with cuff pressures of over 50 mmHg.

## Discussion

Comparison of values obtained by continuous transcutaneous measurement of fetal scalp $PO_2$ and by continuous monitoring of fetal arterial oxygen tension shows good agreement during normoxemia and hypoxemia in the absence of fetal head compression. This confirms the previous reported accuracy of the transcutaneous and intravascular $PO_2$ transducers used in this study (5,15). Jansen *et al,* (3), who were the first to compare these two methods of continuous monitoring of oxygenation in the fetal lamb, found a disparity betweenn $P_{tc}O_2$ and $PaO_2$ at low arterial oxygen tensions, which they attribute to peripheral vasoconstriction in response to hypoxemia. Such a divergence was not observed in our experiments, but exposure to low oxygen concentrations was only of brief duration, and the general anaesthesia may have modified the level of peripheral vasoconstriction and redistribution of fetal cardiac output that is known to occur in hypoxemic conditions (11).

To our knowledge, this is the first experimental study in which the effect of 'labour-like' equatorial compression of the fetal head on $P_{tc}O_2$ was investigated. A different approach was used in another experimental study in fetal sheep, in which varying weights were placed on a ring, 3.5 cm in diameter, around the fetal scalp electrode (4). Weights of 300-500 g reduced $P_{tc}O_2$ to zero, but the published data do not allow a quantitative comparison with our results. We observed that $P_{tc}O_2$ starts to fall at pressures of 25 mmHg applied around the equator of the fetal head and becomes zero at pressures of 40-50 mmHg, whereas intravascular $PO_2$ remains unchanged. The fall in $P_{tc}O_2$ can most likely be attributed to compression of the scalp capillary bed. The measured fetal systolic arterial blood pressure is in the order of magnitude of 50-60 mmHg. Since pressure in the scalp capillary bed will be somewhat lower under optimal conditions of local heating, an equatorial compressive force of 40-50 mmHg can be expected to occlude the scalp circulation completely. The demonstrated significant positive correlation between the duration of application of stable cuff pressures of more than 25 mmHg and the resulting progressive fall in fetal $P_{tc}O_2$ may be explained by the oxygen consumption of the tissue and of the electrode itself, in the presence of reduced oxygen availability.

On the basis of these experiments we cannot exclude the possibility that a decreased intracranial oxygen delivery due to the fall in carotid artery flow which occurs during fetal head compression may in part be responsible for the fall in $P_{tc}O_2$ . However, no change in fetal $P_{tc}O_2$ was observed at cuff pressures between 10 and 25 mmHg, when carotid artery flow already showed a marked drop in all cases. The fall in carotid artery flow appears to be due to the rise in intracranial pressure with an increase in cerebral vascular resistance, which occurred in these experiments because part of the fetal head was outside the uterus. Under physiological conditions of uterine contractions, when the whole fetus is subject to the increase in amniotic presure, it is to be expected that little true increase in fetal intracranial pressure will occur.

Patterns of fetal $P_{tc}O_2$ as illustrated in Figure 4 are observed during human labour in relation to uterine contractions, including a delay of approximately 50-60 seconds between the onset of the contraction and the beginning of the decrease in $P_{tc}O_2$ (2,12,13, 14). In the same clinical studies a positive correlation between peak pressures of uterine contractions and the fall in $P_{tc}O_2$ was observed. The authors postulate that these findings must be explained by the decrease in placental perfusion which occurs during uterine contractions and may affect transplacental oxygen exchange and fetal oxygenation. Such a mechanism cannot be excluded on the basis of our experiments. On the other hand, it has been shown that during human labour a complete ring of equatorial pressure develops between the fetal head and the cervix or vagina during uterine contractions. The resulting equatorial pressure may be three times or more the amniotic pressure, in particular after rupture of the membranes (6). Under physiological circumstances, the whole fetus is subject to the increase in amniotic pressure during uterine contractions, except for the part of the scalp below the cervical-vaginal compression ring which remains at atmospheric pressure. In the presence of a fetal mean arterial blood pressure in the order of magnitude of 50 mmHg, as related to atmospheric pressure, a uterine contraction of, for example, 30 mmHg would raise fetal arterial blood pressure to 80 mmHg relative to atmospheric pressure. An amniotic pressure of 30 mmHg may result in equatorial head-to-cervix pressures of up to 120 mmHg (6), which would be high enough to squeeze and completely occlude the capillary circulation in the fetal scalp. The degree of fetal head compression during human labour within one individual and between individuals is variable, depending on the balance between the force of the uterine contractions and the compliance of the birth canal (6).

Although the data obtained in our animal experiments cannot be quantitatively extrapolated to the situation during human labour, the above evidence suggests that similar biophysical mechanisms could be operative. Therefore, we conclude that compression of the fetal head during labour may lead to variable local changes in the oxygenation of the fetal scalp, as a result of which fetal scalp $P_{tc}O_2$ will cease to reflect fetal arterial oxygen tension. This so-called 'tonsure effect' (9) raises serious questions with regard to the reliability of transcutaneous $PO_2$ monitoring as a method of intrapartum fetal surveillance.

## References

1. Huch A, Huch R, Schneider H and Rooth G. Continuous transcutaneous monitoring of fetal oxygen tension during labour. *British Journal of Obstetrics and Gynaecology,* 84, suppl.1, 1-39 (1977).
2. Huch A, Huch R, Schneider H and Peabody J. Experience with transcutaneous $PO_2$ ($tcPO_2$ ) monitoring of mother, fetus and newborn. *Journal of Perinatal Medicine,* 8, 51-72 (1980).
3. Jansen C A M, Bass F G, Lowe K C and Nathanielsz P W. Comparison of continuous transcutaneous and continuous intravascular $PO_2$ measurement in fetal sheep. *American Journal of Obstetrics and Gynecology,* 138, 670-676 (1980).
4. Jansen C A M and Nathanielsz P W. Pressure-related changes in fetal transcutaneous $PO_2$ measurements. *Journal of Physiology,* 308, 28P (1980).
5. Jansen T C, Kwant G, Lafeber H N, Oeseburg O, Visser H K A and Zijlstra W G. Construction and performance of a new catheter-tip oxygen electrode. *Medical Biological Engineering and Computing,* 16, 274-277 (1978).
6. Lindgren L. The concept of pressure in biology and pressure transducers. *Acta Obstetrica Gynaecologica Scandinavica,* suppl. 66, 87-123 (1977).

7. Loefgren O, Henriksson P, Jacobson L and Johansson D. Transcutaneous $PO_2$ monitoring in neonatal intensive care. *ActaPaediatrica Scandinavica,* 67, 693-697 (1978).
8. Loefgren O. Transcutaneous oxygen measurement in adult intensive care. *Acta Anaesthesiologica Scandinavica,* 23, 534-544 (1979).
9. O'Connor M C, Hytten F E and Zanelli G D. Is the fetus 'scalped' in labour? *Lancet 2,* 947-949 (1979).
10. O'Connor M C and Hytten F E. Measurement of fetal transcutaneous oxygen tension - problems and potential. *British Journal of Obstetrics and Gynaecology,* 86, 948-953 (1979).
11. Peeters L L H, Sheldon R E, Jones M D, Makowski E L and Meschia G. Blood flow to fetal organs as a function of arterial oxygen content. *American Journal of Obstetrics and Gynecology,* 135, 637-646 (1979).
12. Rooth G, Fall O, Huch A and Huch R. Distribution of observed patterns in fetal transcutaneous oxygen tension. *American Journal of Obstetrics and Gynecology,* 140, 693-698 (1981).
13. Schneider H, Strang F, Huch R and Huch A. Suppression of uterine contractions with fenoterol and its effect on fetal $T_cPO_2$ in human term labour. *British Journal of Obstetrics and Gynaecology,* 87, 657-665 (1980).
14. Wladimiroff J W, van 't Hoff D B, Verhoeff A, Drogendijk A C and Jansen T C. Preliminary data on the clinical use of a self-constructed transcutaneous $PO_2$ electrode during labor. In: *Continuous Transcutaneous Blood Gas Monitoring,* edited by A Huch, R Huch and J F Lucey, 245-258, New York, A R Liss Inc. (1979).
15. Wladimiroff J W, van 't Hoff D B, Wallenburg H C S and Drogendijk A C. Simultaneous measurement of transcutaneous and central arterial $PO_2$ in acute sheep experiment. In: *Continuous Transcutaneous Blood Gas Monitoring,* edited by A Huch, R Huch and J F Lucey, 615-619, New York, A R Liss Inc. (1979).

Chapter 27

# A technique for continuous measurements of materno-fetal gas transfer using mass spectrometry suitable for non-invasive intrapartum placental function testing in man

**J A D Spencer, D C Anderes, J C Wollner, R Wolton, P Rolfe and P Johnson**

## Introduction

The clinical assessment of fetal respiratory status in early labour depends largely on the interpretation of changes in the continuous fetal heart rate recording (FHR). Labour imposes a variety of endocrine, behavioural and reflex stimuli on the fetal cardio-respiratory system which makes it unlikely that changes in the FHR pattern would have a direct relationship to acid-base status, except when the latter is significantly abnormal. Thus large false positive (1) and false negative (8) rates exist when using FHR alone. The contraction stress test (CST) or oxytocin challenge test has been accepted by many as a means of assessing fetal reserve in late pregnancy, particularly in high risk pregnancy (6). However, this too has significant false positive and false negative rates (7,10). The NIH task force (13) recommended research into new methods of fetal monitoring, and our group has developed a fetal scalp mass spectrometer transducer (9) which, together with a modified industrial magnetic-sector mass spectrometer, has been assessed in labour (11). In an attempt to improve the assessment of fetal reserve in early labour, we have now used the multi-gas sampling potential of the mass spectrometer to make continuous measurements of materno-fetal transfer of oxygen and helium. Animal experiments are currently being used to develop a short, repeatable test using argon, with the expectation of developing a simple test of placental transfer suitable for use in early human labour.

## Methods

### (i) The system

We have modified an industrial mass spectrometer (MM8-80, VG Medical Systems, Cheshire, UK) to accept two inlets maintained at operational vacuum. Two transducers can be used and measurements therefore obtained from the application sites by alternating between the two inlets. The mass spectrometer employs a magnetic sector of 80 degrees with an 8 cm radius. Its good stability results from the ability to tune the instrument to produce broad flat-topped peaks for improved identification of each mass. Under microprocessor control, the instrument automatically locates each mass peak according to programmed settings of the electromagnetic deflection current at a constant acceleration potential. The output voltage of the mass spectrometer is a linear function of the number of gas molecules sampled and hence the gas pressure.

The skin-surface transducer (9) is a gas collecting chamber with an electrically heated perforated metal membrane support. The magnitude of the depletion error is related to the ratio of membrane to skin permeability, and gas throughput is reduced by using a low permeability membrane with large support orifices. Thus local gas consumption from the skin is minimal. However, in order to provide the mass spectrometer with sufficient gas to measure reliably, the membrane area is maximized commensurate with the limitation on overall transducer dimensions imposed by problems of attachment to the fetal scalp. The gas sample is carried to the mass spectrometer through a nylon cannula within a high-density polyethylene tube. This double cannula system minimizes water vapour and ambient oxygen throughput. The membrane used is polyethylene, 37 $\mu$m thick, and the transducer is heated to 43.5°C. After sterilization in gluteraldehyde, tissue adhesive is applied to the annular attachment rings and one transducer is placed onto the cleaned fetal scalp and the other onto the maternal forearm.

For intra-arterial mass spectrometry in animal experiments, we use 45 cm long steel catheters of OD 0.71 mm with five to seven side slots along the distal 2.5 cm. The catheter is covered by a silicone rubber membrane (Silastic, Dow Corning), 0.55 mm thick, sealed at the tip with adhesive.

### (ii) Performance

*In vitro* testing has been performed with the skin-surface transducer in dry tonometers, and with the intravascular probes in a closed system water bath with controlled flow and temperature using saturated saline solutions. The responses of both skin-surface and intravascular devices are linear, and the lag time due to the cannula is 12 to 15 seconds. The 95% response time for both transducers is approximately 60 seconds. The range of the output voltage of the mass spectrometer can be adjusted according to the quantity of gas entering the analyser. Thus readings for transcutaneous gas levels are in the order of $10^{-11}$ volts and for intra-arterial levels are $10^{-10}$ volts.

Calibration of the skin-surface transducers was performed using known concentrations of gases in a dry tonometer. The intravascular probes were calibrated *in vivo* by comparison with conventional blood gas analysis on an ABL3 blood gas analyser (Radiometer).

Drift over 6 to 8 hour study periods was less than 2 mmHg for both $PO_2$ and $PCO_2$.

### (iii) Subjects

Preliminary investigations of maternal-fetal gas transfer were undertaken using intra-arterial mass spectrometry in three pregnant ewes in late pregnancy (125-130 days) and in three women in early normal labour at term using skin-surface transducers on fetal scalp and maternal forearm. Subsequent work, and the development of a 2-minute argon test, was performed in six ewes in late pregnancy.

The skin-surface transducers were attached, one to the fetal scalp after rupture of the membranes, and the other to the mother's forearm. Gas administration was via a one-way valve to a cushioned, close-fitting face mask.

The ewes were studied either acutely under intermittent barbiturate anaesthesia, or chronically following placement of catheters at operation under general anaesthesia. The maternal mass spectrometer transducer was placed in the right carotid or femoral artery and an arterial sampling line was placed in the left carotid. The fetal mass spectrometer transducer was placed in the left femoral artery and a sampling catheter placed in the right femoral artery. Gases were administered via a tracheostomy. Maternal tidal volume was recorded by integrating the pneumotachograph signal of inspiratory flow. Respiratory gas concentrations, were measured using a BOC Medishield respiratory mass spectrometer. Maternal and fetal blood pressure, fetal heart rate and amniotic pressure were also recorded.

## Results

### (i) Oxygen and helium

Continuous administraion of 75% oxygen and 25% helium to an anaesthetized ewe is illustrated in Figure 1. Fetal levels of both gases were recorded simultaneously by fast cycling between the two mass numbers (32 and 4 respectively). Maternal and fetal recordings were alternated every minute or so. The slow rise in fetal levels is clearly illustrated. In early labour, continuous oxygen was given to the mother and Figure 2 shows the rates of rise of maternal and fetal levels. In all cases, fetal $PO_2$ rose significantly.

Figure 3 shows the effect of a short period of inhalation of helium in a pregnant ewe. Maternal and fetal changes were recorded separately and then together with a switch to the fetus when the maternal peak had been reached. Using skin-surface transducers in early labour, similar curves were obtained in the human as shown in

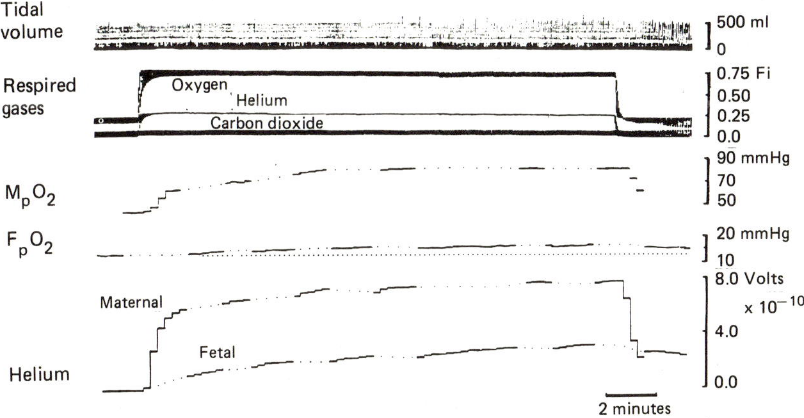


*Figure 1.* Simultaneous mass spectrometer recordings of intra-arterial oxygen and helium levels from mother and fetus alternately during administration of 30% helium in oxygen to an anaesthetized ewe in late pregnancy. Maternal steady state was reached by 10 minutes after an initial rapid rise in levels. Fetal levels rose slowly and did not reach steady state by 20 minutes. The $PO_2$ readings were calibrated in vivo by blood analysis. Helium levels were recorded as mass spectrometer output voltage

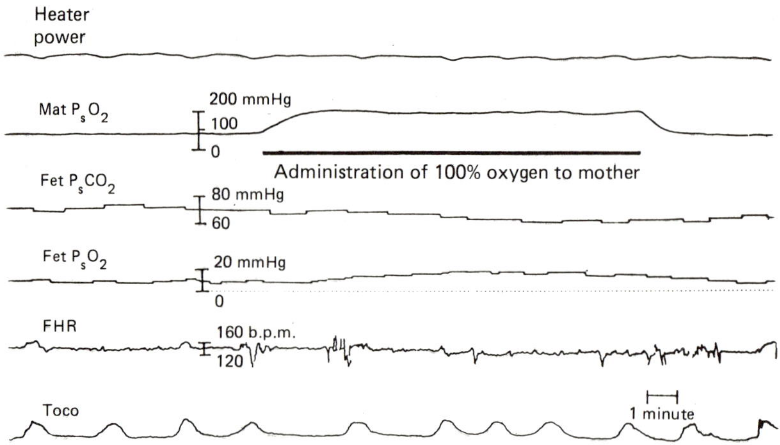


*Figure 2.* Recordings of human fetal scalp skin-surface oxygen (Fet $P_sO_2$) and carbon dioxide (Fet $P_sCO_2$) levels using a single mass spectrometer transducer during administration of oxygen to a mother in early labour. Maternal skin-surface oxygen levels, recorded from the second transducer, rose quickly to reach steady-state level by 3 minutes. Fetal responses were slower; fetal $P_sO_2$ rose significantly in seven of eight cases, and the $P_sCO_2$ fell in two cases. Transducers were calibrated using dry gases of known concentrations.

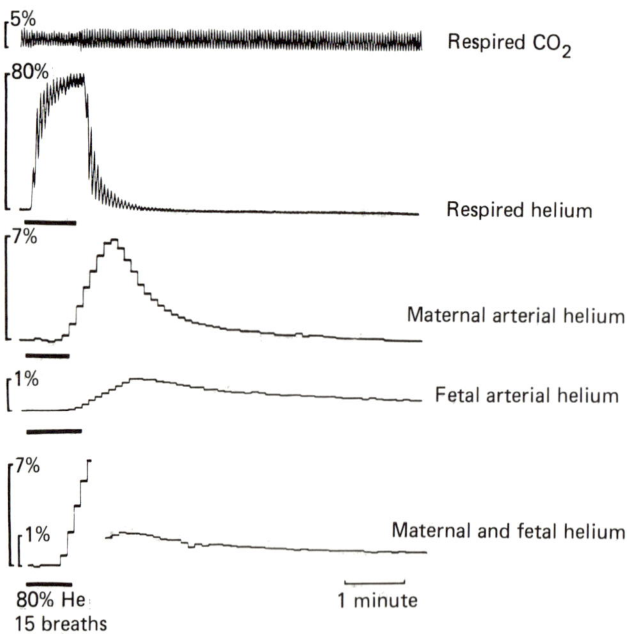


*Figure 3.* Maternal and fetal levels of helium using intra-arterial mass spectrometry following administration of 80% helium in oxygen (black lines) to a ewe in late pregnancy. Two recordings show separate maternal and fetal curves, and the lower trace shows a combined recording where a switch from maternal to fetal recording was made after the maternal peak. Calibration of the probes used dry helium of known concentrations

Figure 4. Higher levels were obtained as a result of instructing the mother to take deep breaths, and consequently the time course of these curves is longer. Such variables as duration of administration, concentration of gas, depth of inspiration and breathing pattern, maternal and fetal circulation times and placental transfer itself all influence the levels obtained in mother and fetus.

Despite these factors, the similarity of the shape of the curves in both the human and animal suggest the validity of the non-invasive human measurements, and standardization of some of the above factors was attempted in developing the 2-minute argon test.

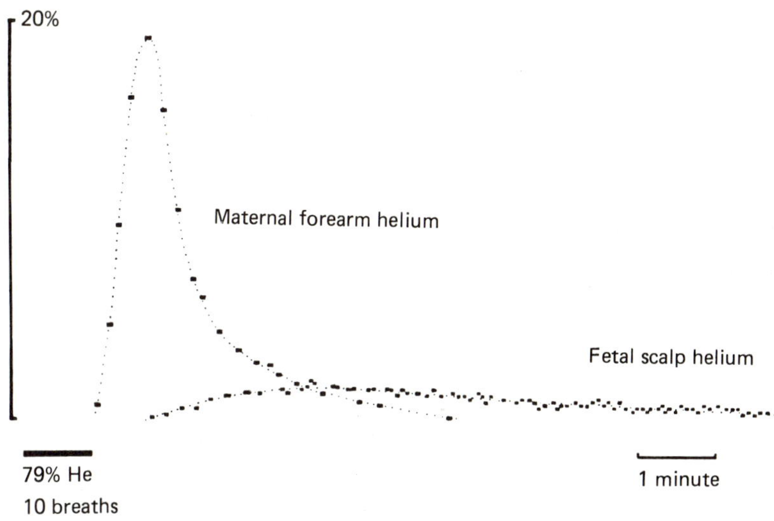


*Figure 4.* Human maternal and fetal skin-surface (SS) helium levels following inhalation of 79% helium in oxygen (black lines) in early labour. The discontinuous lines join readings obtained by alternating between maternal and fetal mass spectrometer transducers.

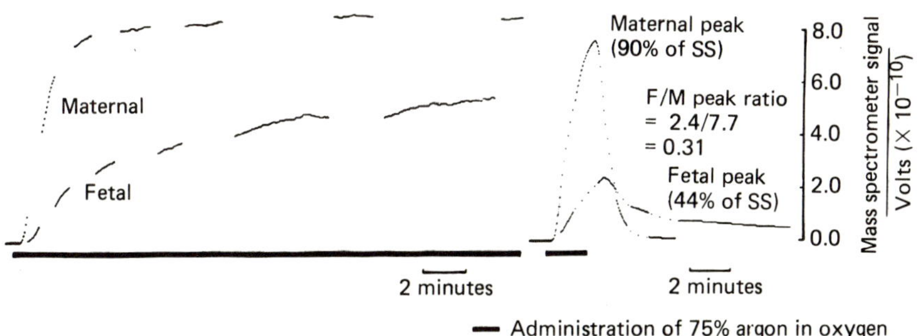


*Figure 5.* Maternal and fetal intra-arterial argon levels during administration of 75% argon in oxygen to a non-anaesthetized ewe in late pregnancy. The peaks after a 2-minute inhalation 'bolus' are compared with 20 minutes' continuous administration where the maternal level reached steady state by 4 minutes but the fetal level was still rising at 20 minutes. The fetal/maternal peak ratio is the fetal to maternal peak level ratio following 2 minutes inhalation of argon by the mother

## (ii) Argon

To be of use in labour, it is essential that any test be shorter than the time taken to reach steady state equilibrium (greater than 20 minutes in the fetus). The relationship between 2 minutes administration of 75% argon in oxygen and continuous administra-

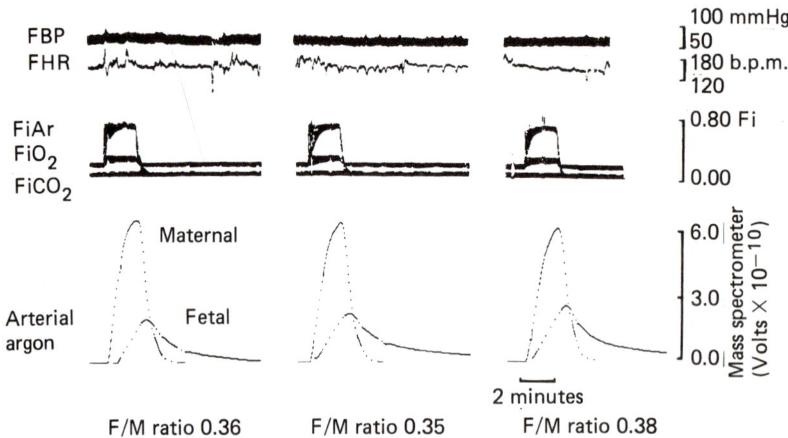


*Figure 6.* Three 2-minute inhalation 'bolus' administrations of argon to a non-anaesthetized ewe in late pregnancy to show the reproducibility of the fetal to maternal peak of argon levels. Note the spontaneous changes in fetal heart rate variability probably indicative of behavioural state changes

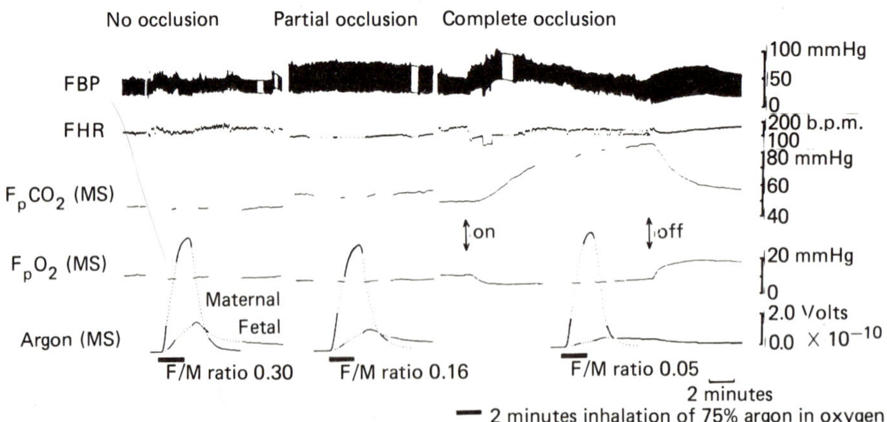


*Figure 7.* Progressive uterine artery occlusion in a non-anaesthetized ewe in late pregnancy. Simultaneous intra-arterial mass spectrometer (MS) recordings of fetal carbon dioxide, oxygen and argon levels are shown, together with the maternal intra-arterial argon level. Partial uterine artery occlusion produced a stable situation with a raised fetal pulse pressure and reduced fetal heart rate variability. The fetal carbon dioxide ($F_pCO_2$) remained slightly elevated, but the small reduction in fetal oxygen ($F_pO_2$) was within normal limits. However the fetal-maternal argon peak ratio was reduced by 50%. Complete uterine artery occlusion resulted in an immediate fetal bradycardia and onset of hypertension which occurred 10 seconds before the fetal $PCO_2$ began to rise sharply and the $PO_2$ fell. The fetal-maternal argon peak ratio was reduced to one sixth but returned to normal immediately after release of the occlusion. This compares with a rebound rise in $PO_2$ and pulse pressure, and a mild tachycardia following release of the uterine artery occlusion

tion for 20 minutes is illustrated in Figure 5. The maternal peak reached 90% of the steady state level and the fetal peak reached 44% of the near-steady state level, producing a fetal to maternal ratio (FMR) of 0.31.

The maternal peak height occurs at 135 seconds and the fetal peak occurs at 175 seconds. The ratio is therefore available within 3 minutes and is consistent with 2-minute inhalations of 60-75% argon. It takes approximately 15-20 minutes for the fetal argon to clear and the test can then be repeated. Figure 6 shows the reproducibility of the maternal/fetal relationship of argon peak levels.

Three different methods of causing fetal hypoxia were used in order to assess the value of this fetal/maternal ratio. Progressive uterine artery occlusion produced a progressive reduction in the fetal level of argon (decreased FMR). Figure 7 shows that partial occlusion also produced a small rise in fetal $PCO_2$ and a small fall in fetal $PO_2$. The pulse pressure was increased and the fetal heart rate variability was reduced. Fetal blood gas changes were more pronounced with complete uterine artery occlusion, and fetal bradycardia occurred immediately. Although cardio-respiratory recovery took approximately 30 minutes after this 15 minute asphyxic insult, the FMR returned immediately to 'normal', confirming the dependence of the fetal argon peak level on uterine artery flow. A rebound rise in fetal $PO_2$ following release of the uterine artery occlusion was noted. Complete umbilical cord occlusion resulted in no fetal argon being recorded, a situation also seen after fetal death. Figure 8 shows this in an anaesthetized ewe at the end of an acute experiment, where fetal argon levels were initially lower as a result of a relative maternal hypoventilation (barbiturate anaesthesia) and reduced uterine blood flow resulting from the supine position.

Maternal isocapnic hypoxaemia produced by administering 6% oxygen and 5% carbon dioxide resulted in fetal normocapnic hypoxaemia. The fetal pH fell to 7.12 over 90 minutes. Repeated 2-minute argon tests were performed and Figure 9 shows the effect on the FMR. The fetal argon level increased during the fetal hypoxic period

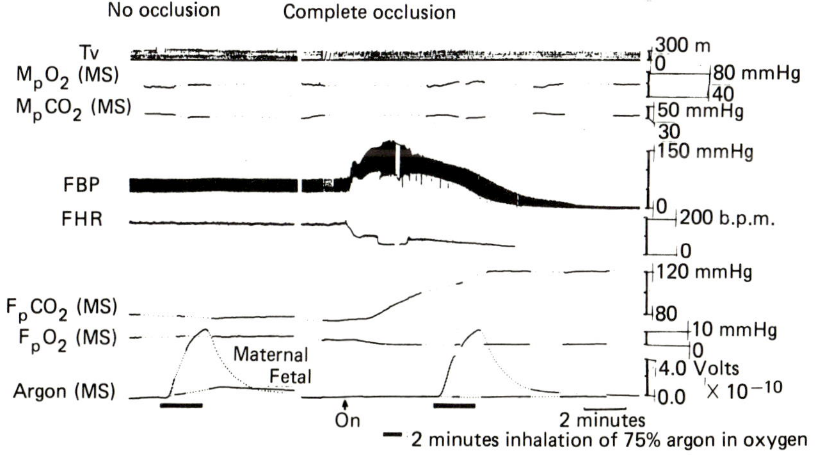


*Figure 8.* Umbilical cord occlusion in an anaesthetized ewe in late pregnancy showing simultaneous intra-arterial oxygen, carbon dioxide and argon levels recorded from maternal and fetal probes alternately at the end of an acute experiment. Fetal $PO_2$ was low and the fetal argon peak was also low due to a combination of maternal hypoventilation (barbiturate) and the supine position. Total occlusion of the cord produced a fetal bradycardia with acute hypertension, followed by a fall in $PO_2$ and a rise in $PCO_2$. No argon was recorded in the fetus (MS – mass spectrometer recordings)

and remained elevated for 2 hours after return of maternal and fetal $PO_2$ levels to normal. The possible explanations for this relative increase in fetal argon are an increase in uterine artery blood flow, an increase in placental transfer and/or circulatory changes in the fetus such as peripheral vasoconstriction and/or increased umbilical blood flow. We are planning direct flow measurements in order to help clarify these questions.

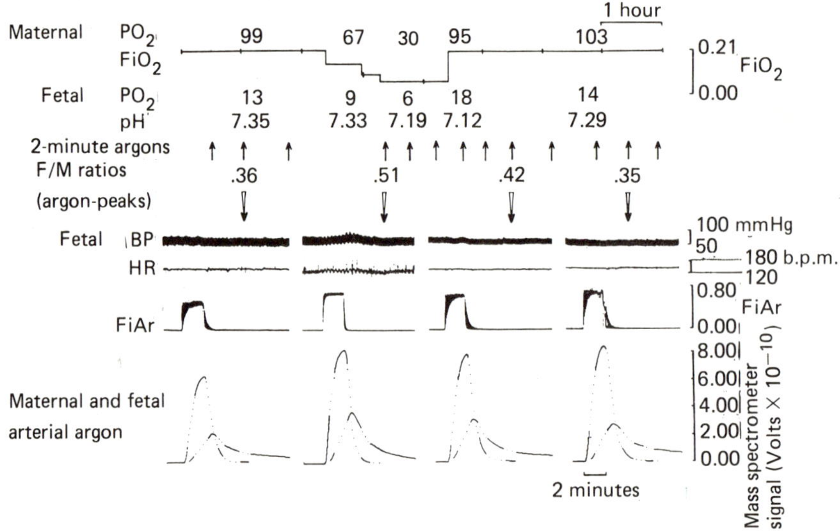


*Figure 9.* Maternal normocapnic hypoxaemia in a non-anaesthetized ewe in late pregnancy produced fetal hypoxaemia with an increased fetal to maternal argon peak ratio of 0.51. This increased ratio persisted for 90 minutes after the hypoxia before returning to the pre-hypoxic ratio of 0.36. An increase in fetal argon may have resulted from one or more of the following factors: increased uterine artery perfusion, improved maternal-fetal transfer and/or fetal peripheral vasoconstriction

## Discussion

Fetal respiration remains poorly understood and its monitoring during human labour is limited to non-invasive skin surface measurements. The first use of skin surface mass spectrometry was described by Delpy and Parker (1975) (5) and the advantage of such a system is the ability to measure multiple gases using a single transducer. Our work has included performance comparisons between intra-arterial and skin surface devices and we find the similarity between readings very encouraging.

Some of the factors involved in maternal-fetal transfer have been determined previously by invasive intermittent sampling with experimental animals (2). Because of this limitation, theories on the regulation of placental transfer have remained semi-quantitative (4). Some investigators have assumed that measuring changes in oxygen transfer across the placenta would be a means of quantifying placental transfer. We feel this is unlikely since oxygen and carbon dioxide are actively involved in metabolism which is a changing factor. Our studies indicate this to be the case particularly in situations such as labour where a restriction to the fetal supply causes a metabolic debt which takes a considerable time to be cleared. The administration of an inert gas, for example, argon or helium, gives an immediate index of delivery rate across the placenta to the fetus at that time. A relationship between oxygen and argon transfer 'rates' by the combination of enriched oxygen with argon may offer a valuable guide to just such discrepancies which are at the very heart of the dynamics of labour.

It has only recently been appreciated from chronic fetal studies that a reduction in uterine blood flow of up to 50% results in isocapnic hypoxaemia with no change in pH (12). Thus the relationship between $PO_2$, $PCO_2$, pH and our 'measure' of placental transfer is not going to be a simple one. Experiments of chronic fetal growth retardation have shown that only the $PO_2$ is slightly altered from control levels (3). Thus there is good reason to believe that measurement of fetal heart rate changes and/or blood gas status is unlikely to detect an initial reduction in placental reserve, whereas materno-fetal transfer of argon or helium, despite its complex components, may be a useful investigative clinical test.

It should be noted that the fetal bradycardic response to uterine artery occlusion occurred before the change in oxygen or carbon dioxide could have been perceived by arterial chemoreceptors. Althought the reflexes involved with such a response are not known, it indicates that non-chemical influences on fetal heart rate are various.

We believe this to be the first description of a method of measuring placental transfer using continuous simultaneous measurements from mother and fetus. It has the advantage that the measurements are immediately available and are easily repeatable. The 2-minute argon test of placental transfer has yet to be tried in human labour. Factors to be verified are the mode and duration of delivery to the mother in order to obtain reproducible maternal and fetal levels under stable conditions. Preliminary results in ewes indicate that such measurements may be of value by being an indication of both utero-placental flow and placental transfer as a combined 'factor' in influencing the fetal-maternal ratio of argon levels. Such a reflection of fetal cardio-respiratory function may well be a more reliable indication of 'reserve' as assessed in early labour than observations of FHR alone.

## Acknowledgements

We acknowledge support for this work from the Medical Research Council, the Department of Health and Social Security, the National Fund for Research into Crippling Diseases and the Oxford Medical Research Fund.

## References

1. Beard R W, Filshie G M, Knight C A and Roberts G M. The significance of the changes of the continuous fetal heart rate in first stage labour. *Journal of Obstetrics and Gynaecology of the British Commonwealth*, 78, 865-881 (1971).

2. Blechner J N, Makowski E L, Cotter J R, Meschia G and Barron D H. Nitrous oxide transfer from mother to fetus in sheep and goats. *American Journal of Obstetrics and Gynecology*, 105, 368-373 (1969).

3. Clapp J F, Szeto H H, Larrow R, Hewitt J and Mann L I. Umbilical blood flow response to embolization of the uterine circulation. *American Journal of Obstetrics and Gynecology*, 138, 60-67 (1980) 4. Dawes G S. A theoritical analysis of fetal drug equilibration. In *Fetal Pharmacology*, edited by L Boreus, pp.381-399. Raven Press, New York (1973).

5. Delpy D T and Parker D. Transcutaneous measurement of arterial blood gas tensions by mass spectrometry. *Lancet*, 1, 1016, (1975).

6. Freeman R K, Anderson G and Dorchester W. A prospective multi-institutional study of antepartum fetal heart rate monitoring. *American Journal of Obstetrics and Gynecology*, 143, 771-781 (1982).

7. Gauthier R J, Evertson L R and Paul R H. Intrapartum fetal heart rate observation and newborn outcome following a positive contraction stress test. *American Journal Obstetrics and Gynecology,* 133, 34-39 (1979).

8. Low P A, Cox M S, Karchmar E J, McGrath M J, Pancham S R and Piercy W N. The prediction of intrapartum fetal acidosis by fetal heart rate monitoring. *American Journal of Obstetrics and Gynecology,* 139, 299-305 (1981).

9. Rolfe P, Burton P J, Crowe J A et al. A fetal scalp mass spectrometer transducer. *Medical and Biological Engineerng and Computing,* 20, 375-382 (1982).

10. Staisch K J, Westlake J R and Bashore R A. Blind oxytocin challenge test and perinatal outcome. *American Journal of Obstetrics and Gynecology,* 138, 399-403 (1980).

11. Sykes G S, Molloy P, Johnson P et al. The non-invasive transcutaneous measurement of fetal blood gases during labour using a mass spectrometer. *European Journal of Obstetrics, Gynaecology and Reproductive Biology,* 15, 438-441 (1983).

12. Wei G, Parer J T and Jones C T. Fetal tachycardia: the role of catecholamines during experimental asphyxia. Presented at the *Tenth World Congress of Obstetrics and Gynaecology,* California, October, (1982).

13. Zuspan F D, Quilligan E J, Iams J D and Van Geijn H P. Predictors of intrapartum fetal distress: the role of electronic fetal monitoring. Report of the National Institute of Child Health and Human Development Task Force. *American Journal of Obstetrics and Gynecology,* 135, 287-291 (1979).

Part 4

# Ultrasound and Fetal Cardiography

Chapter 28

# Measurement of human umbilical venous blood flow *in utero*

R W Gill

## Introduction

The circulation of fetal blood through the umbilical cord and the placenta is clearly a vital link in the intrauterine support of the fetus. A number of methods have been used to study this circulation, both in animals and in man. Thus, in the human fetus, Stembera and McCallum have used local thermodilution to measure blood flow rates in the umbilical cord immediately following delivery at term (14, 17), whilst Assali and Rudolph and their co-workers have measured umbilical flow rates in preterm fetuses during abortion by hysterotomy, using respectively an electromagnetic flowmeter and radioactive microspheres (1, 16). These methods, however, all suffer from the limitation that they require either exposure of the vessel under study or the insertion of one or more catheters into it. This has precluded study of the umbilical circulation in the intact human fetus - until the recent introduction of Doppler ultrasonic methods (4, 6, 7).

## Theoretical basis of Doppler flow measurement

Pulsed ultrasound has been used to produce images of structures within the body for over 25 years. The ultrasound pulse is produced by a piezoelectric transducer and directed into the body along a known line of sight. Partial reflection or scattering of the ultrasound occurs each time an acoustic discontinuity is encountered, and a portion of the scattered sound is picked up by the transducer and converted back into electrical signals. Because ultrasound travels at a known velocity in the body, the time of arrival of each signal (relative to the transmitted pulse) can be directly interpreted as the depth of the scattering structure within the body.

If the scattering object is moving (relative to the transducer), a small change in the frequency of the received signal can be detected. This is the Doppler shift, familiar to us in the form of the astronomer's 'red shift'. The amount of the frequency change is directly proportional to the speed of movement of the object, being given by:

$$\text{Doppler shift} = 2(v/c)(\cos\theta)f$$

where $v$ is the speed of movement of the object, $\theta$ is the angle between the ultrasound beam and the direction of the object's movement, $c$ is the velocity of propagation of

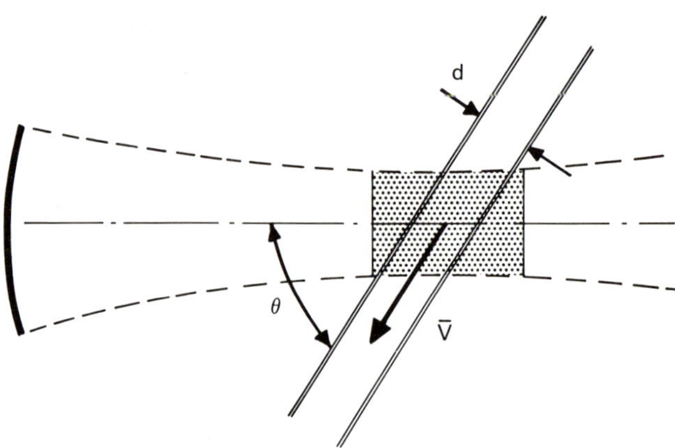


*Figure 1.* Configuration used to measure the rate of blood flow in a vessel using pulsed Doppler ultrasound. The sample volume (shown shaded) is made sufficiently large that it encompasses the entire cross-section of the vessel. The diameter *d* and the angle $\theta$ are measured using ultrasonic imaging. Flow is then computed from the mean Doppler shift, as described in the text

ultrasound in the medium (approximately 1550 metres per second in tissue), and *f* is the frequency of the ultrasound (typically 1.5-10 MHz). Given that the speed of movement of objects within the body rarely exceeds 1-2 metres per second, it can be seen that the Doppler shift is 0.1% or less of the ultrasonic frequency and that it therefore falls within the range of audible frequencies. Thus it is possible to use the considerable signal-processing power of the human ear and brain (in the first instance) to analyse the Doppler signals.

In a pulsed Doppler system a short burst of ultrasound is generated by a focused transducer and transmitted into the body. Scattered signals are detected by the same transducer (acting as a receiver), converted to electrical signals and amplified. A 'range gate' selects the signals at a particular time delay after each transmit pulse, and they are compared with the frequency originally transmitted. The result is a Doppler-shift signal which corresponds to movement only within a limited sample volume, whose distance from the transducer is determined by the delay of the range gate. The dimensions of the sample volume are determined by the width of the ultrasound beam, the length of the transmitted burst and the length of the range gate. Although the beamwidth is normally fixed for a given instrument, the length of the sample volume can be adjusted to suit the requirements of the situation.

For the measurement of blood flow, the scattering objects are simply the moving erythrocytes within the blood. The sample volume is made sufficiently large that it spans the entire vessel cross-section at the point of measurement, as shown in Figure 1. This 'uniform insonification' of the vessel ensures that Doppler-shifted signals are received equally from all points across the lumen. It can then be shown that the *mean* Doppler shift (i.e. the normalized first moment of the Doppler shift spectrum) is proportional to the *average* blood velocity in the vessel at each instant, according to the equation given above (7, 15). Thus the problem of averaging the spatial distribution of blood velocities across the vessel lumen is replaced by the more tractable one of averaging the frequency distribution within the Doppler spectrum (8).

Once the mean Doppler shift has been estimated, two other parameters are required for calculation of the rate of blood flow in the vessel. These are the angle of approach of the ultrasound beam to the vessel ($\theta$) and the cross-sectional area of the vessel.

Both can be estimated from the conventional B-mode images taken in the course of locating the vessel and positioning the sample volume. Note, however, that for accurate measurement of these parameters the ultrasound beam should strike the vessel walls at approximately 90 degrees, whilst for accurate Doppler measurement the angle of approach should be less than 65 degrees (10). These conflicting requirements have been resolved to varying extents in different instruments, as will be discussed below.

## Instrumentation

A wide variety of ultrasound instruments has been designed or adapted for Doppler measurement. A number of these, including the original 'duplex' scanner shown in Figure 2a (2), are aimed at sampling the blood *velocity at a point,* and they therefore have a sample volume which is too small for accurate measurement of flow. Our instrument is the UI Octoson, a multitransducer water-bath scanner (12), with a pulsed Doppler unit incorporated into it (Figure 2b). The use of special dual-frequency transducers allows the beamwidth to be separately tailored for imaging (at 3 MHz) and for Doppler flow measurements (at 1.5 MHz), whilst the ability to select independently any of the eight transducers for imaging and for Doppler measurement allows suitable angles of approach to be chosen for each part of the examination. The linear array system shown in Figure 2c is similar to that described by Eik-Nes *et al* (4) and is now used by several groups for measuring fetal blood flow. This arrangement

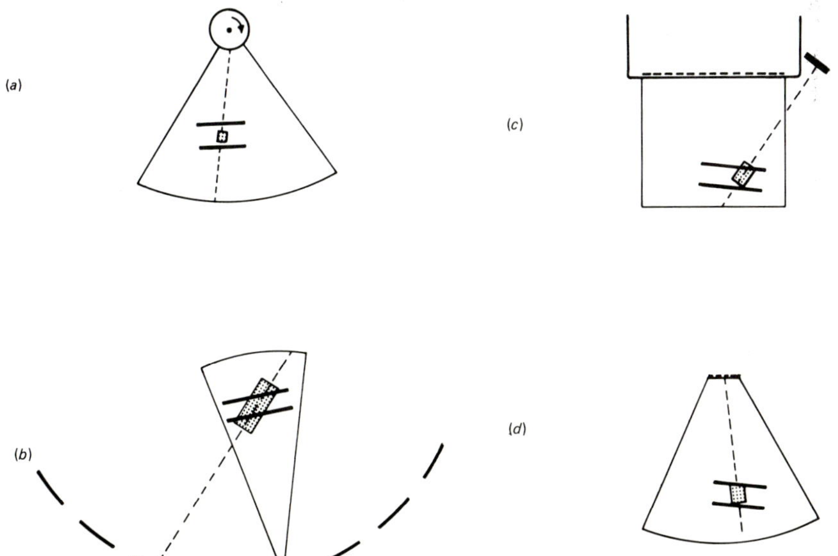


*Figure 2.* Various arrangements of ultrasound B-mode scanners with pulsed Doppler. (*a*) Rotating sector scanner, as in the original 'duplex' scanner. The scanner stops, and one of the imaging transducers is used for the Doppler measurement. (*b*) The UI Octoson, a water-bath scanner with eight transducers. One transducer is selected for imaging the vessel, another for the Doppler measurement. (*c*) Linear array scanner with a Doppler transducer at one end. (*d*) Phased array sector scanner, where the same transducer is used for both imaging and Doppler measurement

also permits optimization of the beamwidths and angles of approach for the B-mode and Doppler examinations, but it does require the vessel to be approximately parallel to the body surface. The configuration shown in Figure 2d, where the same transducer is used to produce the image and to make the Doppler measurement, is not satisfactory because it is impossible to satisfy simultaneously the requirements on the angle of approach for good imaging and for accurate Doppler measurements.

The procedure followed by the operator in using our equipment is as follows. The umbilical vein within the fetal trunk is first located and imaged in axial section. Caliper markers are positioned to determine both the diameter and the orientation of the vein at the point of measurement. The operator then selects one of the eight transducers for the Doppler measurement and activates the pulsed Doppler unit. The angle of approach of the ultrasound beam to the vessel is automatically calculated, and the rate of blood flow is computed and displayed continuously, with the operator having the ability to freeze the display and to make detailed measurements on selected portions of the flow trace at any time.

A Doppler examination consists of five to ten individual measurements, each consisting of two to five seconds of flow record. The calipers are reset for each measurement to reduce random errors, and at least two transducers with different angles of approach are used wherever possible. The Doppler examination adds approximately 15 minutes to a standard obstetric B-mode examination, and there is little or no discomfort for the patient. Successful studies are obtained in 90-95% of patients, with failures usually occurring in highly mobile fetuses or in multiple pregnancies. Flow measurements are made only during periods of apnoea because fetal breathing is known to affect the umbilical circulation.

## Limitations and accuracy

The standard range-velocity limitations of pulsed Doppler instruments are not significant where venous flow is involved. However, more serious limitations are set by considerations of accuracy. Thus, for example, analysis of the errors introduced during the measurement of the diameter and orientation of the vessel shows that these errors become severe for vessel diameters of less than 4 mm and for angles of approach greater than 65 degrees. Similarly, analysis of the effect of non-uniform insonification (in large vessels) on the accuracy of the flow estimate shows that for an error of 5% or less the diameter of the vessel should be no greater than the diameter of the ultrasound beam (where the beamwidth is measured at its -6 dB points) (10). For the UI Octoson operating at 1.5 MHz, this sets an upper limit on the diameter of the vessel of 10 mm for accurate measurements. The human umbilical vein rarely exceeds this size.

In addition, the effect on the flow estimate of high-pass filtering the Doppler signal must be recognized. It has been shown that this filtering, which is necessary to suppress reflections from stationary and slow-moving objects such as the vessel walls and surrounding tissues, causes overestimation of flow by a relatively constant amount (8). The effect of this is kept to a minimum by using a cutoff frequency which is as low as possible (100 Hz in the Octoson), and by introducing a correction factor for the offset.

The principal source of random error in this method of flow measurement is the estimation of the diameter and orientation of the vessel. For the UI Octoson, examination of the repeatability within and between operators indicates that the standard errors of measurement for individual estimates of the diameter and orientation are 0.4 mm and 3 degrees respectively. Calculation of the net effect of these errors on the flow estimate (assuming them to be independent) indicates that, for a typical umbilical vein of 6 mm diameter with an angle of approach of 45 degrees, the predicted standard error of the flow estimate would be 13%. In a recent series of 50 patients, the standard deviation of the flow estimates was calculated for each patient. The result was an average standard deviation of 14%, indicating that the errors attributable to the diameter and angle estimates account for the bulk of the observed random error component in the flow estimate. Clearly more accurate and less operator-dependent methods for estimating these quantities must be deveolped.

Experimentally, the absolute accuracy of this method for measuring flow has been investigated in several ways. Tests using a fluid simulating blood flowing at a steady rate in relatively small plastic tubes (3.8-5.0 mm in diameter) have demonstrated an average error of just 1% and a random error of 14% (7). Recently, further *in vitro* trials have been conducted, using a pump to produce pulsatile flow of human blood through a section of excised human carotid artery. These trials, taken over a flow range of 100 to 320 ml per minute, showed agreement with simultaneous electromagnetic flowmeter measurements to within 4.4%, with a standard deviation of 12%. In addition, comparison of the ultrasonically measured diameter of the artery with the inside diameter as measured with vernier calipers showed agreement to within 0.2 mm.

Eik-Nes and his co-workers, using a surgically exposed pig's aorta, have reported good agreement with no systematic error when Doppler flow measurements were compared with simultaneous measurements made using an electromagnetic flowmeter (5). Although it is not feasible to carry out such animal experiments on the Octoson, we have been able to make two additional sets of *in vivo* observations which help to confirm the accuracy of the method. First, in 21 adult human patients in whom blood flow was measured in both the main portal vein and its left and right branches, the sum of the left and right branch flows was compared with the flow rate in the main portal trunk. The difference averaged 3.5%, with a standard deviation of 13%. Secondly, in six patients with splenomegaly (due to myelofibrosis) it was possible to measure splenic flow in both the splenic artery and the splenic vein. The average difference between the arterial and venous estimates of splenic flow was 5%, with a standard deviation of 4%.

In summary, it has been demonstrated that the absolute error is small (5% or less) for vessels 4-10 mm in diameter and for angles of approach of 65 degrees or less, but that there is a relatively large random error component (of up to 15% for an individual reading), largely attributable to errors in measuring the diameter and orientation of the vessel. As mentioned above, these random errors are reduced by repeating the measurement a number of times and averaging the result.

## Results

Figure 3a shows umbilical venous flow as a function of gestational age in 118 normal pregnancies ranging from 22 weeks' gestation to term (9). The flow rate increases steadily with gestation until a maximum is reached at about 38 weeks, after which there is a reduction. When the flow rate is divided by the estimated fetal weight, the results shown in Figure 3b are obtained. The flow per kilogram decreases steadily from an average of 130 ml/kg per minute at 28 weeks to 70 ml/kg per minute at

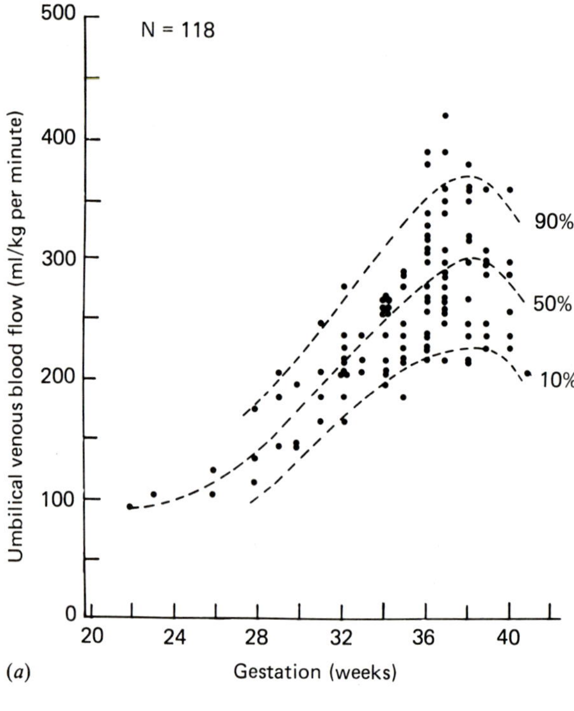


(*a*)

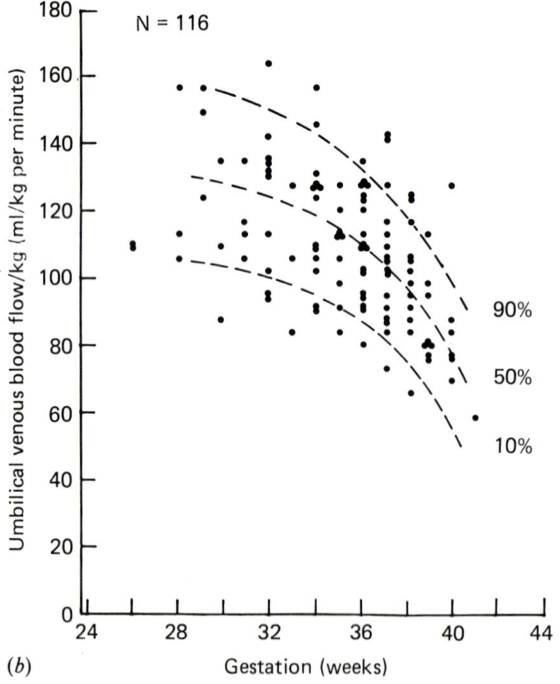


(*b*)

*Figure 3.* (*a*) Umbilical venous blood flow in the human as a function of gestational age. (*b*) Umbilical venous flow per kilogram of fetal weight

**TABLE 1. Umbilical flow per kilogram in normal pregnancies.**

| *Authors* | *Method* | *No patients* | *Gestational age (weeks)* | *Average flow (ml/kg per minute)* |
|---|---|---|---|---|
| Rudolph et al. (1971) | Microspheres (at abortion) | 11 | 10–20 | 110 |
| Assali, Rauramo and Peltonen (1960) | Electromagnetic (at abortion) | 12 | 10–28 | 110 |
| Jouppila and Kirkinen (1983) | Doppler (in utero) | 101 | 30–36 | 100 |
| Kurjak and Rajhvajn (1982) | Doppler (in utero) | 63 | 30–41 | 107 |
| Eik-Nes et al. (1090) | Doppler (in utero) | 20 | 32–40 | 110 |
| Stembera, Hodr and Janda (1965) | Thermodilution (after delivery) | 17 | term | 75 |

term. Other authors have reported values ranging from 75 to 110 ml/kg per minute (Table 1). Where the variation with gestation has been reported, a similar decrease with increasing gestational age has been found (11). In the fetal lamb, the absolute value of the umbilical flow per kilogram is much higher than in the human, but a similar reduction with increasing gestational age has been observed (3).

Umbilical venous flow has been measured in approximately 500 patients attending the ultrasound departments in two hospitals (the Royal Hospital for Women, Paddington, and the Royal North Shore Hospital, St Leonards) for standard B-mode examinations. Of these patients, approximately 40% were inpatients who had been admitted because of poor obstetric histories or complications of pregnancy; in general this group was studied serially from admission to parturition at weekly or half-weekly intervals. The remaining 60% were outpatients, the majority of whom were examined only once. The flow values measured in these two groups of patients were correlated with the known complications of their pregnancies, and with their outcomes.

Abnormal flow values (defined as values falling outside the normal 10th to 90th percentile range shown in Figure 3a) were obtained in 43% of the patients, whilst 37% had some abnormal values of flow per kilogram. By definition, in a population of uncomplicated pregnancies only 20% of the readings would be expected to fall outside this range.

Follow-up information has been obtained on 234 patients in whom delivery occurred within two weeks of their last flow reading. When the results are analysed, the following observations can be made.

Of the fetuses in which some low values of flow (i.e. below the 10th percentile) were measured, one-third (26 out of 77) were small for dates (i.e. they had birth weights below the 10th percentile for their gestational age), whereas only 8% of the remainder (13 out of 157) were small for dates. Furthermore, if these small-for-dates babies are examined for their perinatal outcome, it is found that the morbidity and mortality rates were 45% (9 out of 20) and 23% (6 out of 26) respectively among those with low flow values, whereas there was no morbidity nor mortality among the remaining 13 small-for-dates babies (in whom only normal flow values were measured). (In this context, fetal morbidity is equated with the baby requiring at least one week's stay in the intensive care nursery.) These results strongly suggest that the population of small-for-dates babies, a group known for its high level of perinatal morbidity and mortality, can be divided into high-risk and low-risk subsets on the basis of whether the umbilical flow rates are normal or not.

This raises the question of whether the population of non-small-for-dates babies can be similarly divided into high- and low-risk groups on the basis of umbilical flow. Indeed, the perinatal morbidity and mortality rates of these patients were 6% (5 out of 81) and 7% (6 out of 87) respectively among those with some abnormal flow values, and 4% (4 out of 108) and 0% (0 out of 108) among those with normal flow rates.

It therefore appears possible to categorize a pregnancy as 'high risk' on the basis of umbilical flow, regardless of whether the fetus is small for dates or not. This is significant for two reasons. First, the diagnosis of 'intrauterine growth retardation' is not made with anything approaching 100% accuracy using present methods and, secondly, there are a number of pregnancies with perinatal complications where the fetus is not small for dates. Also of considerable practical significance is the timing of deviations of flow from the normal range relative to other indicators of fetal risk. Abnormal flow values have been observed an average of one week before size measurements indicated the onset of fetal growth retardation, and before fetal cardiotocograph recordings produced 'abnormal' traces. If further results substantiate these observations, a significant impact on patient management could result.

## Discussion

The physiological mechanisms responsible for the abnormal umbilical flow values observed in compromised fetuses have yet to be elucidated. Low flow values appear in association with a variety of maternal complications (hypertension, pre-eclampsia, diabetes, etc), and the relationship between reduced flow on the one hand and reduced fetal growth and perinatal morbidity and mortality on the other is readily acceptable. High flow values have been observed in association with Rh-isoimmunization and other fetal haemolytic disease; where fetal death has occurred, extremely high flow values have been observed. Here the increased flow rate may represent an attempt at compensation for the reduced oxygen-carrying capacity of the blood. Clearly, however, there is need for a great deal of further work in this area.

## Acknowledgements

The assistance and encouragement of my colleagues at the Royal Hospital for Women, the Royal North Shore Hospital and the Ultrasonics Institute are gratefully acknowledged. In particular, the support provided by Drs Peter Warren and William Garrett, and the uncountable hours spent by Ms Adrienne Stewart in gathering data, have been invaluable.

## References

1. Assali N S, Rauramo L and Peltonen T. Measurement of uterine blood flow and uterine metabolism. VIII. Uterine and fetal blood flow and oxygen consumption in early human pregnancy. *American Journal of Obstetrics and Gynecology,* 79, 86-98 (1960).
2. Baker D W, Johnson S L and Strandness D E. Prospects for quantitation of transcutaneous pulsed Doppler techniques in cardiology and peripheral vascular disease. In *Cardiovascular Applications of Ultrasound,* edited by R S Reneman, 108-124, Amsterdam, North-Holland (1974).

3. Dawes G S. *Fetal and Neonatal Physiology,* 68, Chicago, Year Book Medical Publishers (1968).
4. Eik-Nes S H, Brubakk A O and Ulstein M K. Measurement of human fetal blood flow. *British Medical Journal,* 280, 283-284 (1980).
5. Eik-Nes S H, Marsal K, Kristoffersen K and Vernersson E. Transcutaneous measurement of human fetal blood flow. Methodological studies. In *Recent Advances in Ultrasound Diagnosis 3,* edited by A Kurjak and A Kratochwil, Amsterdam, Excerpta Medica (1981).
6. Gill R W. Quantitative blood flow measurements in deep-lying vessels using pulsed Doppler with the Octoson. In *Ultrasound in Medicine,* Vol. 4, edited by D N White and E A Lyons. 341-348, New York, Plenum (1978).
7. Gill R W. Pulsed Doppler with B-mode imaging for quantitative flow measurement. *Ultrasound in Medicine and Biology,* 5, 223-235 (1979).
8. Gill R W. Performance of the mean frequency Doppler demodulator. *Ultrasound in Medicine and Biology,* 5, 237-247 (1979).
9. Gill R W, Trudinger B J, Garrett W J, Kossoff G and Warren P S. Fetal umbilical venous flow measured in utero by pulsed Doppler and B-mode ultrasound. I. Normal pregnancies. *American Journal of Obstetrics and Gynecology,* 139, 720-725 (1981).
10. Gill R W. Accuracy calculations for ultrasonic pulsed Doppler blood flow measurements. *Australasian Physical and Engineering Sciences in Medicine,* 5, 51-57 (1982).
11. Jouppila P and Kirkinen P. The role of fetal blood flow measurements in obstetrics. In *Measurement of Fetal Blood Flow,* edited by A Kurjak, Rome, CIC (1983).
12. Kossoff G, Carpenter D A, Radovanovich G, Robinson D E and Garrett W J. Octoson: a new rapid multi-transducer general purpose water-coupling echoscope. In *Proceedings of Second European Congress on Ultrasound in Medicine,* edited by E Kazner, M deVlieger, H R Muller and V R McCready, 90-95, Amsterdam, Excerpta Medica (1975).
13. Kurjak A and Rajhvajn B. Ultrasonic measurements of umbilical blood flow in normal and complicated pregnancies. *Journal of Perinatal Medicine,* 10, 3-16 (1982).
14. McCallum W D. Thermodilution measurement of human umbilical blood flow at delivery. *American Journal of Obstetrics and Gynecology,* 127, 491-496 (1977).
15. Nakayama K and Furuhata H. Necessary requirements for blood flowmetering by ultrasonic Doppler method. *Electronics and Communications of Japan,* 57-C, 85-92 (1974).
16. Rudolph A M, Heymann M A, Teramo K A W, Barnett C T and Raiha N C R. Studies on the circulation of the previable human fetus. *Pediatric Research,* 5,452-465 (1971).
17. Stembera Z K, Hodr J and Janda J. Umbilical blood flow in healthy newborn infants during the first minutes after birth. *American Journal of Obstetrics and Gynecology,* 91, 568-574 (1965).

Chapter 29

# Ultrasonic measurements of the blood velocity and pulsatile diameter changes in the fetal descending aorta

**G Lingman, G Gennser, K Maršál**

## Introduction

Recently, the ultrasonic method in which the pulsed Doppler technique and B-mode imaging are combined has enabled a non-invasive assessment of blood flow in the umbilical vein (6) and in the fetal descending aorta (2) to be carried out. The volume blood flow is calculated from the mean blood velocity and the mean diameter of the vessel. The blood velocity and the vessel diameter, however, cannot be measured simultaneously due to the interference between the two ultrasound techniques. In arteries, the pulsatile changes of the vessel diameter and of the blood velocity are not simultaneous (8); this is not taken into account when measurements of the two parameters are performed subsequently. However, it is unknown to what degree this fact influences the calculated blood flow. This paper describes an attempt to circumvent the problem of the ultrasound interference and to elucidate the relationship between the vessel diameter and the blood velocity in the human fetal aorta.

## Methods and material

The ultrasound measurements of the fetal aortic blood velocity and of the pulsatile changes of the vessel diameter were synchronized using abdominal fetal ECG. In the same fetus, subsequent measurements of the vessel diameter and of the blood velocity were performed on the thoracic descending aorta.

Fetal ECG was obtained from three electrodes placed on the maternal abdomen at the midline. An electrocardiograph with a subtraction system (11) including an ultrasensitive isolation amplifier was utilized.

The aortic blood velocity was measured by the combined pulsed Doppler and real-time ultrasound technique (2). A real-time linear array ultrasound scanner (ADR, Temple, Arizona, 3.5 MHz) was used for the localization of the vessel. The real time transducer was placed parallel to the fetal aorta which was then insonated by the 2 MHz pulsed Doppler instrument (ALFRED, Vingmed, Norway). The Doppler transducer was attached to the real-time transducer at a fixed angle of 45°. This technique enabled a correction of the measured blood velocity for the angle between the ultrasound beam and the blood flow direction. Doppler shift signals were analysed with a spectrum analyser (DAISY, Vingmed, Norway) and the mean and maximum blood velocities were automatically estimated on-line (7). The analogue signals of the blood velocities were recorded on a polygraph simultaneously with the fetal ECG signals.

The pulsatile changes of the aortic diameter were recorded by a pulsed ultrasound echo tracker using a phase-locked loop system (Teltec, Lund, Sweden) built into the real-time linear array scanner. The spatial resolution of the system was 30 μm at 1.28 kHz repetition frequency (4). The aortic diameter signals were recorded simultaneously with the fetal ECG signals.

The fetal QRS complexes were used for the calculation of the fetal heart rate (FHR), the selection of the equal beat-to-beat intervals (maximum allowed difference 5%) and for the synchronization of the blood velocity and the aorta diameter curves.

The synchronized diameter and mean blood velocity signals were analysed with a microcomputer including a digitizer. The blood velocity signals were corrected for the delay of 20 ms caused by the mean velocity estimator. The time relations between the velocity and diameter curves were studied. The aortic stroke volume was calculated by the formula:

$$Q = \frac{T\int v \cdot d^2 \cdot \pi}{4 \cdot \cos 45} \qquad 1$$

(Q = aortic stroke volume; V = blood velocity; d = diameter of the aorta). The calculations were performed for 8 cardiac cycles in each fetus by integrating 50 synchronized sections per cycle of the diameter and of the blood velocity traces. The aortic stroke volume (Q) was also related to the fetal weight estimated from the ultrasonically measured fetal head and abdominal diameters (1).

From the values of the volume blood flow ($Q_l$) in ml/minute ($Q_l$ = Q.FHR) based on the synchronized calculations and from the values of the time-average mean velocity ($\overline{V}$), an 'effective' diameter ($D_{eff}$) was obtained according to the formula:

$$D_{eff} = \frac{4 \cdot Q^1}{\overline{v} \cdot \pi \cdot 60} \qquad 2$$

The 'effective' diameter was then compared with the systolic and diastolic diameters measured with the echo tracker.

Student's t-test for paired observations was used for statistical evaluations.

The measurements were performed on the descending aorta of 10 normal term fetuses. The level of the measurement was just above the fetal diaphragm. The gestational age of the fetuses was between 36 and 40 weeks as ascertained by ultrasound fetometry in early pregnancy.

## Results

The mean FHR based on the beat-to-beat intervals of the measured cardiac cycles was 135.5 (s.d. ± 4.9) beats/minute. The time-average mean velocity was 33.0 (± 4.4) cm/s. The average systolic and diastolic diameters were 7.3 (± 1.1) and 6.3 (± 1.1) mm, respectively.

The time relation between the synchronized aortic diameter and the blood velocity traces is schematically presented in Figure 1. The onset of the diameter change

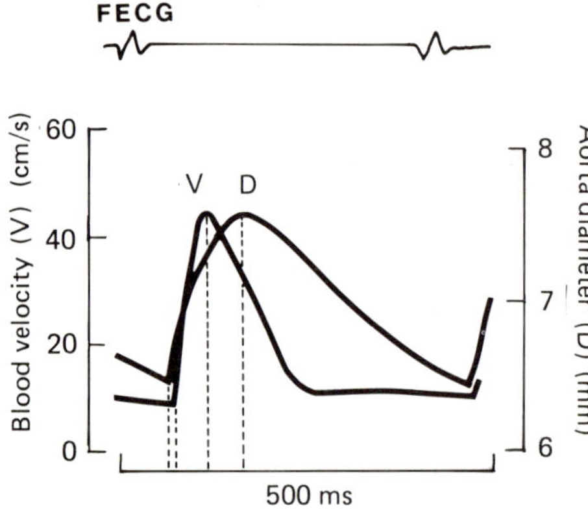


*Figure 1.* Course of the mean blood velocity (V) and the vessel diameter (D) during one cardiac cycle in the thoracic descending aorta of the human fetus. The schematic picture is based on measurements in 10 term fetuses. The subsequent measurements of the two parameters were synchronized by the external fetal electrocardiogram (FECG)

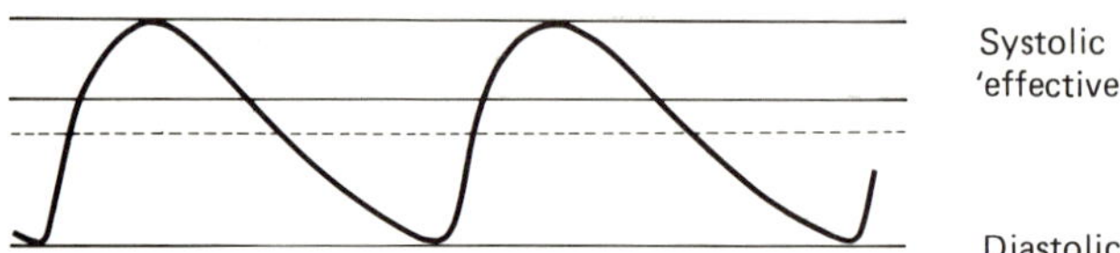


*Figure 2.* Schematic diagram of the pulsatile changes of the aortic diameter in term fetus. The 'effective' diameter of the aorta was calculated from the blood flow values based on the synchronized measurements of the blood velocity and the diameter and from the mean blood velocity values. The 'effective' aortic diameter was significantly larger than the mean diameter (broken line) calculated as the average of the systolic and diastolic diameters

preceded the onset of the velocity increase on average by 7 (± 9) ms (n.s.). The systolic diameter occurred 37 (± 13) ms after the velocity had reached its peak (p less than 0.01).

The mean aortic stroke volume (Q) was 5.4 (± 1.6) ml and the relative aortic stroke volume was 1.8 (± 0.5) ml/kg.

The average 'effective' aortic diameter ($D_{eff}$) was 7.0 (± 1.1) mm which was significantly higher (mean difference 0.21 (± 0.07) mm (p less than 0.01) than the mean aortic diameter calculated from the diastolic and systolic diameter values (Figure 2).

## Discussion

The recently developed ultrasonic method for the measurement of human fetal blood flow (2,6) is an important contribution to the problem of evaluating the fetal circulation *in utero* . However, when using the combined pulsed Doppler and real-time method for fetal blood flow measurements, it is necessary to be aware of the limitations and pitfalls (3). One of the main drawbacks of the method is the impossibility to measure simultaneously blood velocity and the vessel diameter because of ultrasound interference. This is especially disadvantageous when measuring pulsatile arterial flow. At the present time, the technical difficulties of the simultaneous use of the two techniques have not been overcome. This paper gives an indirect solution to the problem by subsequent ECG-synchronized recordings of the fetal blood velocity and the vessel diameter. A similar method was used by Tonge *et al* (10) for the calculation of the aortic stroke volume. In our study, we also analysed the time relation between the diameter changes and velocity curves (Figure 1). The mean time lag between the onsets of the two curves (7 ms) was close to the time resolution limit of the digitizer used for the computerized curve analysis. Thus, the onsets of the vessel expansion and the flow velocity were probably almost simultaneous or at least with a minimum time lag. However, the peak blood velocity occurred before the peak diameter, the time lag being significant. A similar relationship was described for the blood flow and the blood pressure courses in the abdominal aorta (9) and femoral artery (8) in animal experiments.

The calculation of the fetal volume blood flow from the ultrasonically derived blood velocity data and the diameter of the vessel is open to many errors (3,5). The main source of error seems to be the measurement of the vessel diameter (2). The use of a time-distance recorder for the dynamic measurement of the fetal aortic diameter (2) takes acccount of the pulsatile character of the aortic flow and decreases the possibility of error. However, the time lag between the velocity and the diameter courses occurring within one cardiac cycle has not been previously considered. Our present results show that the difference between the 'effective' and the mean aortic diameter measured above the level of the fetal diaphragm was 0.21 mm. This difference causes an error of 6% in the resulting volume blood flow. Before any conclusion can be reached of whether or not to correct the volume blood flow results for the time lag between the two curves, it is necessary to confirm our preliminary results in more studies at various gestational ages and in measurements at different sites on the fetal aorta.

The aortic stroke volume calculated by us was slightly higher than that given by Tonge *et al* (10). The gestational age of the fetuses and their aortic diameters were similar in the two studies. Thus, the difference in the aortic stroke volume was probably due to the differences in the mean blood velocity. A possible explanation for this might be the use of different high-pass filters for filtering the Doppler shift signals (100 Hz in the present study versus 150 Hz in the study by Tonge (10)).

The synchronization of the ultrasound recordings of the fetal aortic blood velocity and the fetal aortic diameter by the external fetal ECG proved to be a suitable method for increasing the accuracy of the fetal blood flow measurements. However, the method is laborious and can hardly be used in a clinical situation. Nevertheless, it can be recommended for physiological and experimental studies on human fetal circulation.

## Acknowledgements

The expert technical help by Mrs Ann Thuring Jönsson, Miss Lena Berg and Mr Anders Zederfeldt is gratefully acknowledged.

The study was supported by grants from the Swedish Medical Research Council (Grant B84-17X-05980-04), The Swedish Tobacco Company (Grant No 8313) and the First of May Flower Annual Campaign for Children's Health.

## References

1. Eik-Nes S H, Grøttum P and Andersson N J. Estimation of fetal weight by ultrasound measurement. II. Clinical application of a new formula. *Acta Obstetrica et Gynaecologica Scandinavica*, 61, 307-312 (1982).

2. Eik-Nes S H, Maršál K, Brubakk O, Kristoffersen K and Ulstein M. Ultrasonic measurement of human fetal blood flow. *Journal of Biomedical Engineering*, 4, 28-36 (1982).

3. Eik-Nes S H, Maršál K and Kristoffersen K. Methodology and basic problems related to blood flow studies in the human fetus. *Ultrasound in Medicine and Biology*, in press (1984).

4. Gennser G, Lindström K, Dahl P, Benthin M, Sindberg Eriksen P, Gennser M and Lindell S. A dual high-resolution two-dimensional ultrasound system for measuring target movements. In *Recent Advances in Ultrasound Diagnosis 3*, edited by A Kurjak and A Kratochwil, 71-75, Amsterdam, Excerpta Medica, (1981).

5. Gill R W. Pulsed Doppler with B-mode imaging for quantitative blood flow measurement. *Ultrasound in Medicine and Biology*, 5, 223-235 (1979).

6. Gill R W and Kossof G. Pulsed Doppler combined with B-mode imaging for blood flow measurement. *Contributions to Gynecology and Obstetrics*, 6, 139-141 (1979).

7. Hatle L and Angelsen B A J. *Doppler Ultrasound in Cardiology - Physical Principles and Clinical Applications*, SINTEF Report No STF 48A810128, Norwegian Institute of Technology, Trondheim (1981).

8. McDonald D A. *Blood flow in arteries*, 2nd edition, Southampton. The Camelot Press Ltd, 118-145, (1974).

9. Spencer M P and Denisson A B Jr. Pulsatile blood flow in the vascular system. In *Handbook of Physiology, Section 2, Circulation, Volume II*, edited by W F Hamilton and P Dow, 839-864, Washington, American Physiological Society (1963).

10. Tonge H M, Struyk P S, Custers P and Wladimiroff J W. Vascular dynamics in the descending aorta of the human fetus in normal late pregnancy. *Early Human Development*, 9, 21-26 (1983).

11. Wheeler T, Murrils A J and Shelley T. Measurement of the fetal heart rate during pregnancy by a new electrocardiographic technique. *British Journal of Obstetrics and Gynaecology*, 85, 12-17 (1978).

Chapter 30

# Non-invasive investigations of fetal and maternal haemodynamics

**J M Arnold, J Sheddon, P N Burns and J M Evans**

## Introduction

The development of the ultrasound duplex pulsed Doppler and real-time scanner has enabled more detailed study of cardiovascular haemodynamics in both the normal and diseased state, and its role in the diagnosis of arterial disease in the adult is well established (4,8). More recently, attention has been focused on the developing fetus as the importance of biophysical parameters in the assessment of fetal well-being is appreciated. Doppler ultrasound provides a safe and non-invasive method for these investigations in pregnancy.

## Background

The aetiology of intrauterine growth retardation (IUGR) is not well understood but it has been suggested that the process involves changes in the fetoplacental circulation.

Physiological changes occur in normal pregnancy in the spiral arteries supplying the placental bed, leading to progressive dilation of these vessels. In IUGR these changes are less evident and occlusive lesions in these arteries have been described. (3,9).

Estimations of blood volume flow in the umbilical vein have been made in normal and complicated pregnancies. Reduced values for umbilical flow rates have been found in cases with IUGR (5,6).

Chronic intrauterine hypoxia is thought to be more common in this group, and may account for the increased perinatal mortality and morbidity rate. Animal studies have shown that in the hypoxic fetus there is cerebral vasodilation and peripheral vasoconstriction, leading to redistribution of blood flow, with increased flow to the brain, heart and adrenal glands (1,2).

To investigate changes in human pregnancy we have studied a group of normal patients and a group 'at risk' for developing IUGR. Blood volume flow in the fetal descending aorta and umbilical vein have been calculated. Changes in peripheral vascular resistance have been investigated by analysing arterial waveform patterns in the fetal descending aorta, fetal carotid artery, umbilical arteries and the maternal uterine artery.

## Method

Fifty normal obstetric patients and 70 'at risk' for developing IUGR were included in the study. Informed consent was obtained from all patients.

Initially all patients attended at 28 weeks' gestation, but in the latter half of the study the patients were seen from 20 weeks' gestation. The normal group were seen every 4 weeks, unless complications arose, and the study group every 2 or 4 weeks depending on maternal and fetal well-being. Routine antenatal examinations were performed at each visit.

Ultrasound examinations were performed with the patient in the left lateral tilt, and using a real-time duplex scanner (ATL 500). Static ultrasound measurements included the bi-parietal diameter, abdominal diameters and head : abdomen ratio. These measurements were made available to the consultant in charge of each patient.

Doppler signals were obtained by first visualizing the vessel under examination in the real-time mode. The path of Doppler beam was represented by a line on the screen, and this plus the position of the sample volume could be adjusted by controls on the transducer. The Doppler beam was introduced by means of a footswitch. When obtaining signals from the fetal aorta and umbilical vein, care was taken to visualize an adequate length of the vessel to allow accurate angle measurement. Controls on the pulsed Doppler were optimized for best signal quality, and the video and heterodyned audio signals recorded on a U-matic recorder to allow off-line analysis. Vessel diameter was measured by using T-M mode, the Doppler beam being positioned at right angles to the vessel.

A real-time spectrum analyser (Radionics 8000), which provides a mean frequency output, was connected to a microcomputer (Apple) to calculate volume flow averaged over 6-9 cardiac cycles. Angle and diameter measurement extracted from the ultrasound and T-M mode scans were entered at the keyboard.

## Calculation of volume flow

Where the angle of insonation of the ultrasound beam to the vessel can be measured, estimation of the mean Doppler frequency shift of the signal will allow the velocity of the blood flow to be calculated. This is done by using the accepted Doppler equation:

$$\Delta f = \frac{2fv \cos\theta}{c} \quad (v << c) \qquad 1$$

where:

$\Delta f$ = mean Doppler frequency shift
f = frequency of emitted ultrasound
c = speed of ultrasound in blood
$\theta$ = angle of insonation of Doppler beam
v = velocity of blood.

Hence:

$$v = \frac{\Delta fc}{2f \cos\theta} \qquad 2$$

In vessels of a suitable size blood volume flow may be calculated as:

$Q = \bar{v} A$

where:

$Q$ = volume flow
$\bar{v}$ = mean velocity of blood
$A$ = cross-sectional area of vessel lumen.

When estimating volume flow there are a number of possible sources of error to be considered. Errors can be incurred in the measurement of the angle $\theta$, vessel diameter (hence lumen area) and mean Doppler frequency shift.

Measurement of the angle is critical. This is measured directly from the screen, and allowing for errors with this method plus registration errors, we feel an error margin of plus or minus 5° to be realistic. With angles of insonnation greater than 55° this will give a wide error margin.

Errors in vessel diameter measurement can be reduced using T-M mode. However, at the frequencies used, the resolution is such that errors may be still up to plus or minus 5 mm.

Analogue methods of mean frequency estimation are cheaper and easier to use, but digital methods are generally more accurate even with optimal signals. If the signals are noisy digital analysis is far superior but more time consuming.

In applying the Doppler principle we make an assumption that the signal received originates from energy scattered equally by all elements of the moving blood. This assumption is incorrect. The shape of the beam is most intense at its centre, thus a greater proportion of the received signal will be from this area where the blood is moving faster. This will tend to overestimate the mean Doppler frequency shift.

Sample volume size is also important. A narrow beam with a short sample volume will cause large errors in the mean Doppler frequency shift. Increasing the length of the beam will reduce these errors. With a longer beam a greater proportion of the signal will originate from the vessel wall area, where the blood is moving more slowly. This will tend to underestimate the mean Doppler frequency shift but in so doing will tend to compensate for errors involved in the non-uniformity of the beam shape.

Having discussed the problems it can be seen that although some may be overcome, others cannot, and studies on blood flow should be looked at critically in view of these errors. Volume flow values are in the process of being analysed and will take into account these criticisms.

## Waveform shape analysis

The arterial waveform pattern is representative of many variables of the arterial system, for example vessel wall elasticity, lumen diameter, pulse pressure and peripheral vascular resistance. Changes in the character of the waveform in relation to altered peripheral vascular resistance have been demonstrated.

The signals are processed through a real-time spectrum analyser (Angioscan 1) and video hard copies made of each waveform. Using a graphics tablet connected to a microcomputer (Apple 2), the maximum frequency outline was traced by hand and averaged over three cardiac cycles. Various parameters, including the pulsatility index (PI) were calculated:

$$\frac{\text{Peak-to-peak height of waveform}}{\text{Mean cardiac cycle}}$$

## Results

One hundred and twenty babies delivered of whom 15 (12.5%) were between the 5-10th centile, corrected for maternal height and weight, and the sex and rank of the baby; 14 (11.66%) were less than the 5th centile (corrections made as above).

The results for the PI are shown in Tables 1-4. There was no significant difference noted between the two groups. Patients 'S' and 'R' were tabulated separately. In the former the fetus was severely growth retarded from 24 weeks gestation, and at 34 weeks antenatal cardiotocograhy showed type II dips. Emergency Caesarean section was performed. The fetus was in good condition at birth. In the second case, intrauterine growth retardation was diagnosed at 28 weeks. Oligohydramnios was

**TABLE 1. Fetal aorta PI.**

| *Gestation* (weeks) | *Normal* | *5–10th centile* | *<5th centile* | *R* | *S* |
|---|---|---|---|---|---|
| 20 | 1.78 | 1.9 | 1.63 | | |
| 24 | 1.8 | 1.97 | 1.98 | | |
| 28 | 1.84 | 1.93 | 1.8 | | |
| 30 | 1.78 | 1.74 | 1.75 | 4.32 | 2.06 |
| 32 | 1.84 | 1.95 | 1.88 | | 1.79 |
| 34 | 1.83 | 1.79 | 2.04 | | 2.03 |
| 36 | 1.84 | 1.87 | 1.84 | | |
| 38 | 1.75 | 1.84 | 1.77 | | |
| 40 | 1.83 | 1.62 | 2.11 | | |

R=Severe IUGR with intrauterine fetal death.
S= Severe IUGR with antenatal fetal distress.

**Table 2. Umbilical artery PI.**

| *Gestation* (weeks) | *Normal* | *5–10th centile* | *<5th Centile* | *R* | *S* |
|---|---|---|---|---|---|
| 20 | 1.3 | 1.43 | 1.4 | | |
| 24 | 1.23 | 1.11 | 1.3 | | |
| 28 | 1.18 | 1.21 | 1.21 | | |
| 30 | 1.13 | 1.36 | 1.00 | 5.32 | 1.60 |
| 32 | 1.04 | 1.18 | 1.18 | | 1.74 |
| 34 | 0.95 | 1.06 | 0.98 | | 2.00 |
| 36 | 0.92 | 0.98 | 1.02 | | |
| 38 | 0.88 | 0.91 | 0.98 | | |
| 40 | 0.83 | 0.97 | 0.96 | | |

R=Severe IUGR with intrauterine fetal death.
S= Severe IUGR with antenatal fetal distress.

**TABLE 3 Fetal carotid PI.**

| *Gestation* (weeks) | *Normal* | *5–10th centile* | *<5th centile* | *R* | *S* |
|---|---|---|---|---|---|
| 20 | 1.74 | 1.79 | 1.87 | | |
| 24 | 1.99 | 1.82 | 1.88 | | |
| 28 | 2.05 | 2.05 | 2.08 | | |
| 30 | 2.08 | 1.53 | 1.79 | 2.06 | 1.68 |
| 32 | 2.12 | 2.15 | 2.1 | | 2.05 |
| 34 | 2.05 | 2.17 | 1.78 | | 1.48 |
| 36 | 2.1 | 2.18 | 2.07 | | |
| 38 | 2.13 | 1.83 | 1.56 | | |
| 40 | 2.14 | 2.03 | | | |

R=Severe IUGR with intrauterine fetal death.
S= Severe IUGR with antenatal fetal distress.

**TABLE 4. Uterine PI.**

| *Gestation* (weeks) | *Normal* | *5–10th centile* | *<5th centile* | *R* | *S* |
|---|---|---|---|---|---|
| 20 | 0.71 | 0.93 | 0.72 | | |
| 24 | 0.63 | 0.96 | 0.66 | | |
| 28 | 0.63 | 0.63 | 0.62 | | |
| 30 | 0.68 | 0.68 | 0.44 | 1.60 | |
| 32 | 0.57 | 0.62 | 0.69 | | 0.28 |
| 34 | 0.57 | 0.63 | 0.67 | | 0.37 |
| 36 | 0.59 | 0.58 | 0.58 | | |
| 38 | 0.51 | 0.55 | 0.61 | | |
| 40 | 0.58 | 0.8 | 0.78 | | |

R=Severe IUGR with intrauterine fetal death.
S= Severe IUGR with antenatal fetal distress.

present and the fetal kidneys and bladder could not be identified ultrasonically even after maternal intravenous frusemide. Because a diagnosis of renal agenesis had been made no action was taken when a 30 weeks' gestation antenatal cardiotocography showed signs of fetal distress. The baby died 48 hours later. A post-mortem examination revealed a severely growth retarded, but otherwise normal female fetus. In both cases cord PI values were significantly elevated, and in the latter case, where intrauterine death occurred, the uterine PI was significantly raised.

## Conclusions

A method of waveform shape analysis using pulsed Doppler ultrasound has been presented. Normal values have been established from 20 weeks' gestation using the pulsatility index. These results have been compared with those obtained from intrauterine growth retarded fetuses and no significant difference has been found between the three groups studied.

However, in the two cases of severe intrauterine growth retardation with evidence of fetal distress, significant differences in cord PI values were found suggesting increased peripheral resistance in the umbilical circulation in these fetuses. In one case, with intrauterine death, values for uterine PI were also significantly raised.

Further analysis of our PI values in the study group, excluding these two cases, showed that the levels were above normal in 18 cases. Eight were less than the 5th centile for birth weight, and nine between the 5th and 10th centile. In eight cases abnormal cardiotocography was noted in the first stage of labour. In the remaining 10 cases where the PI values were normal, abnormal cardiotocography was noted in only two cases.

Although we have shown no significant value of arterial waveform shape analysis in the prediction of intrauterine growth retardation, its relationship with antepartum fetal distress and abnormal cardiotocography in labour has been demonstrated and warrants further investigation.

## Acknowledgements

We thank R Skidmore, A Midwinter and P N T Wells for their interest and encouragement and the Medical Research Council and the South Western Regional Commitee for financial support.

## References

1. Berhman R E, Lees M H, Peterson E N, de Lannoy C W and Seels A E. Distribution of the Circulation in the Normal and asphyxiated fetal primate. *American Journal of Obstetrics and Gynecology*, 108, 956-969 (1979).

2. Cohn H E, Sacks E J, Hetrmann M A and Rudolph A M. Cardiovascular responses to hyperoxemia and acidemia in fetal lambs. *American Journal of Obstetrics and Gynecology*, 120, 817 (1974).

3. de Wolf F, Brosens I and Renaer M. Fetal growth retardation and maternal arterial supply of the human placenta in the absence of sustained hypertension. *British Journal of Obstetrics and Gynaecology*, 87, 678-685 (1980).

4. Fitzgerald D, Gosling R and Woodcock J. Grading dynamic capability of arterial collateral circulation. *Lancet*, 1, 66-67 (1971).

5. Gill R W, Garrett W J, Warren P S, Trudinger B J and Kosoff G. Monitoring blood flow in the fetal umbilical vein. *International Congress Series no 505 Ultrasound in Medicine and Biology. Proceedings of 2nd meeting of World Fed for US in Medicine and Biology*, Miyanyaki, 22-27 July, (1979).

6. Gill R W, Warren P S, Griffiths K A, Garrett W J and Kossoff G. Umbilical blood flow in high risk pregnancy. Recent advances in Ultrasound diagnosis: 3, 220-225. *International Congress Series 552. 4th Congress Ultrasonics in Medicine, (1981).*

7. Gosling R G, Dunbar G, King D H *et al.* The quantitative analysis of occlusive peripheral arterial diseases. *Angiology*, 22, 52-55 (1971).

8. Johnston K W, Marizzo B and Taraschuk I *Non-invasive Clinical Measurement*, (ch. 7), edited by D E M Taylor. Pitman Medical, Tunbridge Wells (1977).

9. Sheppard B L and Bownar J. An ultrastructural study of utero-placental spiral arteries in hypertensive and normotensive pregnancy and fetal growth retardation. *British Journal of Obstetrics and Gynaecology*, 88,695-705 (1981).

Chapter 31

# An improved echo-tracker for studies on pulse waves in the fetal aorta

**K Lindstrom, G Gennser, P Sindberg Eriksen, M Benthin, P Dahl**

## Introduction

The pulsatile behaviour of arteries has long tried the inquiring mind of medical scientists. At the beginning of the 19th century, Young defined the relation between the elasticity of vessel walls and the pulse wave velocity (PWV) (24). Several physical properties of the pulse wave were clarified in the 1920s and 1930s. With external kymographic devices estimations of the PWV were performed along the human aorta, and its dependence on blood pressure and age was established (1, 7). The distortion of the pulse wave during its passage along the vascular tree was appreciated (6) and the contraction of the vascular smooth muscle was found to raise the PWV (15). Pulse waves were also utilized in attempts to quantify the cardiac stroke volume (11) as well as for studying degenerative processes in arteries (3).

In clinical studies, PWV has usually been investigated over long segments of the arterial tree, which therefore have come to include several types of vessels with different characteristics. The available methods for measuring pulse waves have previously been based upon volume changes caused by pressure pulsations. These methods, including plethysmography and oscillography, monitor changes in tissue volume outside and peripheral to the vessel of interest; they have the disadvantages of modifying the pulse wave in its passage from the vessel to the skin surface by compression of the enclosed tissue and of being unable to study selectively pulse waves in particular segments of chosen vessels.

In animal studies, the possibility arose to quantify PWV invasively with strain gauges over short vessel segments which included several advantages: the greater accuracy in measuring the length of the particular vessel segment and the similarity in the shape of the pulse wave at the recording sites facilitating the recognition of similar reference points in the curves.

As early as 1878 Moens (16) formulated the mathematical equation for the propogation velocity of the front of the pulse wave appearing along the arteries. This included gravity, the elasticity coeffieicnt and the thickness of the arterial wall, the density of blood, and the diastolic diameter of the vessel lumen. For practical purposes the benefit of Moens expression has been disputed (7) as three of its factors have been inaccessible quantities *in situ.*

The introduction of the TD-recorder concept (12, 13, 14) and the subsequent refinements of its signal detection processing (4, 10, 19) has now produced an instrument with prospects of monitoring the movements of vessel pulsations directly *in situ* . The pulse wave method for the investigation of the vascular system differs in many respects from the presently available diagnostic ultrasound methods, i.e. combinations of Doppler ultrasound and real-time ultrasonography. First, it is possible, non-invasively, to obtain information about quite new physiological parameters, such as the segmental pulse wave velocity and thereby the regional elastic properties of the vascular system. Secondly, conventional diagnostic ultrasound is extremely sensitive to the exact positioning of the ultrasound transducer for reproducible and consistent results. The pulse wave method, on the contrary, can easily detect a variation in the PWV anywhere along the vessel between the two measuring sites. It is thus relatively insensitive to the exact positioning of the ultrasound transducer and eminently suited to recurrent screening of large populations.

Despite the technical development of the TD-recorder, the measurement procedure was difficult and required much time and patience. In order to facilitate the operation in clinical practice, an improved easy-to-use instrument has been designed which includes a newly developed 'auto-lock' digital phase-locking facility and two independent, simultaneous measuring sites for direct PWV determination.

As data of arterial pulse waves contain a wealth of information concerning cardiovascular function, non-invasive measurement of these pulses is of particular interest in the human fetus, where direct measurements are not applicable. Preliminary work on pulse wave recording has therefore been performed on the aorta in the human fetus.

## Technical description

The improved echo-tracker is basically a TD-recorder (12), equipped with a recently developed automatic version of the automatic range tracking feature (22). It was first applied to one-dimensional ultrasound in the zero-crossing phase-locked system by Hokanson et al, (9), the TD-recorder in analogue form ($\lambda/4$-tracing) by Korba et al (10) and in high-speed digital form ($\lambda/2$-tracing) by Gennser et al (4), and Rapoport and Cousin (19). A block diagram of the equipment is shown in Figure 1. The echo-tracker is interfaced to a commercial real-time scanner with a linear array transducer. The line computer is able to excite the crystals of the ultrasound transducer in any order. The order is determined by a programmable read only memory (PROM). This method allows the selection of crystals in two frames or more, before the same sequence reappears. The interlaced scanning scheme makes it possible to maintain a high frame rate together with a high pulse repetition frequency of the crystals along which beam tracking is performed. The scanning scheme is normally programmed for two different sets of echo-trackers, which allow the vessel to be monitored simultaneously at two different levels; the distance between the levels is measured in steps of 2 mm with a linearity of 0.1 mm.

When measuring within 20 cm from the transducer, the crystals are excited 2560 times per second, i.e. each measuring line will be excited 853 times per second. The phase-locked loop tracker concept is restricted by a few physical and/or practical limitations. The target may not move more than a certain fraction of a wavelength between each emitted ultrasound pulse in order to remain locked by the tracker. This means that the use of a transducer of higher ultrasound frequency will result in a reduced tracking velocity. Therefore, the lateral resolution must be reduced when fast moving objects are to be followed. For the digital echo-tracker, the echo may not

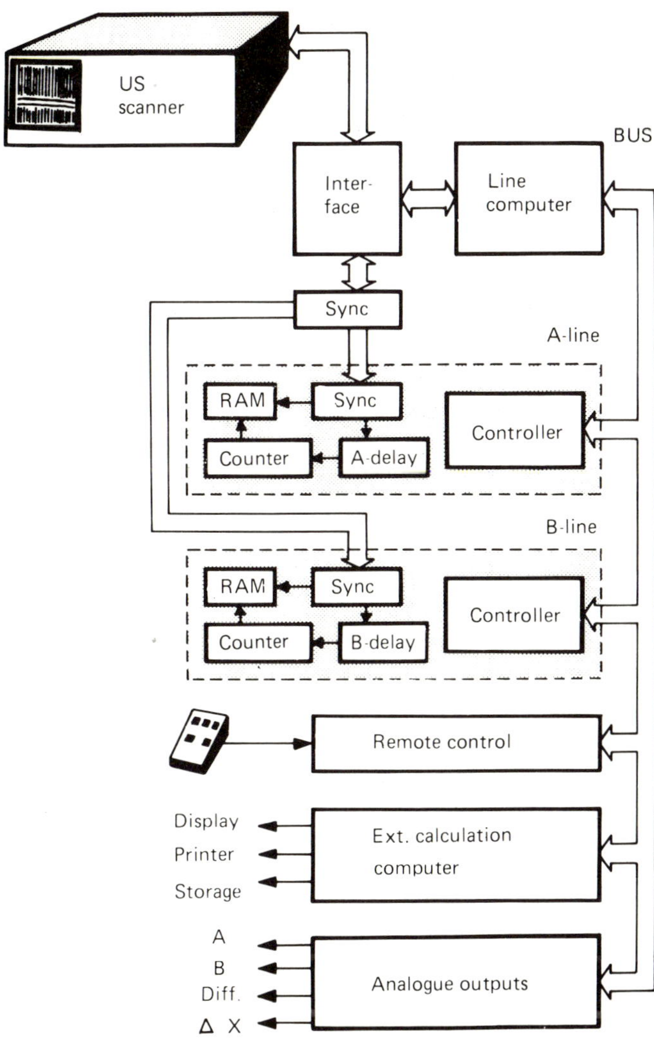


*Figure 1.* Block diagram of the new two-channel, 'auto-lock' echo-tracker

move more than one half wavelength between two samples, i.e. the target may not move more than one quarter of a wavelength. For a 3.0 MHz ultrasound transducer, the wavelength is 0.513 mm and the maximum tracking velocity will be 853 times one quarter of 0.513 mm or 109 mm/second. By reducing the penetration depth from 200 mm to 100 mm, the maximum pulse repetition frequency as well as the maximum tracking velocity can be doubled.

An automatic searching capacity, 'auto-lock', is provided by the instrument as shown in Figure 2. A double marker is placed within the two-dimensional image of the vessel lumen. After initiating the echo search, microcomputers choose two appropriate echoes as the markers are moving laterally and lock in opposite vessel walls to the third negative zero-crossing of echo signals according to given conditions.

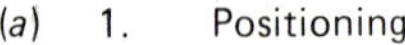


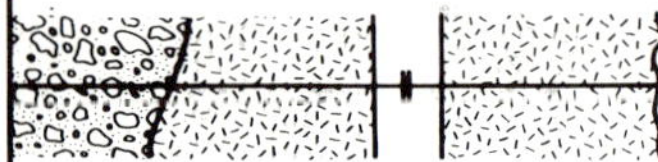



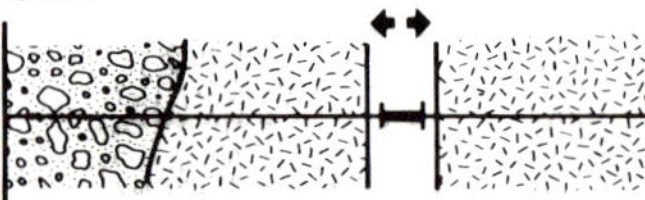



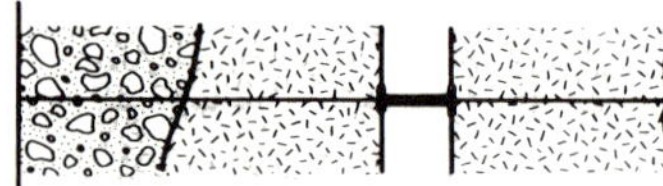



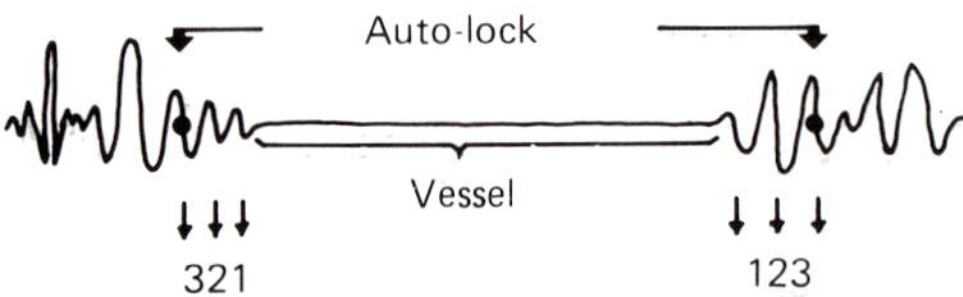


*Figure 2.* (*a*) The auto-locking sequence. A double marker is placed within the two-dimensional image of the vessel lumen. When echo search is started, an internal microcomputer chooses two echoes as the markers are moving lateral-wise. The diameter measured is indicated by an intensified line on the display. (*b*) The minicomputer selects to lock to echoes from opposite vessel walls at the third negative flank zero-crossing

The spatial resolution of the echo movement measurement depends on the measuring clock frequency used, and the standard integrated circuits available today put an upper limit to this frequency. We are presently using 60 MHz, which results in 15 μm resolution. The selected video line information is recorded on-line in digital form with a sampling frequency of 60 MHz and stored in a random access memory. The signal processing is thereafter performed 'off-line' between each ultrasound pulse.

The output signal from each measuring site is the difference between the simultaneous measurements of two opposite vessel walls. The DC-component is automatically removed from the output in order to keep an amplified signal within the range of the pen recorder used. The amplitude of this excluded component is, however, presented on a digital display.

## Pulse wave velocity

The principle for the determination of PWV is shown in Figure 3. When the ultrasound transducer is applied to the patient, two measuring sites (beam A and B) are selected at a mutual distance $\Delta x$. The auto-lock markers are positioned within the vessel walls on the respective beams. When auto-lock is initiated, the four phase-locked echo-trackers automatically lock onto the vessel wall echoes. This is indicated on the

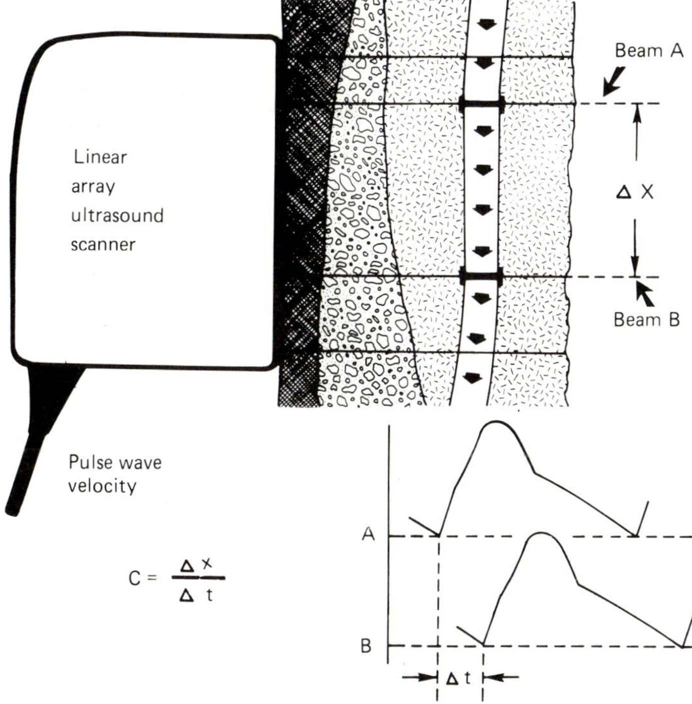


*Figure 3.* The principle for pulse wave velocity (PWV) measurement. Two measuring sites are selected at a mutual distance Δx. PWV is calculated as Δx divided by the pulse wave transit time Δt

ultrasound scanner display as the beam-lines are intensified between the respective locking-sites.

Analogue outputs of Δx, A- and B-signals, automatically adjusted for the recorder used, are then immediately available from the echo-tracker. PWV is then calculated as the mutual distance, Δx, divided by the pulse wave transit time, Δt, along the vessel between the measuring sites.

A first intuitive approach to determine the transit time, Δt, could be to measure the time difference between the front of the pulse wave at the respective measuring sites. However, the accuracy of such a measurement is reduced due to the presence of interfering noise, when the measurement is made in one particular point on the propagating pulse wave only. A better method, often used in radar technology, is to shift a replica of the first pulse waveform along the time axis and find the position for which the integrated squared differences between this shifted waveform and the second pulse wave plus noise are minimum. This is equivalent to simultaneously comparing all points on the two waveforms and establishing a solution which results in a 'best fit'.

Additional problems are created by the fact that the pulse wave changes considerably in shape as it propagates along the vessel. Such distortion is discussed for example by Wiggers (23) and is produced by a number of effects, some of which are:

(a) velocity dispersion, i.e. various frequency components of the pulse wave travel at different speeds;

(b) frequency dependent attenuation of the propagating pulse waves;
(c) non-linear elastic behaviour of the vessels with increasing distension;
(d) the effects of increasing elastic stiffness of arteries with increasing distance from the heart together with the narrowing of the vessels as they branch; and
(e) the basal vascular tone can vary during the recording time.

This makes an accurate estimation of the arrival of the pulse wave an arduous task. The problem is similar to the use of indicators, such as dye, radioisotopes, heat and saline in medicine for physiological measurements. When a mass of indicator traverses a system,its many particles become spread with respect to distance along the vascular system and therefore also spread with respect to time of arrival at the outflow.

To be able to calculate the mean transit time (MTT) of indicator particles in a flowing system, an expression can be derived based on the 'centroid of revolution' about the concentration-time function. If the indicator concentration-time function represents the total distribution of particle transit times, then at some point there will occur a time representing MTT ($\bar{t}$) for all the particles, given by

$$\bar{t} = \frac{{}_{T}\int t \cdot c(t) \cdot dt}{{}_{T}\int c(t) \cdot dt}$$

where c(t) is the indicator concentration as a function of time and T the terminal time of the indicator concentration curve. This method for determining MTT (t) is practically attractive because it deals directly with the dependent variable c(t) and the independent variable t, in a straightforward fashion. The calculation can be performed relatively easily on-line with an interfaced mini or microcomputer. This calculation is similar to the calculation of the centre of gravity of an object.

As shown in Figure 4, the same approach can be used to calculate MTT on pulse waves, if c(t) is exchanged for the radial dilatation of a vessel as a function of time. This results in a calculation which makes use of all parts of the pulse waveform and thus can be automatically calculated, and with limited sensitivity to interfering noise. We are presently using both the time of the wavefront ($t_{1f}$) and the MTT ($t_{1c}$) to find out if there is a significant difference between the methods, which in turn motivates the somewhat more complicated MTT-method for use in clinical work.

The strong influence on the shape of the pulse wave by the elastic properties of the vessel and surrounding tissue also has some benefits. Much useful information about normal and pathological conditions will probably be extracted in the near future from a careful analysis of the pulse waveform alterations. Some examples may be:

(a) The velocity dispersion has been considered theoretically and experimentally in hydraulic models (15) where it was found to be due to the viscosity of the liquid within the tube and to the viscous component of the visco-elastic walls.
(b) The apparent broadening of the pulse waveform as it travels along the vessel is often not due to velocity dispersion but rather to the result of differential attenuation of the frequency components of the pulse wave. If we assume a pulse wave relationship in the standard form $A = A_0.\exp(-K.x)$, the attenuation coefficient, K, is shown to be frequency dependent. It often increases linearly with frequency, $K = \alpha.f$ (17). Estimation of $\alpha$ might become an important parameter for quantitative differentiation between normal and pathological vascular tissue, in a way similar to 'tissue attenuation slope' in diagnostic ultrasound (2).

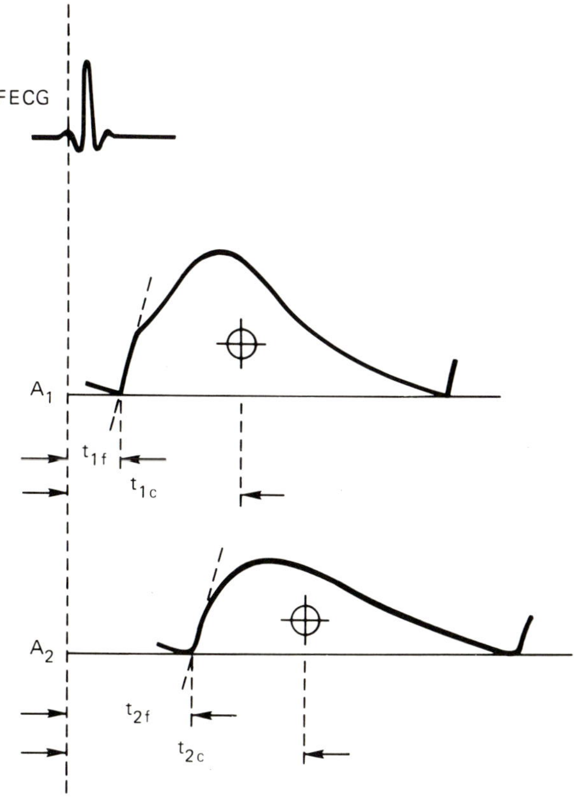


*Figure 4*. Two different ways to determine the pulse propagation time ($\Delta t$): the standard time difference between pulse wave fronts ($t_{2f}$–$t_{1f}$) and the mean transit time (cf. centre of gravity) ($t_{2c}$–$t_{1c}$) for use when the pulse wave has been distorted during the passage between the two measuring sites

(c) The pulse wave velocity is dependent on the blood pressure. There is evidence that the wave velocity of arterial segments increases proportionally with the diastolic pressure (18). This relationship might very well develop into a possible method for continuous non-invasive pressure-monitoring *in vivo* .

## Clinical performance

Using an early version of the auto-lock echo-tracker with measuring capacity at only one level at a time, the accuracy of the output signals was tested *in vitro* against an independent optical measuring method (5). A correlation coefficient of 0.99 was found between the results obtained with the two methods. This echo-tracker was further utilized to study the physiological characteristics of the diameter pulse waves in the fetal descending aorta during the last trimester of normal gestation. The mean amplitude of the pulsations remained unchanged throughout the period, but due to a continuous growth of the diastolic diameter, the pulsatile increment of the cross-sectional area increased with advancing gestational age. The diastolic diameter was reduced and the amplitude of the diameter pulsation increased when the previous

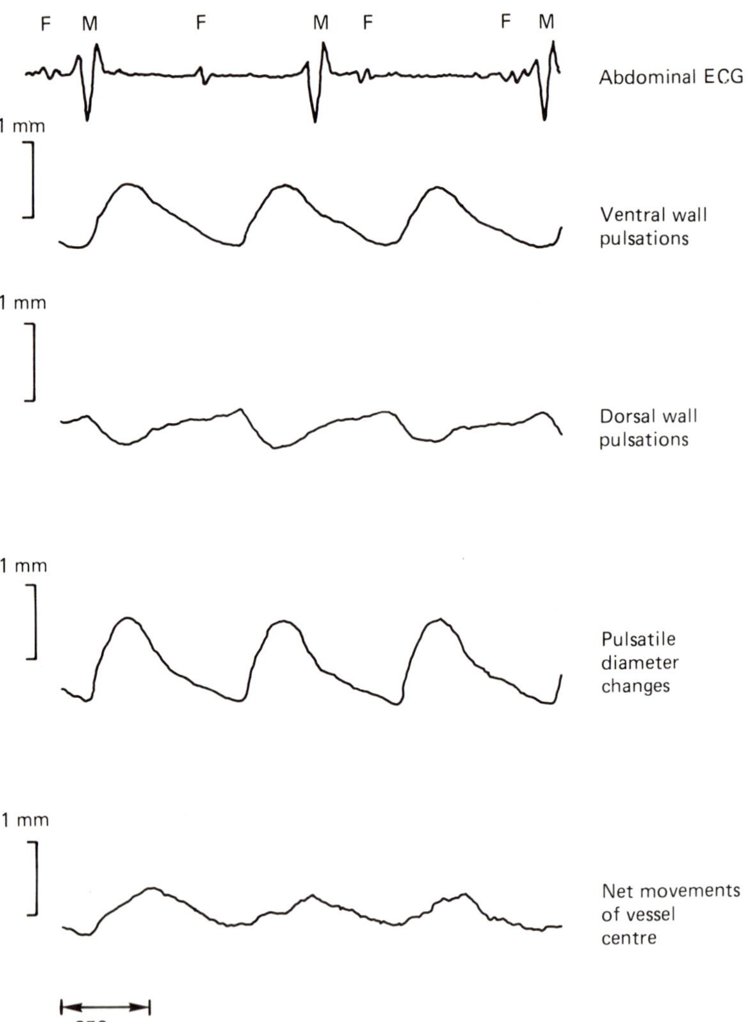


*Figure 5.* Pulse wave recording of the aorta, where not only the differential movement is shown, but also the separate movements of the vessel walls. Due to tethering, the movement of the aorta wall close to the spinal column is markedly reduced. As a consequence, the pulsation of this vessel also includes a net movement of the vessel centre

beat interval was prolonged, thereby giving evidence of an effective Frank-Starling mechanism in the human fetus. The PWV was positively correlated to the gestational age and ranged from 1.35 to 2.89 m/second. As a sign of distortion of the pulse wave along its passage through the aorta, the incremental phase of the pulse curve diminished in duration and its maximum slope increased with increasing distance from the heart (20).

In response to the pregnant woman smoking one cigarette (after an abstinence period of at least 12 hours) the fetus in the last gestational trimester displayed a typical increase of its heart rate (21). In parallel with this increase, consistent changes in the level and waveform of the pulse curves occurred. The diastolic diameter and the pulse amplitude increased, the ascending phase of the curve increased in slope and decreased in duration and the interval from the onset of the Q-wave in the fetal ECG to the arrival of the pulse wave at the site of recording was reduced. These observations demonstrate acute effects of maternal smoking on the dynamics of the fetal aorta suggesting, for example, an increased afterload in the fetal circulation.

From separate monitoring of the movements in the ventral and dorsal wall (performed as an optional programme by the echo-tracker) it also became evident that tethering was present in the aortic wall adjacent to the spinal column. As a consequence, the pulsation of this vessel, apart from the systolic dilatation, also included a lateral dislocation of the longitudinal axis (Figure 5). This is one example of how the echo-tracker, by virtue of its ability to lock to echoes from any selected level of the vessel, can help to clarify detailed physiological features in circulatory dynamics.

## Discussion

The velocity of propagation of the pulse waves created by ventricular ejection represents an important parameter in the analyses of the behaviour of the arterial tree (15). However, its clinical value has until now been limited due to the practical difficulties in making adequate pulse wave recordings. Most authors have discussed pulse waves in terms of the travel of the flow or the travel of the pressure wave, whereas most actual pulse wave recordings have utilized pressure waves only. The common denominator of all present methods to obtain high-quality pressure recordings is the necessity to introduce the measuring device directly within the vessel, ie invasive measurements. Furthermore, for small vessels an annoying source of error becomes significant: if the pressure measurement is performed using a catheter with a diameter comparable to the vessel diameter, the flow pattern can be highly disturbed and thereby seriously affect the local pressure.

With the introduction of the new dual, auto-lock echo-tracker presented in this paper, pulse wave velocity measurements using radial dilatation as a parameter is, for the first time, within reach of becoming a clinical routine. The method is reproducible, accurate, non invasive and safe. Thereby, real-time measurements of the segmental pulse wave velocity can be performed over extended periods of time, permitting continuous surveillance of the elastic properties of the vascualr system.

## References


1. Bazett H C and Dreyer N B. Measurements of pulse wave velocity. *American Journal of Physiology,* 63, 94-116, (1922).
2. Berger G and Perrin J. Attenuation principles and measurement for tissue characterization. In *Ultrasonic Tissue Characterization,* edited by J M Thijsen, 177, Brussels, Stafleus Scientific Publishing Company (1980).
3. Eliakim M, Sapoznikov D and Weinman J. Pulse wave velocity in healthy subjects and in patients with various disease states. *American Heart Journal,* 82, 448-457 (1971).
4. Gennser G, Lindstrom K, Dahl P et al. A dual high-resolution 2-dimensional ultrasound system for measuring target movements. In *Recent advances in Ultrasound Diagnosis 3,* edited by A Kurjak and A Kratochwil, 71-75, Amsterdam: Excerpta Medica, (1981).
5. Gennser G, Lindstrom K, Benthin M et al. Pulse wave measurements using a 2-dimensional, real-time ultrasound scanner with dual phase-locked echo trackers. *Proceedings of the 5th Nordic Meeting on Medical and Biological Engineering,* 2, 376-378, Linkoping, Sweden, (1981).

6. Hamilton W F, Remington J W and Dow P. The determination of the propagation velocity of the arterial pulse wave. *American Journal of Physiology,* 144, 521-535, (1945).
7. Hallock P. Arterial elasticity in man in relation to age and evaluated by the pulse wave velocity method. *Archives of Internal Medicine,* 54, 770-798, (1934).
8. Haynes F W, Ellis L B and Weiss S. Pulse wave velocity and arterial elasticity in arterial hypertension arteriosclerosis and related conditions. *American Heart Journal,* 11, 385-401, (1936).
9. Hokanson D E, Mozersky D J, Sumner D S and Strandness D E Jr. A phase-locked echo tracking system for recording arterial diameter changes in vivo. *Journal of Applied Physiology,* 32, 728-733 (1972).
10. Korba L W, Cobbold R S C and Cousin A J. An ultrasonic imaging and differential measurement system for the study of fetal respiratory movements. *Ultrasound in Medicine and Biology,* 5, 139-148, (1979).
11. Kouchoukos N T, Sheppart L C and McDonald D A. Estimation of stroke volume in the dog by a pulse contour method. *Circulation Research,* 10, 778-781, (1970).
12. Lindström K, Maršál K, Gennser G, Bengtsson L, Benthin M and Dahl P. Device for measurement of fetal breathing moements -I, the TD-recorder. A new system for recording the distance between two echo-generating structures as a function of time. *Ultrasound in Medicine and Biology,* 3, 143-151, (1977).
13. Marsal K, Gennser G and Lindstrom K. Real-time ultrasonography for quantified analysis of fetal breathing movements. *Lancet,* 2, 718-719, (1976).
14. Maršál K, Ulmsten U and Lindström K. Device for measurement of fetal breathing movements - II, accuracy of in vitro measurements, filtering of output signals, and clinical application. *Ultrasound in Medicine and Biology,* 4, 13-26 (1978).
15. McDonald D A. *Blood Flow in Arteries,* 2nd edition, London, Edward Arnold, (1974).
16. Moens A L, Die Pulskurve, Leiden (1878), quoted in McDonald D A *Blood Flow in Arteries,* 2nd edition, London, Edward Arnold (1974).
17. Newman D L, Penney S J and Greenwald S E. Pulse propagation characteristics by an impulse method. *Medical and Biological Engineering and Computing,* 21, 515-517, (1983).
18. Nichols W W and McDonald D A. Wave-velocity in the proximal aorta *Medical and Biological Engineering,* 10, 327-335, (1972).
19. Rapoport I and Cousin A J. New phase-lock tracking instrument for foetal breathing monitoring. *Medical and Biological Engineering and Computing,* 20, 1-6, (1982).
20. Sindberg Eriksen P, Gennser G and Lindstrom K. Physiological characteristics of diameter pulses in the fetal descending aorta. *Acta Obstetrica et Gynaecologica Scandinavica,* in press, (1984).
21. Sindberg Eriksen P and Gennser G. Acute responses to maternal smoking of the pulsatile movements in the fetal aorta. *American Journal of Obstetrics and Gynecology,* (in press) (1984).
22. Terman F E. Radar and radio aids to navigation. In *Electronic and Radio Engineering,* 1015-1055, New York, McGraw-Hill (1955).
23. Wiggers C J. *The Pressure Pulses in the Cardiovascular System,* London, Longmans (1928).
24. Young T. On the functions of the heart and arteries. The Croonian Lecture. *Phil. Transactions of the Royal Society* , 99, 1-31 (1809) Quoted in McDonald D A *Blood Flow in Arteries,* 2nd edition, London, Edward Arnold (1974).

Chapter 32

# Clinical value of prenatal cardiac investigation in high risk pregnancies

P A Stewart, J W Wladimiroff, P M Tonge, M F Niermeijer

## Introduction

Congenital heart disease occurs in about 0.8% of live births. Many of these abnormalities can be corrected by surgery. However, approximately half of these patients have major structural abnormalities, some of which are inoperable or have a very high operative risk. Prenatal detection of congenital heart disease may avoid delays in diagnosis and this may influence the outcome for an affected infant. Moreover, chromosomal abnormality is often associated with structural defects of the heart ranging from a few to 100% in specific syndromes, with trisomy 13 and 18 (100%) and trisomy 21 (40-50%) being the most striking (6). Prenatal detection of an abnormal karyotype and congenital heart disease may profoundly alter the further management of an affected pregnancy. Since recent improvements in ultrasound equipment it is not surprising that increasing attention is being paid to the prenatal detection of cardiac abnormalities in high risk patients (1,5,8,9,10,12).

## Methods

Between 1 January 1982 and 1 March, 1984, 540 patients were referred to our fetal cardiac abnormality screening programme. Of these 70% (Group 1) were referred because of increased risk, e.g. hereditary predisposition, maternal age above 40 years, juvenile diabetes and exposure to possible cardiac teratogens. The remainder (Group 2) were sent to exclude cardiac disease in the present pregnancy, e.g. fetal arrhythmia, ascites, severe growth retardation, polyhydramnios, maternal connective tissue disorders, exposure to rubella or other viruses early in gestation and other fetal pathology such as renal disease or omphalocele. Four methods of investigation were used to assess the fetal heart.

### Two-dimensional real-time sector scanning

Two-dimensional (2D) real-time sector scanning (Diasonics Cardio Vue 100 or Hewlett Packard 77020A Ultrasound Imaging System) with a 3.5 MHz or 5 MHz transducer was used to assess fetal size, structure (with particular attention to the heart), placental location and amniotic fluid compartment. With 2D ultrasound techniques the motion of the fetal heart can be observed at around 6 weeks of gestation, although structural analysis is not possible until approximately 16 weeks of gestation. However, the heart is still rather small at this stage and is best imaged between 18 and 24 weeks of gestation. The heart of the fetus may be viewed from other planes than in postnatal life as the lungs are fluid filled and present no obstruction to the ultrasound beam.

A number of transverse and longitudinal planes are obtained but the examination is, in fact, a continuous sweep allowing each scanning plane to proceed to another in an attempt to demonstrate normal cardiac anatomy.

The position of the fetal head and spine is first sought as a reference. The fetal four chamber view, which is the easiest to recognize is obtained in the transverse axis at the level of the fetal thorax. The right ventricle is closest to the chest wall and its coarser trabeculations and moderator band are typical landmarks. The tricuspid valve is seen to insert more apically than the mitral valve. Pulmonary venous connections to the left atrium are visible as is the movement of the foramen ovale within the left atrium. Demonstration of this view will exclude hypoplasia of the right or left ventricle, absence of an atrioventricular connection and various atrioventricular septal defects. Tilting the transducer towards the left shoulder will reveal the left ventricular long axis plane. The aortic root can be seen connected to the left ventricle, with the anterior wall of the aorta in continuity with the intraventricular septum and the posterior wall continuous with the anterior leaflet of the mitral valve. The right ventricle is seen in an anterior position. Slight rotation of the transducer toward the pulmonary valve area will visualize the long axis of the pulmonary trunk and confirm ventriculo-arterial concordance. The pulmonary trunk may be followed to its branches and via the ductus arteriosus to the descending aorta. More sagittal angulation shows the aortic arch with vessels to the head and neck. Scanning in the longitudinal axis will identify the superior and inferior vena cavae connected to the right atrium, the tricuspid valve connected to the right ventricle and the pulmonary valve which is anterior and cranial to the aortic root. Identification of these views will exclude pulmonary or aortic atresia, truncus arteriosus and transposition of the great vessels, and confirm atrioventricular and ventriculo-arterial concordance, thereby excluding major abnormalities. However, mild degrees of outflow stenosis or obstruction, or small atrial or ventricular septal defects may be missed due to the inherent limitations of the technique.

## 2D directed M-mode echocardiography

2D directed M-mode facilities are essential for the analysis of disturbances of cardiac rate and/or rhythm in the fetus and assessment of chamber sizes.

Fetal arrhythmia is usually discovered in routine prenatal care by auscultation and it is vital (10,12) that every fetus with arrhythmia be carefully examined by ultrasound to exclude possible congenital malformation as a cause for the disturbance of rate or rhythm. M-mode echocardiography may predict the focus of extrasystolic events and elucidate the precise nature of brady- and tachyarrhythmias. Correct assessment of a fetal arrhythmia is vitally important in the prognosis and further management of the fetus. M-mode echocardiography, especially in conjunction with 2D examination provides the means to evaluate early signs of cardiac compromise, e.g. right heart enlargement or pericardial effusion, and the effects of prenatal treatment or tachyarrhythmias can be followed.

## Fetal transabdominal electrocardiography

Recording of the fetal transabdominal electrocardiogram is also attempted (Corometrics Medical Systems Inc 112 Fetal Monitor) when an arrhythmia is diagnosed but provides only limited information as only ventricular depolarization is obtained. However, it may be useful for the timing of ventricular events. It may be more difficult to record the fetal QRS-complex between 28 and 34 weeks due to interference caused by the vernix caseosa which further limits its usefulness during this period of pregnancy.

## Pulsed-wave Doppler analysis of fetal blood flow

Pulsed-wave Doppler in combination with 2D real-time ultrasound is used to measure human fetal blood flow at the lower thoracic level of the fetal descending aorta in the third trimester of pregnancy.

First, after locating the fetal aorta using the real-time transducer placed parallel to the vessel, mean blood flow velocity in the aorta descendens is measured using a pulsed Doppler system (PEDOF) as described by Eik-Nes *et al* (2,3). The mean blood flow velocity is measured over ten consecutive cardiac cycles.

Second, using a dual-time distance recorder similar to that described by Sindberg Eriksen (7), the pulsatile vessel diameter changes at the same site are recorded, again over ten consecutive cardiac cycles.

Due to interference between the real-time and the Doppler transducers, mean blood flow velocity and pulsatile vessel diameter profiles cannot be measured simultaneously.

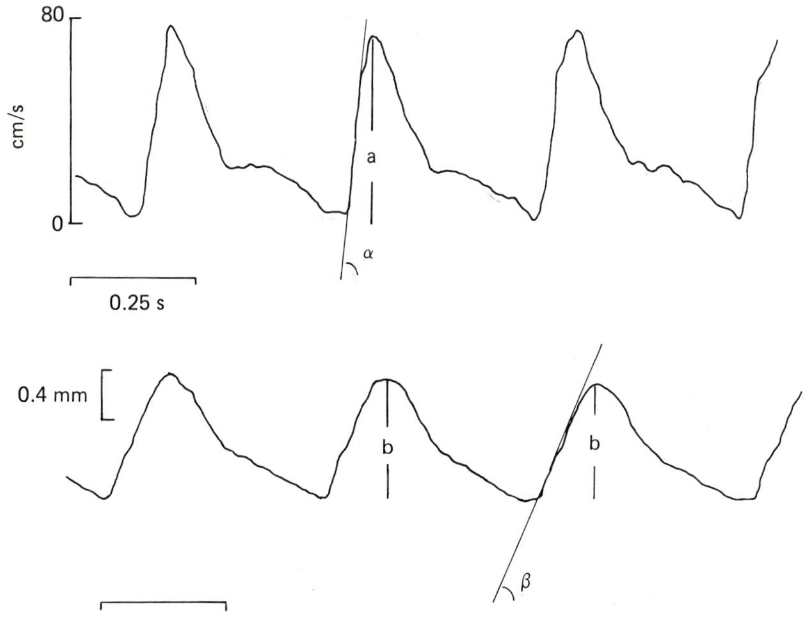


*Figure 1.* Tracings of normal mean flow velocity and pulsatile diameter profiles in the third trimester of pregnancy. a = peak mean velocity (cm/sec); b = maximum diameter change (%); $\alpha$ = acceleration of mean flow velocity (cm/sec$^2$); $\beta$ = rate of vessel wall expansion

Therefore, these two parameters are compared in cardiac cycles of equal R-R intervals as obtained by external fetal ECG (11). The tracings obtained are shown in Figure 1.

Each cardiac cycle in both the mean blood flow velocity profile and pulsatile vessel diameter profile is divided into ten equal points, and at each of these points blood flow is calculated using the formula:

$$\frac{Q = V.A}{\cos \alpha}$$

where Q = flow, V = mean blood flow velocity, A = vessel luminal area, $\alpha$ = angle between the real-time and Doppler transducer (fixed at 45°).

Hence a mean blood flow waveform can be constructed for ten cardiac cycles. Improved accuracy in present investigations will be made possible by the introduction of a computer program that samples mean blood flow velocity, pulsatile vessel changes and the fetal ECG every 5 ms, i.e. 200 samples per second. This enables a very complete mean blood flow waveform to be plotted. In current studies, normal values and normal waveform patterns are still being established. Early blood flow measurements (11) when compared with blood flow measurements of high risk pregnancies, e.g. congenital heart disease, fetal arrhythmia, have provided additional information about fetal well-being.

The techniques described are of major clinical importance in providing a cardiovascular profile of fetuses with cardiac disorder thereby allowing delivery of an infant in optimal condition.

## Results

In the study period, 540 fetuses were referred for fetal cardiac investigation. All 540 fetuses underwent 2D structural cardiac analysis. Where possible, when abnormalities of cardiac structure, rate or rhythm were observed all the methods of examination described above were attempted.

There were 19 structural abnormalities detected in fetuses with a gestational age ranging from 20-37 weeks (Tables 1-3).

Further investigation showed six fetuses (31%) to have an abnormal karyotype. Four of these were diagnosed prenatally and two postnatally. Severe oligohydramnios was present in one fetus with double outlet right ventricle rendering prenatal karyotyping impossible and the other fetus with polyhydramnios and ventricular septal defect (VSD) had been referred from another hospital and karyotyping was not done until after delivery. Seven of the patients (37%) had associated rhythm and/or rate disturbances. Fifty patients were referred with arrhythmia and seven (14%) had associated structural abnormality.

Blood flow measurement using PWD was performed in seven cases with arrhythmia. These were four cases of complete heart block (CHB), two cases of tachyarrhythmia (one with atrial flutter of ±460 beats per minute and a ventricular response varying from 92-264 beats per minute), and one case of bradycardia associated with a wandering pacemaker and complete atrioventricular septal defect. Doppler analysis showed that below 50 beats and above 250 beats per minute aortic blood flow and stroke volume dropped below normal values (11) suggesting the functional limits of the fetal myocardium to be around these rates.

When cardiac structural defects were diagnosed in the absence of other pathology or an abnormal karyotype, management of the pregnancy proceeded normally with the infant being transferred immediately after delivery to the paediatric cardiology unit for further care. Regular monitoring of abnormalities such as obstructive foramen ovale was carried out to identify early signs of cardiac compromise such as right heart dilatation, pericardial effusion or ascites. Decisions regardng the time and mode of delivery were made according to the findings.

In pregnancies in which complex lesions of the heart alone, or in combination with other structural abnormalities (e.g. omphalocele, Meckel syndrome) or abnormal

**TABLE 1. Group 1 (patients referred with increased risk).**

| | *No. patients* | *False negative* | *False positive* | *True positive* |
|---|---|---|---|---|
| Previous child CHD | 179 | Coarctation | — | — |
| | | muscular VSD | — | — |
| Parent CHD | 64 | — | — | Incomplete AVSD<br>Hypertrophic cardiomyopathy<br>Holt-Oram syndrome |
| Other family CHD | 14 | — | — | — |
| Juvenile diabetes | 47 | — | — | DORV+subpulmonary VSD |
| Epilitic | 39 | — | — | — |
| Drug Addict | 27 | — | — | Coarctation and abnormal tricuspid valve |
| Age above 40 years | 18 | — | — | — |
| | 388 | 2 (0.5%) | — | 5 (1.3%) |

CHD=congenital heart disease; VSD=ventricular septal defect; AVSD=atrioventricular septal defect; DORV=double outlet right ventricle.

**TABLE 2. Group II (arrhythmia).**

| | *No. patients* | *False negative* | *False positive* | | *True positive* |
|---|---|---|---|---|---|
| Ectopics | 31 | — | — | (6.5%) | Univentricular heart<br>Obstr. foramen ovale |
| Various A-V block | 7 | — | — | | RA-tumour |
| | | | | (57%) | Complex CHD, asplenia<br>Complex CHD, asplenia<br>VSD (trisomy 18) |
| Bradycardia | 2 | — | — | | |
| Complete AVSD | | | | | Complete AVSD |
| Various tachyarrhythmias<br>— | 9 | — | — | | — |
| Sinus tachycardia<br>— | 1 | — | — | | — |
| | 50 | — | | | 7 (14%) |

RA=right atrial; CHD=congenital heart disease; VSD=ventricular septal defect; AVSD=atrioventricular septal defect; A-V=atrioventricular

**TABLE 3. Group II (abnormalities in present pregnancy).**

| | *No. patients* | *False negative* | *False positive* | *True positive* |
|---|---|---|---|---|
| Polyhydramnios | 23 | VSD (trisomy 21) | TGV (positional) | Complex CHD (trisomy 18)<br>Incomplete AVSD (Meckel)<br>VSD+MCA (trisomy 18)<br>(1 in arrhythmia group) |
| Ascites | 10 | — | — | (2 in arrhythmia group) |
| Small-for-dates | 23 | — | ASD (positional) | DORV (trisomy 13) |
| Miscellaneous (omphalocele, infections, etc.) | 46 | — | Ventricular inversion (positional) | Obstr. foramen ovale (tricuspid dysplasia)<br>VSD+omphalocele (trisomy 18)<br>Ectopia cordis, DORV, MCA |
| | 102 | 1 | 3 | 7 (6.9%) |

VSD =Ventricular septal defect; TGV=transposition of the great vessels; CHD=congenital heart disease; AVSD=atrioventricular septal defect; MCA=multiple congenital abnormalities; DORV=double outlet right ventricle; ASD=atrial septal defect.

karyotype were diagnosed, termination of pregnancy was offered depending on the gestational age, or surgical intervention in the pregnancy was avoided. In one case (Table 3) in which complex congenital heart disease was diagnosed, karyotyping revealed trisomy 18. However, the result only became available one day prior to spontaneous delivery of the infant and active neonatal assistance was not given. The infant died 30 minutes postpartum. In another case, a patient (Table 2) was referred at 35 weeks of gestation with polyhydramnios and bradycardia. A diagnosis of VSD with 2:1 atrioventricular block was made. Karyotyping was recommended but was not carried out by the referring hospital. Caesarean section was performed at 38 weeks of gestation because of growth retardation and the infant which died shortly afterwards, was found to have trisomy 18.

Diagnosis of disturbances of rate or rhythm in isolation resulted in further care appropriate for the type of arrhythmia found. Extrasystoles, even when of frequent occurrence, had a benign outcome and all arrhythmias disappeared during the pregnancy or shortly after birth. There were two fetuses who had associated structural abnormality (Table 2).

The first, who had obstruction at the level of the foramen ovale with a grossly dilated right atrium and ventricle and paradoxical motion of the interventricular septum continued to have multiple extrasystoles throughout the delivery. At the age of 6 months, the heart size had returned to normal and the electrocardiogram revealed normal sinus rhythm. The second fetus, who had severe growth retardation, was referred to our hospital for possible Caesarean section. Echocardiography revealed a univentricular heart and coarctation of the aorta. This fetus died on the day of admission before any further plans had evolved. However, Caesarean section would not have been performed in view of the cardiac abnormality.

In cases of CHB in the presence of a structurally normal heart the fetus was monitored regularly for signs of cardiac compromise as previously discussed. One fetus whose mother had Waldenström's hyperglobulinaemia was found by PWD to have reduced aortic blood flow at 36 weeks. Caesarean section was performed at 37 weeks of gestation but the infant died 2 days after birth from intractable cardiac failure. Vaginal delivery was attempted in one fetus and although baseline atrial rate remained at 150 beats per minute without appreciable changes relative to uterine contractions, emergency Caesarean section had to be carried out when fetal scalp pH dropped to 7.07. Vaginal delivery was successful in another case. However, elective Caesarean section allows optimal timing of delivery and facilitates smooth transfer of the infant to the neonatologist and paediatric cardiologist.

There was serological evidence of maternal collagenosis in all cases of fetal CHB with a structurally normal heart. One mother developed clinical signs of lupus erythematosus, for the first time, 3 months after the delivery of her infant.

In the structurally normal heart, tachyarrhythmia resulting in severe congestive cardiac failure in a pre-viable fetus poses a serious therapeutic problem, and may result in fetal death. In one fetus first seen at 25 weeks of gestation with severe ascites, polyhydramnios and a ventricular rate of about 240 beats per minute, immediate maternal intravenous administration of 0.75 mg digitalis per day, was given. This continued for 5 days with no effect upon the tachycardia and on the sixth day after a reduction in the dosage of digitalis, procainamide 1 g over 1 hour was given, with 4 g/24 hours as a maintenance dose. On the eighth day verapamil 10 mg was given over 1 hour. However, fetal death occurred the same day. Block dissection of the sino-atrial node revealed no clear abnormality.

Digitalis is known to cross the placenta readily and has been the most commonly used agent in attempting to cardiovert fetal tachyarrhythmias. Results of success have been variable which may be partly explained by administration of non-therapeutic doses or possible resistance in some fetuses. Three other fetuses treated by us with digitalis 0.75 mg daily failed to respond to treatment and all were delivered by Caesarean section and cardioverted by pharamacological means after delivery. One fetus first seen at 38 weeks of gestation with atrial flutter of 440 beats per minute and a ventricular rate of 220 beats per minute was treated by maternal administration of digitalis 2 mg over 24 hours. The fetus was found to have normal sinus rhythm 24 hours later. However, at delivery the cord serum digitalis level was 0.2 ng/ml (therapeutic range 0.5 ng/ml - 2.5 ng/ml).

### Missed diagnoses

Three diagnoses were missed (0.5%). These were a perimembranous VSD in a fetus with duodenal atresia and trisomy 21, a muscular VSD, and coarctation of the aorta. All of these diagnoses may also be difficult to make in postnatal life. Coarctation of the aorta usually occurs in the region of the ductus and as this is wide open in fetal life this defect may be obscured by the ductus. Apparent visualization of the arch of the aorta does not exclude coarctation with certainty for this reason. Obstetric management of these pregnancies would not have been altered in any way if these diagnoses had been made prenatally.

### False positive diagnosis

Three false positive diagnoses were made (0.5%) and were the result of positional problems. A tentative diagnosis of transposition of the great arteries was made in a fetus with gross ascites and hydrothorax. The diagnosis was made in the absence of positive identification of the branching of either vessel on a purely positional basis.

The heart of this fetus was found to be normal. Another fetus with an omphalocele was thought to have ventricular inversion. The parents opted for termination of this pregnancy and the fetus was found to have multiple congenital abnormalities including severe scoliosis. Examination of the heart in situ showed that the scoliosis and the omphalocele had distorted the position of the heart which was found to be normal. The third fetus was referred with severe growth retardation and oligohydramnios. A secundum atrial septal defect was diagnosed. The fetus died in utero and post mortem examination revealed microscopic cystic disease of the kidneys. The primum and secundum septum met in the central fibrous body. This was considered a variant of normal but the variation in position probably resulted in visualization of an apparent defect in this region. In none of these patients did the false positive diagnosis affect the ultimate outcome of obstetric decisions concerning the fetus.

## Conclusion

Evaluation of the heart of the fetus in pregnancies at risk for cardiac abnormalities is becoming of major clinical importance. Reassurance can be given to parents when abnormalities are excluded. When abnormalities are diagnosed a realistic prognosis can be given and appropriate obstetric measures taken according to the degree of disease and expected prognosis. In cases where severe disease is present or cardiac abnormalities in combination with other structural abnormalities and/or abnormalities of karyotype, termination of pregnancy can be offered, depending on gestational age or abstention from surgical intervention in the pregnancy advised.

In cases with a good prognosis careful follow-up may be offered resulting in the delivery of an infant in optimal condition.

At present the use of 2D and M-mode examination provide the most useful means of evaluating the fetal heart. Use of PWD techniques may provide further information concerning the cardiovascular status of the fetus. A combination of these techniques provides a cardiovascular profile of fetuses with cardiac disorders facilitating better management of an affected fetus.

## References

1. Allan L D, Tynan M, Campbell S and Anderson R H. Normal fetal cardiac anatomy - a basis for the echocardiographic detection of abnormalities. *Prenatal Diagnosis,* 1, 131-139 (1981).

2. Eik-Nes S H, Brubakk A O and Ulstein M. Measurement of human fetal blood flow. *British Medical Journal,* 1, 280-283 (1980).

3. Eik-Nes S H, Maršál K, Person P H and Ulstein M K. Ultrasonic measurements of blood flow in the human fetal aorta and umbilical vein. In: *Proceedings of the 7th Congress on Fetal Breathing and Other Measurements,* edited by G S Dawes, 1-8, Oxford (1980b).

4. Kleinman C S, Hobbins J C, Jaffe C C, Lynch D C and Talner N S. Echocardiographic studies of the human fetus: prenatal diagnosis of congenital heart disease and cardiac dysrhythmias. *Pediatrics,* 65, 1059-1067 (1980).

5. Lange L W, Sahn D J, Allen H D, Goldberg S J, Anderson C and Giles H. Qualitative real-time cross-sectional echocardiographic imaging of the human fetus during the second half of pregnancy. *Circulation,* 62, 799-806 (1980).

6. Nora J J, Nora A H and Wexler P. Hereditary and environmental aspects as they affect the fetus and newborn. *Clinical Obstetrics and Gynaecology,* 24, 851-861 (1981).

7. Sindberg-Eriksen P, Gennser G and Lindström G. Characteristics of pulse waves in the fetal aorta descendens. In: *Recent Advances in Ultrasound Diagnosis 3,* edited by A Kurjak and A Kratochwil, 234-240, Amsterdam, Excerpta Medica, (1981).

8. Stewart P A, Wladimiroff J W and Gussenhoven W J. Antenatal real-time ultrsound diagnosis of a congenital cardiac malformation. *European Journal Obstetrics, Gynecology and Reproductive Biology,* 14, 233-237 (1983).
9. Stewart P A, Wladimiroff J W and Essed C E. Prenatal ultrasound diagnosis of congenital heart disease associated with intrauterine growth retardation. A report of 2 cases. *Prenatal Diagnosis,* 3, 279-285 (1983).
10. Stewart P A, Tonge H M and Wladimiroff J W. Arrhythmia and structural abnormalities of the fetal heart. *British Heart Journal,* 50, 550-554 (1983).
11. Tonge H M, Struijk P C, Custers P and Wladimiroff J W. Vascular dynamics in the descending aorta of the human fetus in normal late pregnancy. *Early Human Development,* 9, 21-26 (1983).
12. Wladimiroff J W, Struijk P C, Stewart P A, Custers P and De Villeneuve V H. Fetal cardiovascular dynamics during cardiac dysrhythmia. Case report. *British Journal Obstetrics and Gynaecology,* 90, 573-577 (1983).

Chapter 33

# Pulsed Doppler evaluation of the fetal and neonatal circulation

**Dale C Alverson, Marlowe Eldridge, Terrance Dillon, Thomas Blomquist, William Berman Jr**

## Introduction

Fetal and neonatal well-being, as well as perinatal circulatory physiology, can be assessed through a consideration of oxygen transport. Oxygen delivery must be adequate to meet the metabolic demands of the tissues. The relationship between the oxygen transport and oxygen consumption ($\dot{V}o_2$) is yet to be defined; preliminary studies, however, suggest that the relationship between these two variables reflects a great deal about the adequacy and functional integrity of the perinatal circulation. Systemic oxygen transport (SOT) is dependent upon both blood flow ($\dot{Q}$) and arterial oxygen content ($CaO_2$ ) expressed as SOT = $\dot{Q}$ x $CaO_2$ . Blood flow quantification, therefore, is required for understanding and analysing perinatal circulatory physiology and pathophysiology. Blood flow is dependent upon heart rate, circulatory loading conditions and myocardial function. Because traditional methods of determining blood flow, myocardial contractility and circulatory loading have required invasive techniques, few studies of human perinatal circulatory physiology have been conducted.

Recent advances in pulsed Doppler ultrasound methodology have permitted the non-invasive investigation of blood flow (1-3, 17) in human fetuses and neonates; preliminary studies suggest that myocardial contractility can also be assessed non-invasively (4, 5). We have used pulsed Doppler technology to study the fetal and neonatal circulation in animals and in man. This paper will discuss those applications of pulsed Doppler ultrasound in laboratory and clinical settings.

## Methods

### The Doppler principle

The Doppler principle states that the frequency of sound will be shifted in proportion to the velocity (V) of a backscattering object. This relationship is expressed by the equation:

$$V = \frac{\Delta FC}{2F_o \cos\theta}$$

where V = the velocity of the backscattering object (red blood cells), F = the sound frequency shift, C = the speed of sound in the medium (in tissue C = 1 540 metres per second), $F_o$= the frequency of the sound source, and $\theta$ = the angle of insonance between the sound beam axis and the velocity vector of the moving object. If $\theta$ is less than 15 degrees, cos $\theta$ can be assumed to be 1; otherwise that angle measurement is critical in calculating the true velocity.

Pulsing the sound signal permits range gating, or 'focusing' of the ultrasonic beam in a specific site (the sample volume). The maximum depth of sampling and maximum measurable velocity are determined by the frequency of the applied ultrasound and the pulse repetition frequency (PRF) (18).

## Instrumentation

We have used both custom-designed 20 MHz and 10 MHz pulsed Doppler velocimeters (Craig Hartley, Baylor Research Development Laboratories, Houston, Tx) and commercially available 5 MHz and 3.5 MHz velocimeters (Advanced Technology Laboratories, Bellvue, Wa, and Cardionics Inc, Hayward, Ca) with and without duplex imaging capabilities. A combined ultrasound imaging and Doppler velocimetry system is necessary for fetal flow studies.

Hand-held ultrasound transducers are used for fetal and neonatal investigation. Custom-designed transducer tip number 6 or 8 French catheters (Jerry Davis and John Adams, Lovelace Research Center, Albuquerque, NM) have been used for animal studies to ensure continuous sampling in the desired flow stream.

## Measurement technique

### *Fetal studies*

A 5 MHz duplex scanning system (ATL Mark V), which combines a real-time, two-dimensional sector scanner with a range- gated pulsed Doppler velocimeter, is used. The ultrasonic image defines the orientation and dimensions of the fetal descending aorta and allows for accurate measurement of the insonance angle between the Doppler ultrasonic beam and the vector of the aortic blood flow stream (Figure 1). The flow velocity measurements are obtained quasi-simultaneously upon imaging the vessel. The Doppler audiosignals are analysed with an offset zerocrosser counter (ZCC) to generate velocity waveforms. These waveforms are then integrated off-line with a bit-pad microprocessor to measure a temporal mean velocity. The true mean velocity ($\bar{V}$) is determined by division of the measured velocity by cos $\theta$. The descending aortic diameter is measured directly from the ultrasonic image and the cross-sectional area calculated as $A = \pi d^2/4$. Descending aortic blood flow is then calculated as $\dot{Q}$ = $\bar{V}$ (cm/sec) x A ($cm^2$) x 60 (sec/min).

The imaging and Doppler velocity measurement techniques have also been applied to intracardiac investigation in order to define better anatomical arrhythmic and functional characteristics of the fetal heart.

### *Newborn studies*

Here 3.5, 5, or 10 MHz range-gated pulsed Doppler velocimeters and suprasternal transducer probes are used to obtain ascending aortic flow velocity signals in the

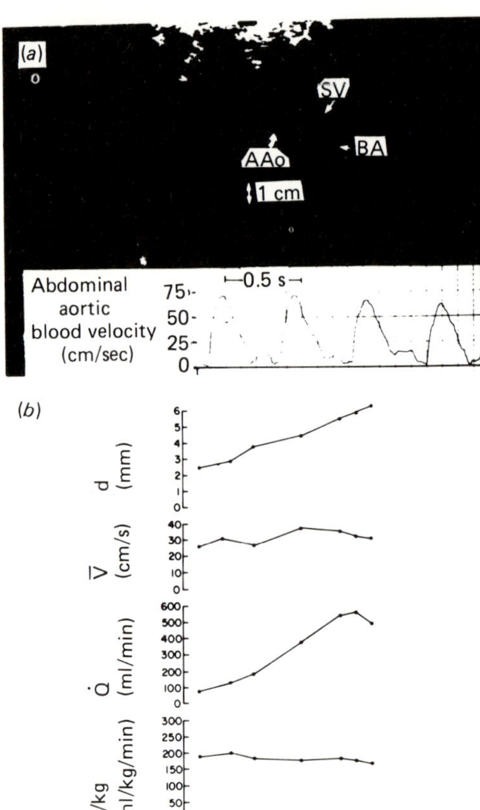


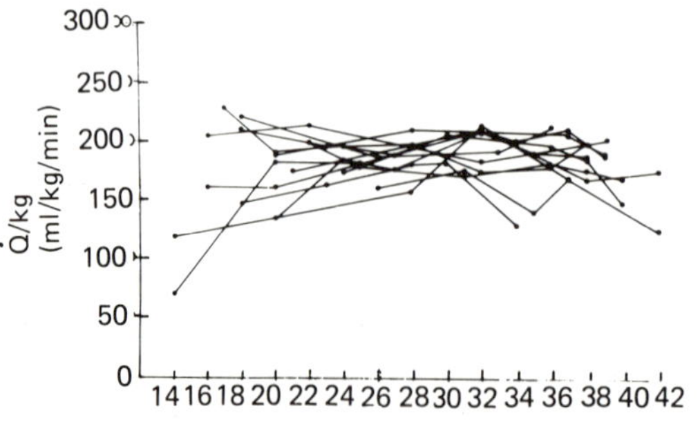


*Figure 1.* (a) The upper photograph demonstrates the real-time ultrasound image of a human fetus showing the abdominal aorta (AAo) with the Doppler ultrasound beam axis (BA) and flow velocity sample volume (SV). The tracing shows the typical aortic blood flow velocity waveforms obtained at the time of study. (b) The middle graphs demonstrate the changes in abdominal aortic diameter (d), mean flow velocity (V), calculated blood flow ($\dot{Q}$) and $\dot{Q}$/kg (estimated fetal weight) in a representative fetus studied from 18 to 40 weeks' gestation. (c) The lower graph shows $\dot{Q}$/kg in the initial study of fetuses in healthy mothers. (From Eldridge and Berman (18) with permission from the editor *Pulsed Doppler Ultrasound in Clinical Pediatrics*)

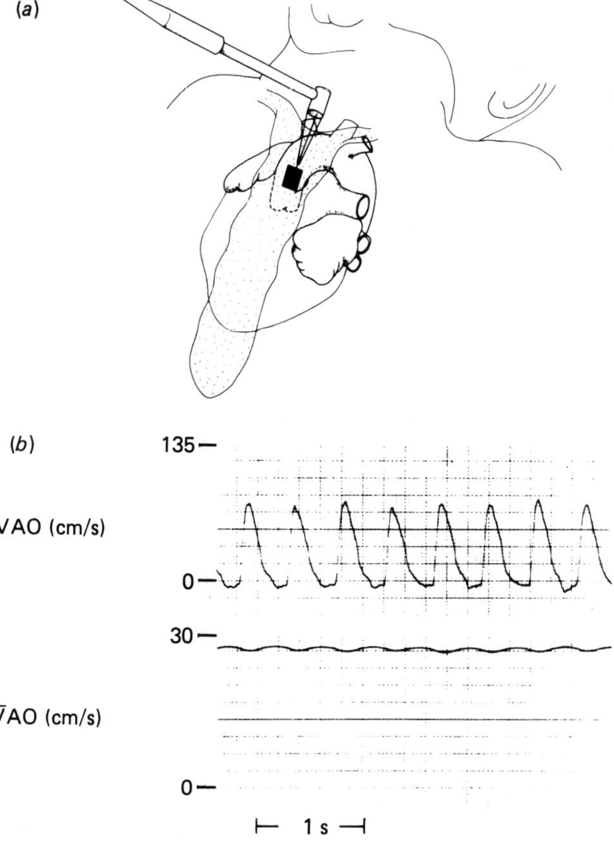


*Figure 2.* (a) The Doppler transducer is placed in the suprasternal notch on a layer of contact gel. The ultrasound beam is directed into the region of the ascending aorta just above the aortic valve leaflets. The sample volume depth is adjusted using the range gate. (b) The lower tracings demonstrate the characteristic phasic and mean ascending aortic blood flow velocity waveforms obtained in the neonate. $\bar{V}_{Ao}$ is then used for calculation of cardiac output as $\dot{Q}_{Ao} = \bar{V}_{Ao} \times A_{Ao}$, where $A_{Ao}$ = the ascending aortic cross-sectional area determined by M-mode echocardiography. (Tracing from Alverson et al (3) with permission from the editor and publisher, *American Journal of Perinatology*)

neonate (1-3). The frequency of ultrasound used depends upon the anticipated depth of sampling (the lower frequencies are used for deeper penetration in larger subjects). The Doppler transducer is positioned in the suprasternal notch on a layer of airless contact gel, and the ultrasonic beam directed into the region of the ascending aorta (Figure 2). The sample volume depth is adjusted using the range gate. After consistently good flow signals are obtained, the mean ascending aortic blood flow velocity ($V_{Ao}$) is measured by electronic integration and compared to an internal calibration signal.

The ascending aortic internal diameter (d) during systole is determined echographically (Irex System II) on each subject. The aortic cross-sectional area is then calculated: $A_{Ao} = \pi d^2/4$ (cm$^2$). Doppler derived left ventricular cardiac output is determined as $Q_{Ao}$(ml/min) = $\bar{V}_{Ao}$(cm/sec) x $A_{Ao}$(cm$^2$) x 60 (sec/min). Flow determinations are normalized to body weight in kilograms.

*Contractility studies*

Doppler derived flow velocity variables were compared to the peak rate of rise of left ventricular pressure (LV $dP/dt_{max}$) in dogs under a variety of inotropic and loading conditions (4, 5). Velocity-related measurements were obtained by using a transducer tip 20 MHz pulsed Doppler catheter (number 6 or 8 French) placed in the ascending aorta via the carotid artery.

A Millar transducer tip pressure catheter was placed in the left ventricle in order to obtain accurate pressures and LV $dP/dt_{max}$, which in turn was used as an index of myocardial contractility (6, 7). A balloon tip Berman catheter was placed in the descending aorta in order to change afterload acutely by balloon inflation and deflation. Inotropic state was changed by continuous intravenous infusion of dobutamine or propranolol (see Figure 3 for the animal model design).

Multiple regression analysis was used to determine a flow velocity variable which correlated closely with LV $dP/dt_{max}$, independent of loading conditions.

## Study populations

*Fetal studies*

Fetal flow velocity data could be obtained consistently after 18 weeks' gestation (17). Maternal consent was obtained prior to study in accordance with procedure at the Lovelace Medical Foundation. Ultrasonically determined fetal biparietal diameter and transverse abdominal diameters were used to estimate gestational age and fetal weight.

Initially, 16 healthy women in the second trimester of pregnancy agreed to fetal flow studies performed at 2- to 4-week intervals until term. A total of 72 examinations were performed on these normal fetuses.

We subsequently studied serially subdiaphragmatic descending aortic flow in 24 fetuses, 19 of non-smoking (NS) mothers and five of smoking (S) mothers. The S mothers smoked more than 10 cigarettes per day throughout pregnancy, but did not smoke for 2 hours prior to study. Studies were done during three periods of gestation: (a) 20-24 weeks, (b) 28-32 weeks, and (c) 36 weeks to delivery.

*Neonatal studies*

All neonates were studied in the nurseries at the University of New Mexico Hospital after parental consent was obtained. Doppler derived ascending aortic flow ($\dot{Q}_{Ao}$) data were collected in healthy preterm and neonates in the first week of life to help establish normal values for Doppler derived left ventricular output in this patient population (3).

We have also used this technique to study $\dot{Q}_{Ao}$ in 18 infants before and after closure of a haemodynamically significant patent ductus arteriosus (PDA) by indomethacin or surgical ligation (2).

Doppler-derived LV output has been studied in five infants with supraventricular tachycardia before and after cardioversion. Additional studies have been done in selected infants with myocardial dysfunction requiring inotropic support, and in infants requiring partial exchange transfusion for polycythaemic hyperviscosity syndrome.

*Contractility studies*

Ten healthy adult mongrel dogs were studied in our animal laboratory facilities at the University of New Mexico. Ketamine was used for anaesthesia and dogs were killed by barbiturate overdose at the conclusion of the study.

## Results

*Fetal studies*

Satisfactory studies were completed in 94% (68 out of 72) of the initial examinations of normal fetuses. Inadequate studies resulted from excessive fetal movement or variations in fetal position. All pregnancies were uncomplicated throughout term gestation. Three deliveries were by caesarean section due to breech presentation. The one-minute Apgar scores were greater than 7 and birthweights were over 2.8 kg in all fetuses studied.

Fetal abdominal aortic diameter (d) increased linearly with gestational age. Mean abdominal aortic flow velocity ($\bar{V}$) increased only slightly until 36 weeks' gestation, with a slight decline near term. Abdominal aortic flow ($\dot{Q}$) increased with gestational age until 38 weeks' gestation and declined slightly thereafter. Weight related flow ($\dot{Q}$/kg estimated fetal weight) remained relatively unchanged throughout pregnancy. Figure 1c shows $\dot{Q}$/kg for the 16 fetuses. Results were relatively constant throughout gestation with a mean of 184 ± 20 (s.d.) ml/kg per minute. Some fetuses had a slight decline in $\dot{Q}$/kg near term. These values are similar to those reported by Eik-Nes *et al* (16) using similar techniques to measure thoracic aortic blood flow in 26 fetuses of 32-40 weeks' gestation.

**TABLE 1. Gestational age period.**

| | | *I* (*20–24 weeks*) | *II* (*28–32 weeks*) | *III* (*36 weeks-term*) |
|---|---|---|---|---|
| Number of patients studied | NS | 16 | 19 | 13 |
| | S | 5 | 5 | 5 |
| FHR | NS | 146±9 | 140±10 | 132±8 |
| | S | 145±6 | 144±11 | 144±8† |
| d | NS | 3.3±0.4 | 4.5±0.5 | 5.8±0.5 |
| | S | 3.3±0.4 | 5.1±0.02 | 5.9±0.3 |
| $\bar{V}$ | NS | 20±5 | 31±8 | 34±7 |
| | S | 36±11** | 46±11* | 46±10** |
| Vp | NS | 36±12 | 60±12 | 68±8 |
| | S | 69±24** | 84±5* | 105±16** |
| $\dot{Q}$ | NS | 97±26 | 317±93 | 522±60 |
| | S | 180±19** | 568±134** | 738±20* |
| $\dot{Q}$/kg | NS | 179±18 | 192±16 | 180±24 |
| | S | 254±68** | 306±12** | 278±36** |
| SV/kg | NS | 1.2±0.1 | 1.4±0.2 | 1.4±0.2 |
| | S | 1.7±0.4** | 2.1±0.2** | 1.9±0.3** |

FHR=fetal heart rate (b.p.m.), d=blood vessel diameter (mm), $\bar{V}$=mean velocity (cm/s), Vp=peak velocity (cm/s), $\dot{Q}$=blood flow (ml/min), $\dot{Q}$/kg blood flow per estimated fetal weight (ml/kg per minute), SV/kg= stroke volume per estimated fetal weight (ml/kg per beat), †=significantly higher ($p<0.01$) than NS fetuses, *=significantly higher ($p<0.005$) than NS fetuses, **=significantly higher ($p<0.001$) than NS fetuses.

A total of 63 additional Doppler examinations were performed to study the effects of smoking on fetal haemodynamics: 48 on fetuses of NS mothers and 15 on fetuses of S mothers. Four examinations were unsuccessful due to fetal movement or unsatisfactory position. All infants were born at more than 38 weeks' gestation. Estimated gestational age and Apgar scores were not significantly different between groups. The mean birthweight of S fetuses (2860 ± 280 g) was significantly lower than NS fetuses (3570 ± 300 g), p less than 0.001. Haemodynamic data of the S and NS groups are shown in Table 1.

Fetal heart rate was not significantly different until the third period, when S fetuses had higher rates. Abdominal aortic diameters were not significantly different except during the second period, when S fetuses had larger diameters. Peak velocity (Vp), mean velocity ($\bar{V}$), $\dot{Q}$, $\dot{Q}$/kg and SV/kg were significantly higher in S fetuses in each period of study. $\dot{Q}$/kg remained relatively constant for NS and S fetuses throughout gestation, averaging 182 ± 20 ml/kg per minute in NS and 276 ± 49 ml/kg per minute in S fetuses, p less than 0.001.

## *Neonatal studies*

Characteristic ascending aortic blood flow velocity signals were obtainable in all neonates studied (Figure 2). In the study of healthy infants, the LV output, represented as $\dot{Q}_{Ao}$, averaged 221 ± 56 (s.d.) ml/kg per minute in the preterm infants and 236

**TABLE 2. Femoral arterial blood flow velocity.**

| | *Preclosure* | *Postclosure* | *P value* | *Normal values* |
|---|---|---|---|---|
| LV output (ml/kg per minute) | | | | |
| Surgical ligation (8) | 320±30* | 224±27 | <0.02 | |
| Indomethacin (12) | 358±19 | 271±21 | <0.001 | |
| Total (20) | 343±16 | 252±17 | <0.001 | 221±20 |
| $V_f$ m(cm/sec) | 3.4 | 10.9 | <0.05 | 9.1 |
| LA/Ao | 1.60 | 1.41 | <0.002 | <1.15 |
| PEP/LVET | 0.25 | 0.34 | <0.001 | 0.36 |

*mean ± s.e.m., LV=left ventricular, $V_f$=mean femoral blood flow velocity, LA/Ao=left atrial to aortic root diameter ratio, PEP/LVET=pre-ejection period to left ventricular ejection time ratio.

**TABLE 3. Cardiac output, haemoglobin concentration and systemic oxygen transport in two infants with polycythaemic hyperviscosity.**

| *Case number* | *Q (ml/kg per minute)* | *Hgb (g/dl)* | *$O_2$ sat (%)* | *$CaO_2$ (ml $O_2$/dl)* | *SOT (ml $O_2$/kg per minute)* |
|---|---|---|---|---|---|
| Pre-exchange | | | | | |
| I | 138 | 23.0 | 93 | 28.7 | 39.6 |
| II | 187 | 24.0 | 99 | 31.8 | 59.5 |
| Postexchange | | | | | |
| I | 230 | 18.0 | 93 | 22.4 | 51.5 |
| II | 237 | 20.0 | 99 | 26.5 | 62.8 |

Q=cardiac output, Hgb=haemoglobin concentration, (%$O_2$ sat)=percent oxygen saturation, ($CaO_2$)=arterial oxygen content, (SOT)=calculated systemic oxygen transport. (In one of the infants studied, as flow increased, blood pressure dropped indicating a decrease in systemic vascular resistance after partial exchange.)

± 47 in the term infants, with an average of 230 ± 50 ml/kg per minute in the 22 infants studied during the first week of life (3). These results compare favourably with values reported by Burnard *et al* (8) using thermodilution and Fick techniques in newborns.

In infants with PDA, the LV output averaged 343 ± 16 (s.e.m.) ml/kg per minute, well above predicted normal values. After closure with indomethacin or surgical ligation, LV output fell significantly to 252 ± 17 (p less than 0.001) (2). Femoral arterial blood flow velocity was much lower than normal when the ductus was patent and rose to normal levels after ductus closure, consistent with presumed improvement in effective systemic blood flow (Table 2).

Flow calculations in the five infants with supraventricular tachycardia averaged 118 ± 14 (s.d.) ml/kg per minute during tachyarrhythmia and rose to 212 ± 17 ml/kg per minute following conversion to sinus rhythm (p less than 0.001). Heart

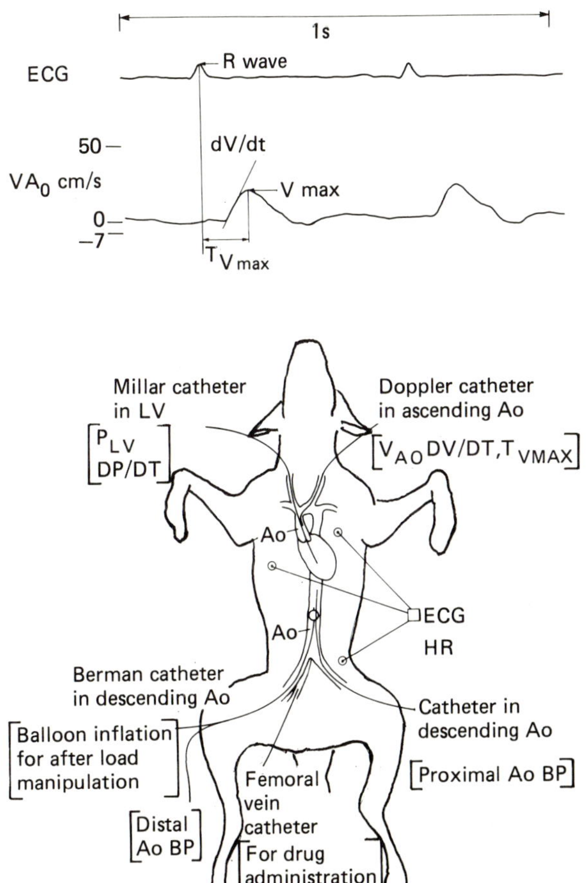


*Figure 3.* The dog model was used to compare dP/dt to Doppler-derived flow velocity variables. The balloon tip catheter in the descending aorta (Ao) was used to change afterload acutely by balloon inflation and deflation. The upper tracing demonstrates how $T_{Vmax}$ was measured and that flow velocity variable correlated closely with dP/dt, independent of afterload changes

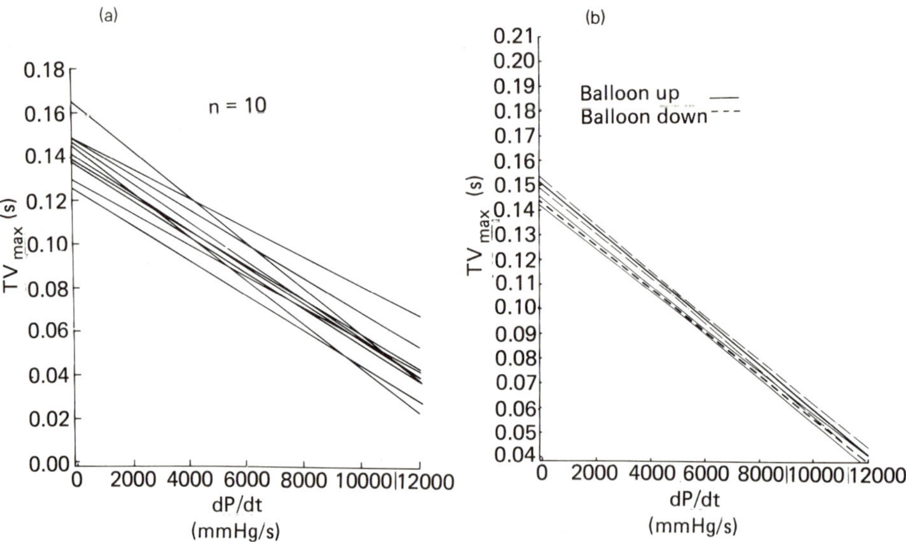


*Figure 4.* (a) This graph shows the linear regression slopes of the 10 individual dogs studied, comparing $T_{Vmax}$ to dP/dt. Slopes and y-intercepts were similar in all dogs. The average correlation coefficient was −0.92. (b) This graph shows the linear regression slopes with 95% confidence limits of all dogs combined, comparing $T_{Vmax}$ to dP/dt with and without balloon inflation. Note that there was no significant difference in the relationship with afterload manipulation

rate fell from 248 ± 22 to 155 ± 13 b.p.m. (p less than 0.002) and stroke volume rose from 0.47 ± 0.1 to 1.35 ± 0.2 ml/kg (p less than 0.001).

Using the Doppler technique, we have been able to assess the effectiveness of inotropic therapy in selected patients with myocardial dysfunction. Left ventricular output, in addition to the more traditional measurements of heart rate, heart size and blood pressure, is used to document drug effect and guide dosage adjustments.

In two infants with polycythaemic hyperviscosity we have noted an increase in cardiac output after partial exchange transfusion and, despite the drop in haemoglobin concentration, an actual increase in systemic oxygen transport (Table 3).

### *Myocardial contractility studies*

Baseline levels of heart rate, vascular pressure, LV $dP/dt_{max}$, LV pressures, aortic flow velocity and dV/dt were within the range reported for dogs under anaesthesia in our laboratory. Interventions used to vary myocardial contractility resulted in levels of $dP/dt_{max}$ ranging from 500 to 11 000 mmHg per second. As shown previously (5, 19), $V_{max}$ and dV/dt varied in parallel with LV $dP/dt_{max}$ following inotropic stimulation. Afterload increase, however, resulted in reductions in those velocity-based variables without a significant change in dP/dt.

Time to peak flow velocity ($T_{Vmax}$) was the single velocity-based variable which correlated highly (r = -0.92) with $dP/dt_{max}$ over a wide range of inotropy, independent of afterload manipulation. $T_{Vmax}$ was measured from the peak of the R wave on ECG to the peak of the aortic flow velocity waveform (Figure 3). The linear regression slopes and y-intercepts comparing $dP/dt_{max}$ to $T_{Vmax}$ were similar in all dogs studied, with no significant effect caused by balloon inflation or deflation (Figure 4).

## Discussion

Pulsed Doppler ultrasound methodology offers the clinician and physiologist a useful tool for characterizing haemodynamic function in the perinatal period. This technique can be used non-invasively to study the cardiovascular system in the fetus and newborn.

Fetal flow studies of the descending aorta reflect blood supply to both the placenta and the lower body of the fetus. Fetal lamb studies have shown that up to 80% of distal abdominal aortic blood flow goes up to the placenta (26). If the same flow distribution exists in the human fetus, then measurements in our study would reflect primarily placental flow. The fact that Q/kg varied little throughout the second and third trimesters of pregnancy suggests that placental perfusion parallels fetal weight during gestation. Previous investigators (14, 21) have speculated that vascular lesions in the placenta may explain the decline in Q/kg near term, a finding seen in 44% of the fetuses we studied. Moreover, since previous animal studies (10-12) have suggested that fetal abdominal aortic blood flow may change acutely with fetal distress, this technique may prove useful in assessing fetal and placental function in high risk pregnancies. In the study of fetuses of smoking mothers, the higher blood flows may result from a redistribution of flow to the vital organs and placenta. This redistribution may reflect decreased oxygenation due to higher fetal carboxyhaemoglobin levels. Changes in flow may also be related to stimulation of catecholamine release, as suggested by Divers *et al* (17), leading both to redistribution of flow and to inotropic stimulation. Our studies illustrate how pulsed Doppler methodology can be used to study the haemodynamic pathophysiology of fetal disorders in a variety of perinatal circumstances.

The Doppler studies in the neonate characterize the status of LV output under a variety of circumstances and demonstrate the usefulness of flow determination in management and understanding of neonatal circulatory distress. It is worth while re-emphasizing the effect of PDA on LV output and the relationship of LV output to effective systemic flow with the ductus patent. Previously published data suggest that during the first few hours of life the ductus arteriosus is patent and transfers approximately one-third of the LV output back into the pulmonary circulation (11, 20). In premature infants, persistent ductal patency is common (13, 20, 22). The high LV output seen prior to PDA closure in our studies is consistent with a large left to right PDA shunt with diminished systemic flow, as suggested by low femoral arterial flow velocities. As the LV output fell toward normal after ductus closure, the mean femoral arterial blood flow velocity rose to normal, suggesting improvement in effective systemic flow (2). Therefore, caution must be taken in interpreting changes in LV output in the presence of a PDA. A change in LV output may reflect only a change in ductus shunting, with no significant change in systemic flow. In these cases, knowledge of right ventricular (RV) output may be more meaningful. Preliminary studies (24) suggest that Doppler derived tricuspid valve flow may be the most reliable method of obtaining RV output and, thereby, systemic flow in these cases.

Other investigators have studied previously the relationship of LV myocardial contractility to aortic blood flow velocity and acceleration, dV/dt (9, 20, 23, 25, 26, 28). Although blood flow acceleration reflects contractile function under a variety of circumstances, most of these investigators have found that variable to be afterload dependent, as shown in our studies. Therefore dV/dt alone cannot be used to predict LV function accurately when afterload is changing. However, the relatively simple measurement, $T_{Vmax}$, has a strong negative correlation with LV dP/dt, independent of afterload, and may be useful in characterizing the myocardial contractile state. With currently available instrumentation, aortic flow velocity and $T_{Vmax}$ can be obtained non-invasively. Additional studies are in progress to determine whether or not these measurements are useful in the evaluation of patients with PDA, in shock, or receiving a variety of drugs affecting both inotropy and vascular resistance.

Further work must be done with Doppler methodology to improve its usefulness and application to the study of fetal and neonatal physiology. This technique has the potential for providing a better understanding of developmental circulatory physiology and perhaps for improving our management of patients with perinatal cardiorespiratory distress.

## Acknowledgements

The authors thank Marilyn Aldrich and Pam Angelus for help in performing the neonatal flow studies, Sue Corlew for performance of neonatal echocardiographic studies, and Jeanette D Sanchez for aid in preparation of the manuscript.

## References

1. Alverson D C, Eldridge M W, Dillon T, Yabek S M and Berman W Jr. Non-invasive pulsed Doppler determination of cardiac output in neonates and children. *Journal of Paediatrics,* 101, 46 (1982).

2. Alverson D C, Eldridge M W, Johnson J D et al. Effect of patent ductus arteriosus on left ventricular output in premature infants. *Journal of Paediatrics,* 102, 754 (1983).

3. Alverson D C, Eldridge M W, Johnson J D, Aldrich M, Angelus P and Berman W Jr. Non-invasive measurement of cardiac output in healthy preterm and term newborn infants. *American Journal of Perinatology,* 2, 148 (1984).

4. Alverson D C, Berman W Jr, Blomquist T, Eldridge M, Intress C and Christensen D. Assessment of myocardial contractility using pulsed Doppler ultrasound. American Physiological Society 1983 Meetings. *Physiologist,* 26, A-65 (1983).

5. Alverson D C and Berman W Jr. Non-invasive assessment of myocardial contractility with pulsed Doppler ultrasound. In *Pulsed Doppler Ultrasound in Clinical Pediatrics* . Chapter VI, section B, edited by W Berman Jr. Futura, Mt Kisco, NY (1983).

6. Berne M and Levy M N. The cardiac pump. In *Cardiovascular Physiology,* 4th edn., pp 71-93, Mosby, St Louis, Mo (1981).

7. Broughton A and Korner P I. Basal and maximal inotropic state in renal hypertensive dogs with cardiac hypertrophy. *American Journal of Physiology,* 245, 433 (1983).

8. Burnard E D, Granang A and Gray R E. Cardiac output in the newborn infant. *Clinical Science,* 31, 121 (1966).

9. Chung D C W, Chamberlain J H and Seed R G F L. The effect of haemodynamic changes on maximum blood flow acceleration at the aortic root in the anaesthetized, open chest dog. *Cardiovascular Research,* 8, 362 (1974).

10. Clapp J F, Szeto H H, Larrow R, Hewitt J and Mann L I. Umbilical blood flow response to embolization of the uterine circulation. *American Journal of Obstetrics and Gynecology,* 138, 60 (1980).

11. Cohn H E, Sacks E J, Heymann M A and Rudolph A M. Cardiovascular response to hypoxemia and acidemia in fetal lambs. *American Journal of Obstetrics and Gynecology,* 120, 817 (1974).

12. Cohn H E, Piasecki G J, and Jackson B T. The effect of fetal heart rate on cardiovascular function during hypoxemia. *American Journal of Obstetrics and Gynecology,* 138, 1190 (1980).

13. Danilowicz D, Rudolph A M and Hoffman J I E. Delayed closure of the ductus arteriosus in premature infants. *Pediatrics,* 37, 74 (1966).

14. Dawes G S. *Fetal and Neonatal Physiology,* edited by C A Smith and N M Nelson, p 91, Year Book Medical, Chicago (1968).

15. Divers W A, Wilkes M M, Babakina A and Yen S S C. Maternal smoking and elevation of catecholamines and metabolites in the amniotic fluid. *American Journal of Obstetrics and Gynecology,* 141, 625 (1981).

16. Eik-Nes S H, Brubakk A O and Ulstein J K. Measurement of human fetal blood flow. *British Medical Journal,* 280, 283 (1980).
17. Eldridge M W and Berman W Jr. Serial measurement of human fetal aortic blood flow. In *Pulsed Doppler Ultrasound in Clinical Pediatrics* . Chapter VI, section C, edited by W Berman Jr. Futura, Mt Kisco, NY (1983).
18. Eldridge M W, Alverson D C, Howard E A and Berman W Jr. Pulsed Doppler ultrasound: principles and instrumentation. In *Pulsed Doppler Ultrasound in Clinical Pediatrics* . Chapter I, edited by W Berman Jr. Futura, Mt Kisco, NY (1983).
19. Eldridge M W, Alverson D C and Berman W Jr. Non-invasive assessment of left ventricular function using pulsed Doppler ultrasound. *Pediatric Research,* 16, 99A, (abstract) (1982).
20. Emmanouilides G C. Persistent patency of the ductus arteriosus in premature infants: incidence, perinatal factors and natural history. In *Report of the 75th Ross Conference on Pediatric Research,* edited by M A Heymann and A M Rudolph, pp 63-68, Ross Laboratories, Columbus, Ohio (1978).
21. Gill R W, Trudinger B J, Garrett W J, Kossafh G and Warren P S. Fetal umbilical venous flow measured in utero by pulsed Doppler and B-mode ultrasound. *American Journal of Obstetrics and Gynecology,* 139, 720 (1981).
22. Heymann M A and Hoffman J I E. The problem of patent ductus arteriosus in premature infants. *Pediatrician,* 7, 3 (1978).
23. Kezdi P, Stanley E L, Marshall W J Jr and Kordenat R K. Aortic flow velocity and acceleration as an index of ventricular performance during myocardial infarction. *American Journal of Medical Science,* 257, 61 (1968).
24. Meijboom E, Valdes-Cruz L M, Sahn D J, Horowitz S, Scagnelli S, Larson D and Allen H D. Echo Doppler method for calculating volume flow across the triscuspid valve: validation in an open chest canine model and initial clinical studies. *Circulation,* 68, III-331 (abstract) (1983).
25. Nakamura Y, Takahashii M, Hattori S, and Ikeuchi S. The estimation of the ventricular function by means of peak aortic flow velocity - diastolic aortic pressure relationship. *Japan Heart Journal,* 21, 381 (1980).
26. Nutter D O, Noble R J and Hurst V W III. Peak aortic flow and acceleration as indices of ventricular performance in the dogs. *Journal of Laboratory and Clinical Medicine,* 11, 307, (1971).
27. Rudolph A M and Heymann M A. Circulatory changes during growth in the fetal lamb. *Circulation Research,* 26, 289 (1970).
28. VanDen Bos G C, Elzinga G, Westerhof N and Noble M I M. Problems in the use of indices of myocardial contractility. *Cardiovascular Research,* 7, 834 (1973).

Chapter 34

# On-Line monitoring of fetal blood flow velocities using pulsed Doppler ultrasound

**F Fallenstein, A Berec, K Vetter, A Huch, R Huch**

## Introduction

The Kranzbuehler 8130/8105 combination of an ultrasound real-time scanner and pulsed Doppler technique permits qualitative as well as quantitative investigations of blood flow in the fetal aorta and umbilical vein (3,5). In its most recent version this instrument combines a 3 MHz real-time scanner with a 2 MHz pulsed Doppler unit. Doppler shifts generated by flow directions towards and away from the transducer are processed separately in a two channel spectrum analyser. A section of 1.2 seconds of the Doppler spectra is displayed on-line on the video monitor together with the real-time image. Flow measurements are evaluated off-line from frozen images selected so as to show a Doppler signal record with a minimum of artefacts.

Our first experiences with this instrument in clinical research show particularly that the off-line evaluation of the Doppler signal is rather inconvenient for clinical use:

1 The stored data cover only a 1.2 second interval of monitoring time. Therefore only two or, at most, three fetal heart cycles can be investigated.

2 The off-line evaluation includes the positioning of different calipers manually and subsequent calculation of the mean Doppler frequency as a weighted average by an inbuilt microcomputer system. This procedure generally takes 2 minutes, even if an experienced operator is working with the instrument.

Because of these problems, the efficiency with which a patient is examined can be poor, especially when it becomes necessary to adjust the transducer to obtain good signal quality.

In order to overcome some of these problems, we designed a special electronic system which makes it possible to calculate the values of the mean Doppler frequencies on-line and continuously for either flow direction.

## Principle of operation

Assuming P(f) to be the power density function of a frequency spectrum, the mean frequency is expressed by the first moment of P(f), i.e.

$$\bar{f} = \frac{\int f \cdot P(f)df}{\int P(f)df} \qquad 1$$

where the integration has to be performed over the bandwidth of the spectrum (1,2,4).

In practice, the frequency spectrum of a signal is generally obtained by the method of Fast Fourier Transformation (FFT) giving a series of discrete amplitude components $A(ix\Delta f)$ ($i = 0...n$) at equally spaced frequency intervals $\Delta f$. The integrals in equation 1 are then replaced by sums and the power is expressed by the squared amplitude which is in fact the power in one load unit:

$$\bar{f} = \frac{\Sigma i \cdot \Delta f \cdot A^2(i \cdot \Delta f)}{\Sigma A^2(i \cdot \Delta f)} \qquad 2$$

Once the mean frequency of an ultrasound Doppler spectrum is known, the mean velocity can be calculated by

$$\bar{V} = \frac{\bar{f} \cdot c}{2 \cdot f_c \cdot \cos \alpha} \qquad 3$$

with c: ultrasound velocity
$f_c$: ultrasound transmitter frequency
$\cos \alpha$ : angle between ultrasound beam and flow direction.

## Technical design

The spectrum analyser of the Kranzbuehler instrument operates on the principle of FFT and is internally controlled by an MC 6800 microprocessor. The data from the spectrum analyser are digitally available in a bit-parallel word-serial format. A

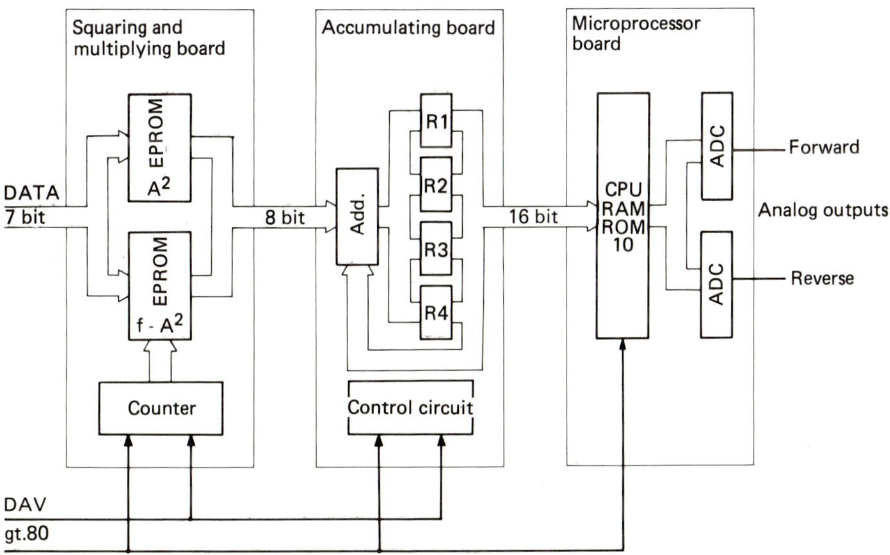


*Figure 1.* Schematic diagram of the on-line mean velocity processor for the use with the Kranzbuehler 8130/8105 US real-time and pulsed Doppler combination

complete spectrum sample consists of 80 values of the forward channel and 80 values of the reverse channel. One value, i.e. the amplitude of a single frequency line, is coded in a 7-bit binary word. Handshaking is performed by two control lines: 'data valid' coming with each data word, and 'greater 80' indicating the completion of one cycle.

Since the cycle rate of the spectrum analyser is 200 Hz, the average data output rate at the interface is 32 kHz, in practice about 40 kHz with short gaps between the cycles.

Using this interface for computing the mean frequency according to equation 2, the ancillary electronics must be able to perform squaring, multiplying and accumulating operations within 25 microseconds. Attempts to solve this solely by software with a conventional microcomputer system would fail because of timing problems. We therefore decided to use special hardware to construct the terms of numerator and denominator in equation 2 and to perform the division at the end of one cycle with a microcomputer which can do this easily within 5 milliseconds.

Figure 1 shows a schematic diagram of our device. It is divided into three functional blocks, each built on a printed circuit board of 100 x 160 mm size.

### 1 Squaring and multiplying board

These operations are performed by a table technique. The interface data lines are connected to the address lines of EPROMs which are programmed in such a way that the appropriate results can be read from the output lines with 8 bit accuracy. The squaring function uses 7 address lines of a 2716 EPROM corresponding to 128 bytes of information. As already mentioned, one cycle consists of 80 frequency lines, thus the binary coding of the frequencies also requires 7 bits. Consequently the multiplying function is performed with a 7 bit by 7 bit table which is programmed into a 27128 EPROM with 14 address lines and 16 kbytes of information. Frequency information is obtained from a binary counter which is incremented by the data valid signal (DAV), and reset to zero after the completion of a cycle by the greater 80 line (gt80).

### 2 Accumulating board

This part consists of a 16-bit binary adder and four 16-bit registers which build up the sums of the numerator (R1) and denominator (R2) from the forward channel Doppler spectra, and in the same way R3 and R4 for the reverse channel. Some additional circuitry controls the appropriate timing of the whole unit. The electronics of this board use bipolar integrated packages.

### 3 Microcomputer board

This is a self developed device for universal use in laboratory instrumentation purposes. Desgined as a minimum configuration with resident program memory, it contains an MCS 6503 8 bit-CPU, 128 bytes RAM, 2048 bytes EPROM, 16 programmable I/O lines, a timer and an automatic power on reset control. In addition, it is equipped with two 8 bit digital-analogue-converters for this special application. As soon as a frequency scan is complete, which is indicated by the gt80 line, the CPU immediately reads the contents of the registers R1 through R4 and saves them in the RAM, taking advantage of the small gap in the data stream from the spectrum analyser. Thus the first two boards are quickly free for processing the next cycle while the CPU has enough time to compute the quotients and to control the output of the results to the digital- analogue-converters.

Noise and artefacts in the Doppler spectra can be increased by the process described above, especially if the original Doppler signals are relatively weak. For this reason, we insert low pass filters between the analogue outputs and the recorder. A cut off frequency of 35 Hz has been found to achieve sufficient noise reduction without flattening physiological patterns significantly. Another pair of low pass filters with a cut off frequency of 1 Hz is provided to allow the recording of the mean blood flow velocity over a series of heart cycles.

The conversion from mean frequency to mean velocity according to equation 3 is only a matter of adjusting the gain of the recording device. For this purpose one can change the input of the spectrum analyser to a sine wave generator with constant frequency. Since ultrasound velocity and ultrasound transmitter frequency are constant, and the angle can be measured with a caliper on the video display of the real-time scanner, one can calibrate the recording in cm/second units by a simple attenuator which is provided with a degree-scale following the $1/\cos\alpha$ function.

The output signals are available in two different modes:

1 The signals of forward and reverse Doppler channels appear separately as positive and negative voltages respectively. This is advantageous if, for instance, one is monitoring venous blood flow in one channel, and noise signals cannot be removed from the other channel. In this case one can select and record only the appropriate channel.

2 The signals of either channel are summed to a single combined signal. This mode would be preferred when flow direction clearly changes in a vessel during one heart cycle, for example, in the *aorta descendens,* of adult subjects.

## Clinical examples

Although we designed our system primarily for fetal monitoring, the first *in vivo* example presented here is the record of the mean aortic blood flow velocity in a healthy male adult subject (Figure 2).

This section, covering 10 seconds, is taken in the combined mode, showing clearly the reversal of flow direction between systolic maximum and diastolic minimum.

Figure 3 is a selection of four fetal measurements in the *aorta descendens* . Each section is 10 seconds long and shows both the mean blood flow velocity curve and the corresponding averaged velocity (smooth lines).

Subject A:

A 40-year-old fifth-gravida, 33 weeks of gestation, anti-c antibodies - with normal amniocenteses so far. The estimated weight of the fetus was 2200 g. The flow

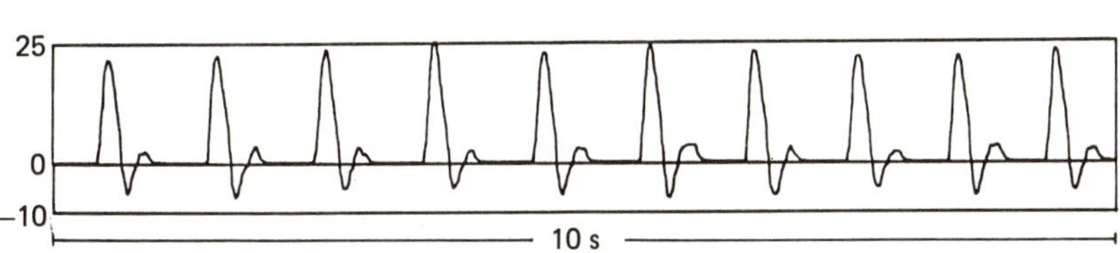


*Figure 2.* Mean blood flow velocity, measured in the descending aorta of a healthy male adult

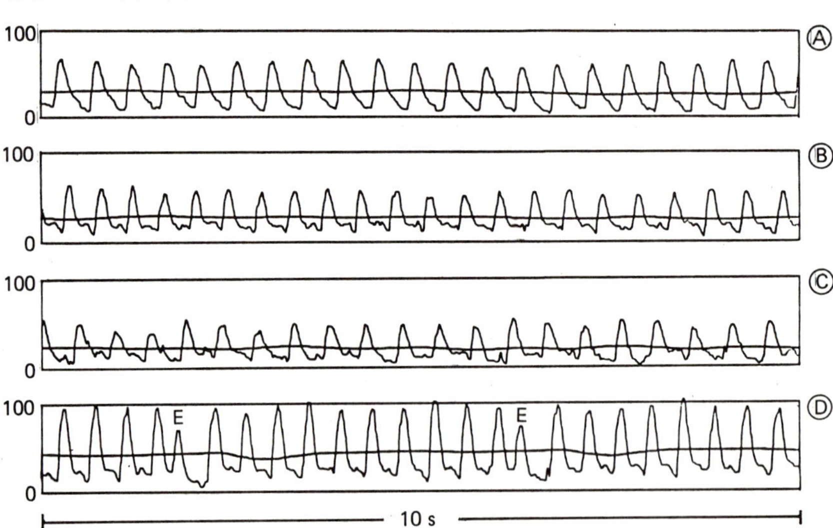


*Figure 3.* Mean blood flow velocity and averaged velocity (smooth lines), measured in the descending aorta of four fetuses (see text for more detailed clinical information)

characteristics were as expected for a normal pregnancy without fetal anaemia. The flow velocity was 30 cm/second, estimated flow was 486 ml/minute or 221 ml/minute per kg.

Subject B:

A 24-year-old primigravida with polytoxicomania in the 33rd week of pregnancy. The baby was born 2 days after this measurement after spontaneous rupture of the membranes. It was a girl of 2490 g with a good adaptation. The flow characteristics were quite normal with a velocity of 29 cm/second and an estimated flow of 514/ml/minute or 207 ml/minute per kg.

Subject C:

A 31-year-old second gravida, at 38 weeks of gestation. The fetus was a somewhat smaller than ideal. The aorta was wider than expected and the flow velocity, at 24 cm/second, was less than in the previous cases. The estimated flow was 654 ml/minute or 242 ml/minute per kg.

Subject D:

A 27-year-old primigravida at 34 weeks of pregnancy. She had premature contractions and was under tocolytic therapy. In addition she has slight diabetes mellitus and a large fetus of the order of 2700 g. The flow data are characterized by a quite high velocity, 44 cm/second, as is expected with beta-2-mimetic agents. Thus the flow is 786 ml/minute or 291 ml/minute per kg. This section of measurement shows two extrasystolic cardiac cycles (E) of the fetus causing a slight temporary decrease in the averaged flow velocity trace.

## References

1. Atkinson P and Woodcock J P. *Doppler ultrasound and its use in clinical measurement.* London, Academic Press, (1982).

2. Eik-nes St et al. Noninvasive Messung des fetalen Blutstromes mittels Ultraschall. In *Ultraschall,* 2, 226-231 (1981).

3. Fallenstein F et al. Probleme bei der quantitativen nicht-invasiven Erfassung von Blutfluessen mit Hilfe der Spektral-alalyse von US-Pulsed-Doppler-Signalen. In *Ultraschalldiagnostik 82,* Interventionelle Sonographie, edited by R Ch Otto and F X Jann, pp. 177-180 Stuttgard-New York, Thieme, 177-180 (1983).

4. Fish J P. Recent advances in cardio-vascular doppler. In *Progress in Medical Ultrasound 2,* edited by A Kurjak, pp. 217-231 Amsterdam, Excerpta Medica (1981).

5. Warnking R et al. Noninvasive Bestimmung des fetalen Blutflussvolumens. In *Ultraschall 2,* 232-234 (1981)

Chapter 35

# Fetal heart rate variability calculated by an external technique during pregnancy

**J Melchior, N Bernard, Ph Magne**

## Comment in response to Professor G S Dawes' Keynote Lecture

Since 1980, in an attempt to obtain more accurate and objective fetal heart rate assessment, we have used a system in which a calculator is connected to a cardiotocograph. In an earlier study, the analogue output of the fetal monitor, model HP 8020, fed a rectangular pulse, synchronous with the QRS-wave peak, to a peripheral unit, then to a calculator, model HP 9825 A. R-R interval measurements were quite accurate, but the system was only working with a direct ECG signal, which restricted its use to intrapartum applications only after the membranes had been ruptured.

Short-term variability has been shown to be one of the most important indicators of fetal well-being, and as we are convinced of its high predictive value, particularly before labour, we wanted to derive this index from an external method. Thus successive antenatal recordings could be compared and fetal risk assessed.

We have found the abdominal ECG technique to be generally unsuccessful, and we had to wait for the development of an improved monitor, model HP 8040, to measure with good accuracy the periodicity of the signals obtained from an external method. This instrument performs a correlation processing technique measuring the periodicity from the Doppler ultrasound signals, as well as from a suitable direct ECG signal. A digital output is available, data being acquired, stored and processed by a calculator, model HP 85.

In order to evaluate the new monitor, we first compared fetal heart rate records obtained simultaneously on the same fetus, from an internal direct ECG and from the external auto-correlated ultrasound signal. The same monitor model (HP 8040) was used for both.

For each trace, the number of epochs to be recorded is chosen, as well as the number of intervals to be measured. The total duration varies from 20 to 30 minutes. The following parameters are calculated for each epoch:

Frequency (bpm)
Oscillations (bpm)
Interval index (from YEH)
Variability (msec)
S.d. variability (msec)
Differential index (from YEH)

Module (from de Haan)
Argument (from de Haan)

If required, an orthochronogram can be plotted from these results using the calculator; the scale is then 15 points/cm.

We are now evaluating the system in all of our routine antenatal monitoring cases so that the best parameter may be defined in terms of its predictive value for the condition of the fetus and its outcome.

Part 5

# Signal Processing

Chapter 36

# Detection of components of autonomic cardiac control by time series analysis of heart rate in lambs: technical report

**A S I Siimes, I A T Välimäki, R T Oja, K J Antila**

## Introduction

The activity of cardiovascular chronotropic control is related to the well-being of fetuses and neonates. Therefore patterns of heart rate (HR) and heart rate variability (HRV) are routinely examined by fetal and neonatal monitoring to detect and predict perinatal hazards. Current knowledge concerning the interaction between vagal and sympathetic cardiac control is rather limited in fetuses (5) and neonates in spite of extensive clinical investigation. In this research project we wanted to study the influence of the autonomic nervous system on heart rate by experiments in chronic lamb models. This report is a description of the operative and computer techniques developed for the HR analysis.

## Signal acquisition

### Experimental procedures

Pregnant sheep of known gestational age (110-136 days, term in Finnish breed 143 days) were operated on under low spinal anaesthesia. Polyvinyl catheters were placed into the maternal femoral artery and vein, into the fetal carotid artery, jugular vein and trachea as well as into the amniotic cavity. Silver electrodes were implanted into the fetal thorax for recording an ECG signal and under one upper eyelid for recording fetal eye movements. Neonatal lambs were operated on under local anaesthesia at the age of 3 days. Catheters were inserted into the carotid artery and jugular vein, and ECG electrodes were implanted bilaterally into the chest wall. The catheters and electrodes were tunnelled under the skin and kept in a nylon pocket, the vascular catheters were filled with heparin solution. The animal was allowed to recover from the operation for at least 3 days. The fetal studies were carried out until the time of delivery and the neonatal lambs were studied until the age of 2 months.

Recordings of ECG through a neonatal monitor (512 Neonatal Monitor, Corometrics Medical Systems Inc, Wallingford, Ct, USA), fetal eye movements, arterial blood pressure, intra-amniotic pressure and intratracheal pressure and/or transthoracic impedance were simultaneously made on paper and magnetic tape by a high quality seven-channel FM tape recorder (Philips Analog 7) under visual control with a four-channel oscilloscope (Figure 1).

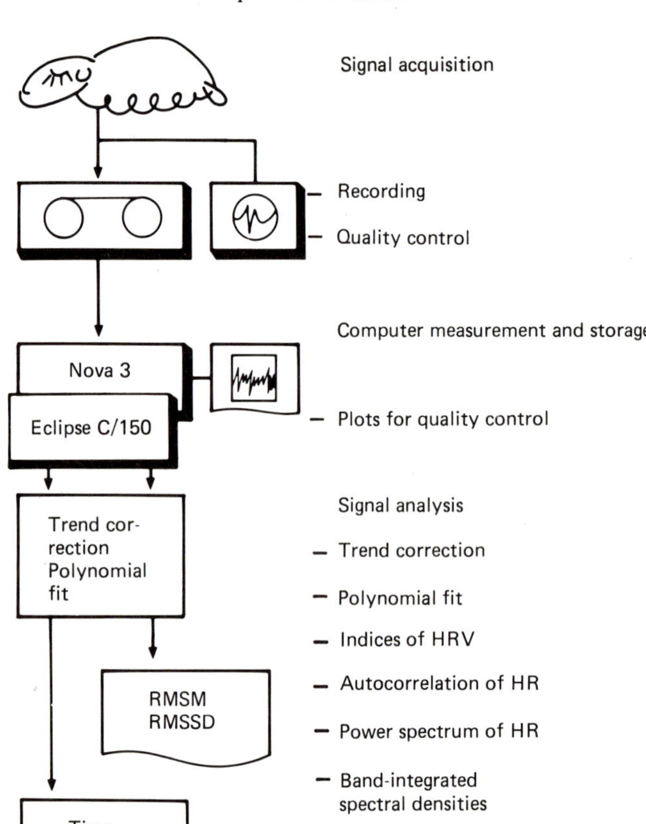


*Figure 1.* Signal acquisition and analysis of heart rate variation

Atropine as sulphate (0.1-0.2 mg/kg), propranolol (1-2 mg/kg) and/or phenoxybenzamine (1-2 mg/kg) were given intravenously to the lamb to generate vagal and/or sympathetic adrenergic blockade. Thereafter the recordings were repeated. Both fetal and neonatal arterial blood were sampled for acid-base and pH measurements. The acid-base remained normal during the experiments.

## HR signal preprocessing

After the series of experiments the records were analysed off-line. The ECG was played back at eight times real-time speed. The ECG was band-pass filtered at the typical frequency range of the QRS complex (8-25 Hz, real-time). An adjustable threshold trigger was used to generate a trigger pulse for each R-wave under visual quality control. This time series was fed into a minicomputer (NOVA 3, Data General Corp, Southboro Ma, USA) through a special-purpose interface which measured the R-R intervals with a resolution of 1 ms (Figure 1). The series of R-R intervals was stored on the computer disc memory for further analyses. These were carried out in a compatible minicomputer with higher processing capacity (ECLIPSE C/150, Data General Corp). Representative stationary records of 90 seconds duration of ECG were selected, short enough to assure a stable sleep state. However, a 90- second period was considered to be the minimum period to obtain adequate signal length. In some cases a longer segment of the signal was measured, for more reliable analysis of low-frequency components of HRV. Records containing ectopic cardiac arrhythmias, noise artefacts or sudden large changes in heart rate were avoided or corrected by an error rejection algorithm.

## Signal analysis

### Indices of HRV

The computer was programmed to identify the mean, the minimum and maximum instantaneous heart rates and to compute the mean R-R interval, the root mean square of the differences from the mean (RMSM, representing the overall variation of HR) and the RMS value of successive R-R interval differences (RMSSD, the beat-to-beat variation of HR). The coefficients of variation, CV (percentage of RMSM from the mean R-R interval) and CVS (percentage of RMSSD from the mean R-R interval) were calculated for indices of relative HRV (1, 11, 12). The indices of HRV were computed before and after detrending the signal with a fourth order polynomial approximation.

### Dynamic plots of HRV

To depict dynamics of cardiac control the instantaneous HRV indices were computed using a moving window technique of 50 successive R-R intervals. The window was moved in steps of one R-R interval through the whole record. For visual display and quality control, both the instantaneous HR signal and the HRV signals were plotted as a function of time to illustrate the stationarity of HR in the record (Figure 2a).

### The use of autocorrelation function (autocorrelogram)

Major periodic components of HRV were investigated by computing an autocorrelation function for each series of R-R intervals (Figure 2b). Linear trends were removed before this computation by computing the linear regression and subtracting it from the original signal. The autocorrelogram was computed up to a lag period needed to visualize three successive periodic components (3).

### Spectral analysis of HR

In order to investigate components of periodic HRV in detail the R-R intervals were low-pass filtered and sampled equally spaced using a SIN(X)/X digital filter. The cut-off frequency was selected on the basis of the lowest heart rate of the signal (cut-off frequency = 1/2 x the lowest instantaneous HR, the Nyquist criterion (6)). To remove slow trends from the signal a polynomial approximation up to a fourth order was used (Figure 2e). A discrete fast Fourier transform was then applied and the power spectrum of the signal was computed from the Fourier transform (Figure 2f).

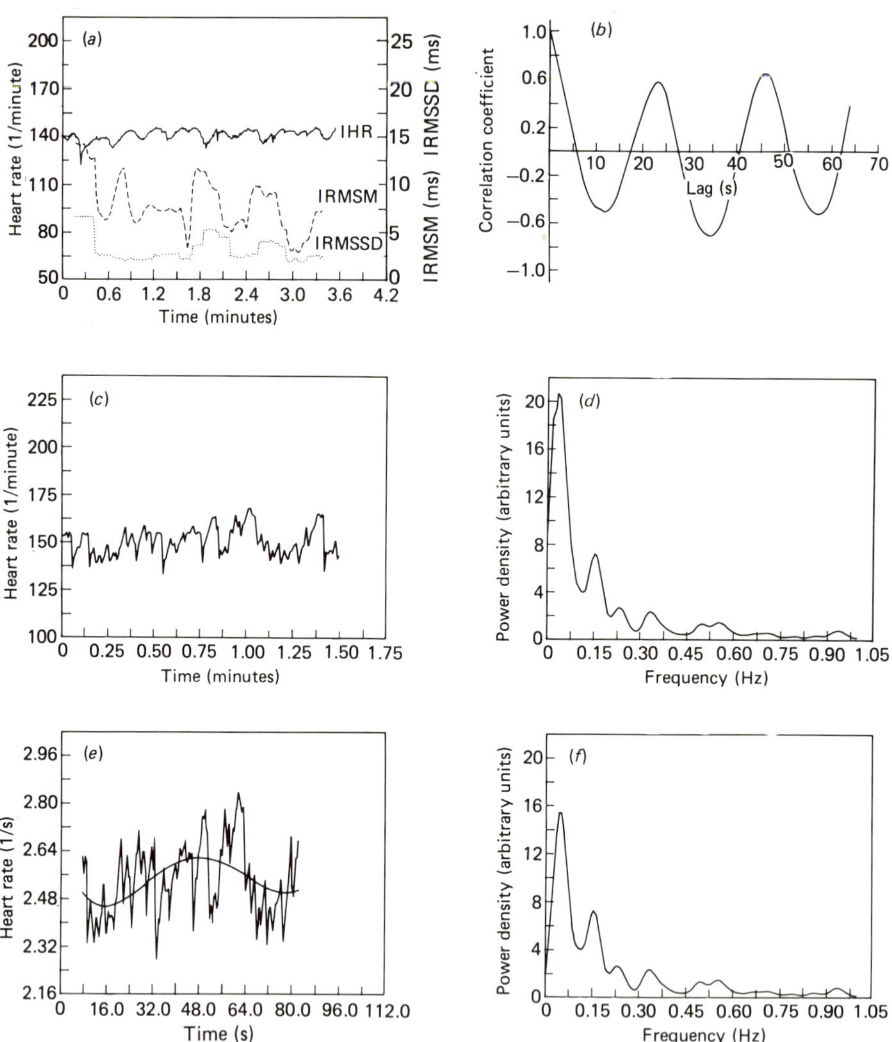


*Figure 2.* (*a*) Instantaneous heart rate (IHR) presenting a sinusoidal pattern and instantaneous HRV indices: IRMSM and IRMSSD computed from a 3.5 minute record of R-R intervals in a fetal lamb (gestation age 122 days) during alpha-adrenergic blockade. Instantaneous indices of HRV were computed using a moving window of 50 successive R-R intervals. (*b*) Autocorrelogram for the same signal presenting one periodic component with a cycle length of 23 s (0.043 Hz). (*c*) Plot of instantaneous HR of a 44-day-old lamb, no medication. (*d*) Power spectrum computed for the signal in *Figure 2c* after using a Sin(X)/X digital low-pass filter and elimination of linear trend. (*e*) Plot of the HR signal in *Figure 2c* after Sin(X)/X filtering. The fourth order polynomial trend approximation is plotted on top of the signal. (*f*) Power spectrum of the heart rate signal in *Figure 2e* after polynomial trend correction

## Spectral bands

The power spectra of individual records were then divided into ten bands from 0 to 1.0 Hz. The power spectrum was integrated over each frequency band to achieve a considerable data reduction (9). Data points representing a certain frequency band of each record were combined to generate average spectral densities for intergroup comparisons (Figure 3).

## Results

### Indices of HRV

In fetal lambs RMSM (after detrending of the signal) was in the range of 2-15 ms, and RMSSD in the range of 1-12 ms. In neonatal lambs RMSM varied from 9 to 45 ms, and RMSSD from 7 to 43 ms. During the period of 6-13 days after birth the mean RMSM ± s.d. was 14.4 ± 3.0 ms, and the mean RMSSD 9.4 ± 2.1 ms, and the corresponding coefficients of variation CV 5.1 ± 1.1% and CVS 3.3 ± 0.7%, respectively (n=20).

### Effect of autonomic blockade on HRV

Figure 4 shows power spectra computed before medication and after adrenergic blockade (alpha- and beta-blockade, phenoxybenzamine 1 mg/kg, propranolol 2 mg/kg i.v.) as well as after the triple blockade (alpha-blockade, beta-blockade and atropine 0.1 mg/kg i.v.) in a 44-day-old lamb. After the triple or complete autonomic blockade RMSM decreased from 16.5 to 1.6 ms, and RMSSD from 12.0 to 1.0 ms. In the power spectrum the remaining HRV was found at the low frequencies of less than 0.1 Hz.

### Intergroup comparisons by band integration

Figure 3 shows averages (±s.e.m.) of band integrated power spectra of eight neonatal lambs (aged from 7 to 31 days) before and after treatment with atropine 0.1 mg/kg i.v. Atropine resulted in a significant decrease of power at high-frequency bands from 0.12 to 1.00 Hz. When the relative distribution of the total power in the frequency bands (%) was computed for each record, the relative amount of the power in the frequency bands below 0.09 Hz was found to be increased while the relative amount of power in the frequency bands from 0.12 to 1.00 Hz was decreased.

## Interpretation and discussion

Because our main interest was the effect of nervous control on sinus rhythm, it was extremely important to remove all artefacts and/or arrhythmias from the signal because they resulted in a large increase in the RMSM and RMSSD and also caused a distortion of the power spectrum. After the use of an automatic error rejection and correction algorithm (1) the signal was inspected visually and corrected manually when needed. The preprocessing of the signals was an interactive procedure requiring a considerable amount of human effort and time. However, it was an absolutely necessary step to obtain error-free data for the analysis.

HRV indices of the original R-R interval series were computed to estimate the total variability of the HR. The detrending of the signal with a fourth order polynomial approximation resulted in a residual HRV and this was seen as a reduction of RMSM. RMSSD did not decrease by detrending the signal.

In most cases the fourth order polynomial trend correction appeared optimal to obtain a sufficient stationarity of the signal without loss of information at the

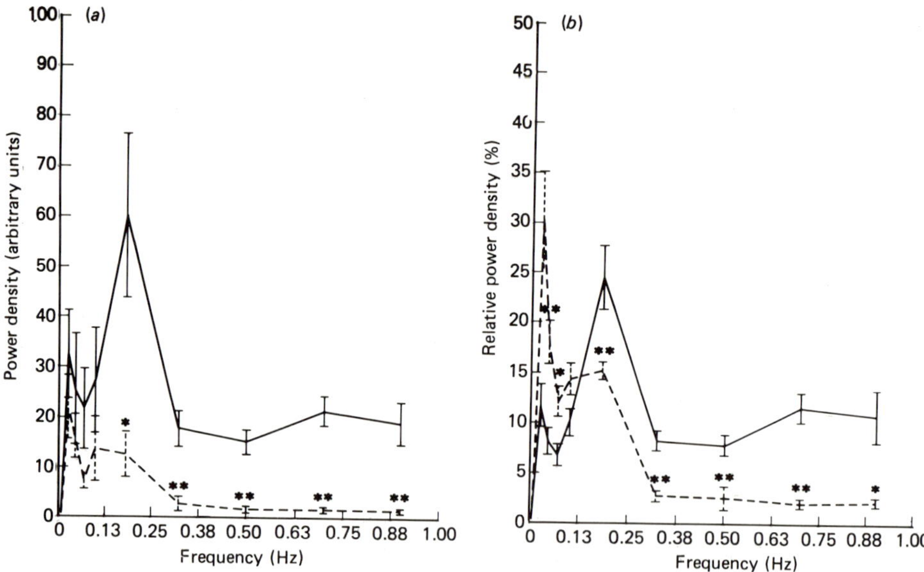


*Figure 3.* (*a*) Average band integrals of power spectra (±s.e.m.) of eight neonatal lambs before and after treatment with atropine. Fourth order polynomial trend correction was used on the signals. (*b*) The same data as in *Figure 3a*, each individual spectrum computed as the relative distribution of power in the spectrum (%). — control; ---- atropine; * p⟨0.05; ** p⟨0.01

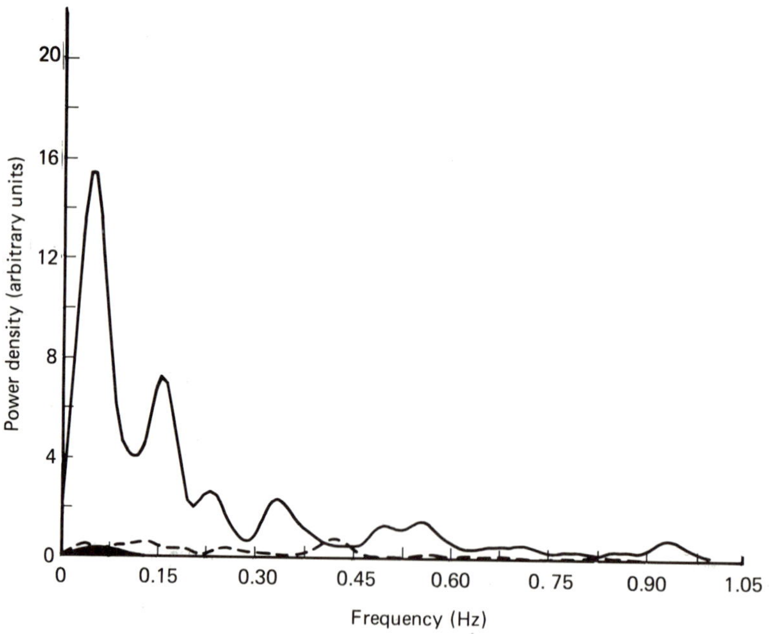


*Figure 4.* Power spectra for the heart rate of a neonatal lamb computed after Sin(X)/X filtering and fourth order polynomial trend correction before medication, after alpha- and beta-adrenergic blockade and after simultaneous sympathetic and parasympathetic blockade. — control; ---- after adrenergic blockade (alpha and beta); ▬ after adrenergic and cholinergic blockade

frequencies of interest, equal to or greater than 0.04 Hz. The components of the signal with a frequency less than 0.02 Hz were removed in the detrending procedure in the records of 90 seconds' duration. The order of the polynomial must thus be decided on the basis of the frequency range of interest and the duration of the sample. SIN(X)/X digital low-pass filtering was used on the signal to sample the original R-R interval sequence equispaced and to prepare it for time series analysis. The filtering caused a reduction of the original signal length by 10 seconds at both ends (window width 20 seconds) and this had to be considered when selecting the length of the original samples.

Before the autocorrelation analysis the data were detrended with linear trend correction. The autocorrelation analysis was found to be convenient in the visual analysis of a process with one to two periodicities in it or in the identification of a random process.

The cut-off frequency was chosen to be incorporated in the computer program on the basis of the longest R-R interval in the original series using the Nyquist criterion to avoid aliasing errors. This results in a different cut-off frequency in each sample. The sampling frequency was chosen to be at least 2.2 times the cut-off frequency. Different sampling frequencies may result in different power densities in the power spectra, and therefore the sampling frequency and cut-off frequency were selected to be fixed, when computing integrated power densities and comparing their values between different animals. The higher heart rate of fetal lambs permitted computation of the power spectrum to a higher frequency than in neonatal lambs with a lower heart rate. Because of this the arrhythmia caused by respiratory movements of the fetus (4) may be visible in the power spectrum (10), in spite of the fact that the fetal respiration rate may be higher than that of the neonatal lamb.

Spectral analysis of the heart rate was the most informative way to display and quantify the different components of the HRV and their changes during autonomic blockade. Computation of the HRV indices showed that by total autonomic nervous blockade the residual HRV after detrending decreased by 90%. Power spectrum analysis of the heart rate indicated that most of the variation left was at the frequencies of less than 0.10 Hz. Based on studies in adult men, it is thought that power around 0.1 Hz results from blood pressure regulation while high-frequency variation results from respiration (7). However, low-frequency components of HRV around 0.02-0.05 Hz may result from the regulation of peripheral vasomotor activity and skin temperature (7,9) or from humoral regulation, possibly mediated by the renin-angiotensin system, as has been described in dogs (2).

The power spectrum analysis of the heart rate in the atropine experiments in neonatal lambs showed that the effect of atropine on the HRV was more pronounced at frequencies higher than 0.12 Hz. This accords with the earlier reports showing that the cholinergic system is capable of causing fast changes in the heart rate (8).

## Conclusions

The impact of autonomic cardiac control on HRV in fetal and neonatal lambs was depicted by time series analysis using time services analysis. Calculation of HRV indices gave the information of the direction and magnitude of the change in HRV, and whether it occurred in overall or beat-to-beat variation or in both. Power spectrum analysis showed in which frequencies the original HRV and the HRV after physiological changes or pharmacological manipulation were found. We conclude that time series analysis, especially the power spectrum analysis, is a valuable method in the investigation of physiological control mechanisms of heart rate during the perinatal period.

## Acknowledgements

This work has been supported by The Sigrid Juselius Foundation, the Academy of Finland and Finnish Cultural Foundation, which is gratefully acknowledged. The bedside Corometric Neonatal Monitor 512 was kindly provided for our use by Kone Instrument Division, Kivenlahti, Finland. We also thank Mr Lauri Halkola, Ms Mervi Julkunen, Ms Ulla Martin and the personnel of the College of Veterinary Medicine for their contribution to the project.

## References

1. Antila K. Quantitative characterization of heart rate during exercise. *Scandinavian Journal of Clinical and Laboratory Investigation,* 153, Suppl 39, 1-68 (1979).
2. Akselrod S, Gordon D, Ubel F A, Shannon D C, Barger A C and Cohen R J. Power spectrum analysis of heart rate fluctuation: a quantitative probe of beat-to-beat cardiovascular control. *Science,* 213, 220-222 (1981).
3. Campbell K. Ultradian rhythms in the human fetus during the last ten weeks of gestation: a review. *Seminars in Perinatology,* 4, 301-309 (1980).
4. Dalton K J, Dawes G S and Patrick J E. Diurnal, respiratory and other rhythms of fetal heart rate in lambs. *American Journal of Obstetrics and Gynecology,* 127, 414-424 (1977).
5. Dalton K J, Dawes G S and Patrick J E. The autonomic nervous system and fetal heart rate variability. *American Journal of Obstetrics and Gynecology,* 146, 456-462 (1983).
6. Jenkins G M and Watts D G. Fourier analysis. In *Spectral Analysis and Its Applications,* 16-56, Cambridge, Holden-Day (1969).
7. Kitney R I and Rompelman O. (Editors). *The Study of Heart Rate Variability,* Oxford, Clarendon Press (1980).
8. Kollai M and Koizumi K. Reciprocal and non-reciprocal action of the vagal and sympathetic nerves innervating the heart. *Journal of the Autonomic Nervous System,* 1, 33-52 (1979).
9. Lindqvist A, Oja R, Hellman O and Välimäki I. Impact of thermal vasomotor control on the heart rate variability of newborn infants. *Early Human Development,* 8, 37-47 (1983).
10. Siimes A S I and Välimäki I A T. Variability of heart rate and respiration rate in fetal and newborn lambs. Preliminary experience. In *Advances in Paediatric Heart-Rate Variability Analysis,* edited by I A T Välimäki and K J Antila. Turku, Finland, Annales Universitatis Turkuensis, Series D (in press).
11. Tarlo P A, Välimäki I A T and Rautaharju P M. Quantitative computer analysis of cardiac and respiratory activity in newborn infants. *Journal of Applied Physiology,* 31, 70-75 (1971).
12. Välimäki I A T, Rautaharju P M, Roy S B and Scott K E. Heart rate patterns in healthy term and premature infants and in respiratory distress syndrome. *European Journal of Cardiology,* 1, 411-419 (1974).

Chapter 37

# Computation and evaluation of heart-rate and stroke volume oscillations in fetal lambs

**J Morgenstern, T Abels, R Leblanc, T Somville**

## Methods and Materials

Date were derived from seven chronically instrumented fetal lambs with weights ranging from 2900-3200 g, and gestational ages from 128-134 days. Up to 16 cardiovascular variables were measured during 60 different study periods and stored on-line on digital tapes. The data could be observed during the digitizing process. There was a total monitoring time of approximately 60 hours, containing 350 000 heart beats. The most commonly selected sampling rate was 2 or 3 ms, and in a few cases this was changed to 5 or 6 ms.

A typical control picture (2 ms sampling rate) for a few heart cycles is shown in Figure 1. The top two traces refer to electromagnetically measured flows in the ascending aorta (AsAo) and the pulmonary trunk (PA), respectively, while the third trace shows the ECG. The subsequent traces are the arterial blood pressure (Pa) in the ascending aorta, the heart sounds and the Pa in the descending aorta (DAo). Traces 4 and 6 are measured with Millar-Catheters while trace 8, the Pa in the AsAo, was also measured with an open-ended catheter. Trace 9 is the electromagnetically measured flow in the DAo. Traces 10, 12 and 14 are the pressure in the inferior vena cava (IVC), pressure in the thorax (THO) and the intra-amniotic pressure (IA), respectively. An interesting ectopic beat occurs which causes a large increase in stroke volume (traces 1, 2 and 9).

## Extraction of oscillations in FHR

Oscillations of fetal heart rate (OSC) are defined by their amplitude and number of complete cycles per minute (3). In order to separate OSC from any trace, two different groups of algorithms were studied: those parameter dependent (2 methods) and those parameter independent (4 methods) . The parameter dependent methods are:
a) moving average over x points
b) convex envelope, i.e. the positive extreme values form an upper borderline, while the negative values form a lower borderline. Each point in a borderline was connected to x/2 previous and x/2 following points within the same borderline. The extreme borders form the convex envelope with the OSCs varying about the line in between.

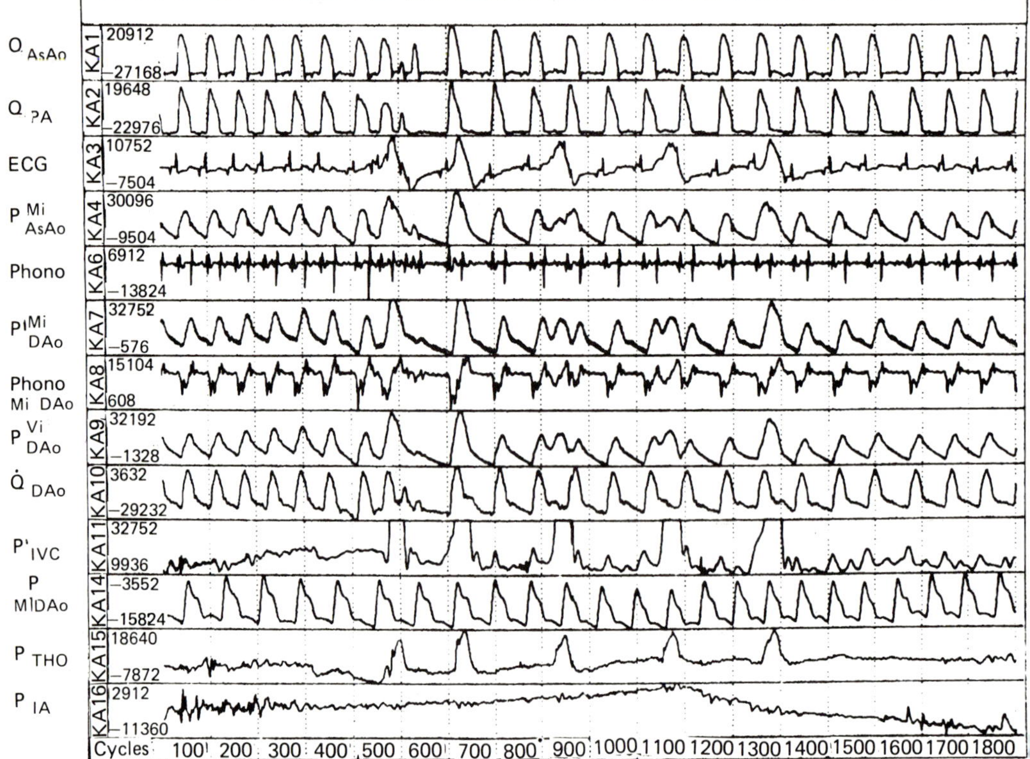


*Figure 1.* Original records during the digitizing process. Q = flow; P = pressure; AsAo = ascending aorta; DAo = descending aorta; PA = pulmonary artery; IVC = inferior vena cava; THO = thoracic; Mi = Millar-catheter; Vi = vinyl-catheter; M = maternal

The parameter independent methods are
c) envelope peak-to-peak, i.e. the line runs in between the upper and lower borderline through the weighted extreme values.
d) extreme-to-extreme, i.e. the line runs through the mean values of two successive extreme values.

Methods c) and d) were modified to e) and f), respectively by taking into account the turning points. It could easily be shown that only parameter independent methods c) to f) give reliable and reproducible results.

Examples of two of these methods are shown in Figure 2. At the top of this figure a 1-minute FHR trace (left) is shown with the corresponding stroke volume (SV) trace (right), calculated from the flow in the ascending aorta. In the middle of Figure 2, these original tracings are now shown dotted, while the solid lines are derived from a a moving average process. In the bottom of the figure, the solid lines were derived from the envelope peak-to-peak including turning points. The differences in these two methods are striking, but overall the total number of OSC does not differ much. The best method - Figure 2, bottom traces - was selected visually by a highly experienced clinician and simultaneously by a method described elsewhere (5).

The number of SV-OSC is higher than FHR-OSC. This fact has a simple explanation. While the FHR-OSCs are only based on the beat-to-beat time periods,

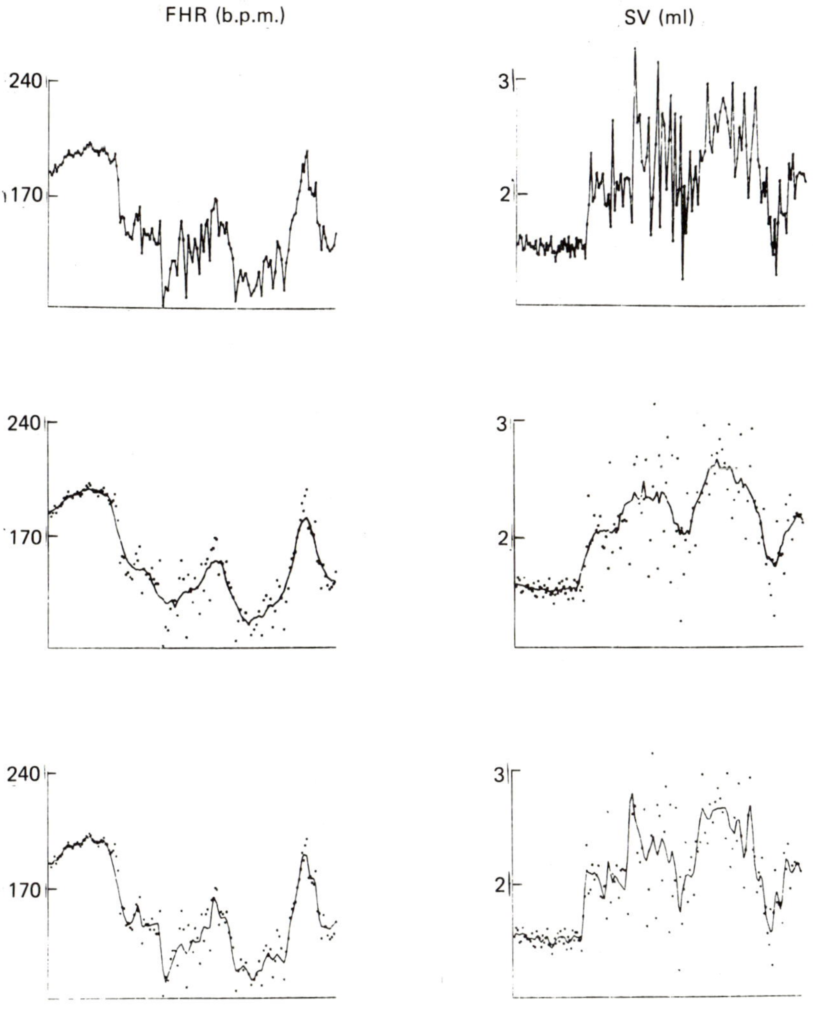


*Figure 2.* Top: one-minute FHR (left) and corresponding SV-traces (right). Middle: moving average (+ 3 beats) with the original trace dotted. Bottom: extreme-to-extreme including turning points with the original trace dotted

the SV-OSCs are based on a beat-to-beat SV pulse integration. (At this point it is worth mentioning that in some episodes the flow zero-line drifted. Therefore for each flow beat an individual flow-zero was calculated.) The SV-values are almost always different and already three beats may form an OSC. Therefore the number of OSCs related to SV is very much dependent on a moving average procedure carried out before starting the actual OSC evaluation. A scatter plot with the number of moving average points versus the number of OSCs shows that the number of OSC declines with the number of moving average points. At about 15 moving average points (beats) both the FHR and SV end up with about 10 OSC/minute.

From each OSC several parameters were calculated: total duration (Dt), duration of the positive shape (Dp), total amplitude (APt), area of the positive shape (Ap)

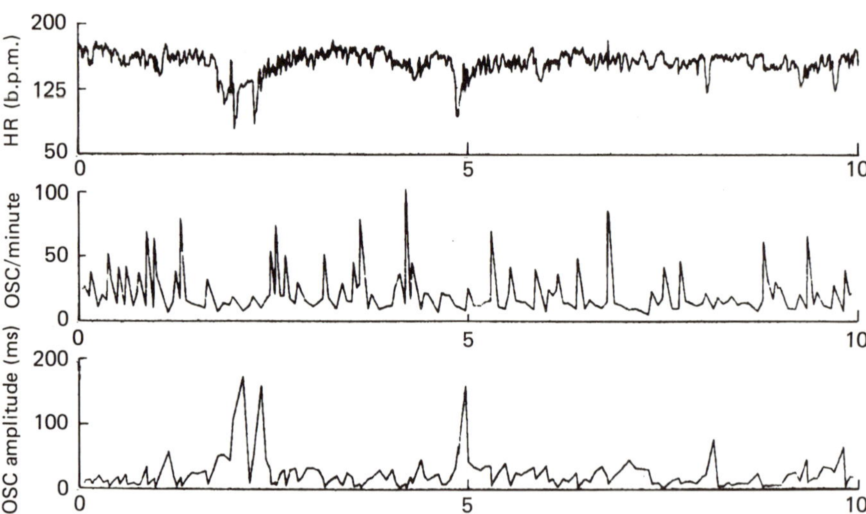


*Figure 3.* From top to bottom: FHR-trace, number of OSC per minute instantaneously calculated from each OSC and the corresponding OSC-amplitude

and the number of heart beats per OSC (N). From these, several other parameters, e.g. the degree of asymmetry concerning the duration and/or amplitude, could be calculated. Furthermore, the new instantaneous parameter, number of OSCs per minute (OSC/minute) was calculated from each Dt, and in the same way the instantaneous FHR in beats per minute (b.p.m.) is calculated from each RR-interval. In Figure 3 (middle trace), this parameter is plotted parallel to the FHR (top trace). The third trace shows the corresponding OSC-APt. These new parameters, which are comparable to summing up absolute values of beat-to-beat FHR differences - defined as rate of alteration speed (2), reflect in a reliable, quick and easy way specific changes in FHR-OSC. Since they are very simple and a real-time evaluation is possible, we would like to recommend them as new on-line FHR parameters.

From 7922 FHR-OSC and 3611 SV-OSC the following results are derived. Since the histograms are not normally distributed, and in order to be able to compare the results with common clinical knowledge and other publications, the median values are calculated and used in addition to the mean values.

In summary, on average 10 (6) heart beats form an FHR-(SV)-OSC, an OSC lasts for 3.5 (2) s, has an At of 6.5 ms (0.27 ml) and about 17 (26) OSC/minute were calculated. Since the total number of FHR- and SV-OSC are not equal and *a priori* the time t(i) when the i-th FHR-OSC starts does not match with the time when the i-th SV-OSC starts, an interpolation procedure was used in order to correlate these time series. This evaluation is still in progress.

## OSC treated as a stationary stochastic process

Sustained OSC may be attributed to the existence of a feedback control system regulating the output. In our approach we made the assumption that many biological feedback control systems, related in specific ways, have an output which exhibits random or fluctuating properties. Thus the observed records could be regarded as a number of an abstract ensemble of functions, called stochastic process. Changes in one of the closed loops may take the system out of its stationarity. Therefore we tried to identify OSC records as random processes, in order to detect typical traces where the process becomes non-random. From a record of such a time series, it is not usually possible to predict future values, except probabilistically from its past values.

The recognition of where the process begins to change its characteristics may be of diagnostic value, since the well accepted clinical knowledge describes, e.g. the FHR-OSC (3) by its amplitude and frequency.

In a certain stationary range, the output is oscillating - generated by a linear aggregation of random shocks - about a line of stability. If such a time series exhibits an instance of non-stationarity in variance, it will need time to return to its starting level, although the cause of generation - the random shocks - have not changed. Thus, even such processes without strictly independent parts, (i.e. where the autocorrelation function (acf) is not zero) could be treated as though they were random (Figure 4, top left).

In Figure 4, a FHR trace of about 30 minutes is shown. This trace was divided into 73 subtraces and the acf and partial autocorrelation function (pacf) were calculated and plotted in one diagram (Figure 4, top left and right). The mean acf and pacf with the corresponding s.d. are shown underneath. Although the mean acf tails down after about 5-7 points and the s.d. is constant overall, there are many sub-acf which do not behave like this. The pacf cuts off very quickly in nearly all cases. In some situations the acf is useful because it contains all the information about a random process that can be extracted from the spectrum, and it gives a visual picture

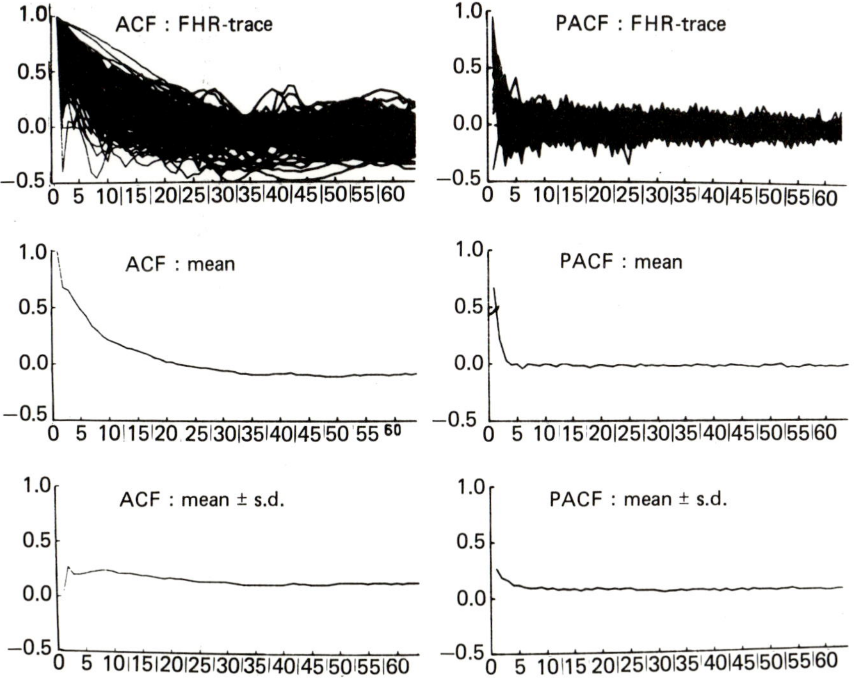


*Figure 4.* From top to bottom: FHR-trace 73 acf and pacf curves successively from the FHR-trace, corresponding mean acf and pacf curves with their s.d. values

of the way in which the dependence in the time series is damped out with the lag between points in the series.

Since the simplest type of stochastic process is a linear process, which can be generated by a linear operation on a purely random process, the two special cases of the linear process - autoregressive and moving average process (ARMA) - were chosen.

The unpredictable distortion mentioned above, which causes a deviation from equilibrium, together with the fact that the distortions are additive with a limited time decay, could be modelled by a moving average (MA) process. If an actual point could be estimated e.g. by a weighted sum of previous points including a distortion $\varepsilon_j$ of a MA-type, an autoregressive part in the model seems reasonable. The $\varepsilon_j$, which represent in this case the OSC, may be regarded as a series of shocks which drive the system.

$$X_t = \sum_{\kappa=1}^{p} \beta_\kappa X_{t-\kappa} + \sum_{\kappa=0}^{q} \alpha_\kappa \epsilon_{t-\kappa}$$

Both processes could be identified by their acf and pacf, respectively.

In MA-processes the acf has a cut-off after p-points and in AR-processes the pacf has a cut-off after q-points. This definition and identification looks easy, but this is deceptive.

The reliability of computed acf in ARMA-processes is usually extremely poor. This problem becomes even more difficult because of the poor iterative calculation methods presently available. These methods can often only provide a rough impression of the system.

The calculation (1) of the initial estimates of an ARMA (p,q)-process is based on the first pq1 acf-values $c_j$, j=O,...,pq. From these the autoregressive parameters are estimated. Using these estimates, the first p1 autocovariances $c_j$, j=0,..,p of the derived series

$$X'_t = X_t - \beta_1 X_{t-1} - \ldots - \beta_p X_{t-p}$$

are calculated. Finally, the autocovariances $c_j$were used in an iterative calculation to compute initial estimates of the moving average parameter, $\alpha$j, j=1,...,q and of the residual variance of $\varepsilon_k$.

(To evaluate the degree of the ARMA-process (5), the so-called $\kappa$ and $\lambda$ matrix, respectively, were used.)

Having estimated the $\alpha_\kappa$, $\beta_\kappa$ and the variance of $\varepsilon_\kappa$, the model could be verified by considering when or where the process runs into non-stationarity. This happens if the residuals of $\varepsilon_\kappa$ are high or if their acf changes significantly.

The FHR trace shown in Figure 5 (top) was simulated by an ARMA (1,1)-process. The middle trace in the figure, marked as 'ERROR', represents the variance of $\varepsilon_\kappa$. The values close to zero in the middle of this trace indicate no change in the degree of randomness, while visual inspection might identify a characteristic change. In spite of the fact that, from the basic assumptions, the squared and added acf of the $\varepsilon_\kappa$ should be $\chi^2$-distributed, the test value RVAL (Figure 5, bottom trace), indicates significant variations.

A change in the autocorrelation function indicates that the process has changed its characteristics, and reflects a possible change in OSC characteristics, while the variance of the original time series did not change significantly.

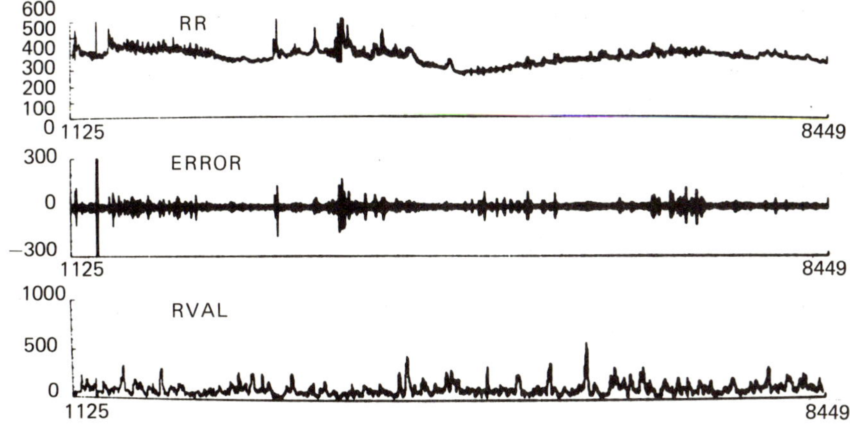


*Figure 5.* Preliminary result of an ARMA(1,1) process. From top to bottom: FHR-trace, the 'ERROR' of the model and a test value RVAL

## Acknowledgements

The surgeries were performed by A M Rudoph, MD and MA Heymann MD; Cardiovascular Research Institute, University of California, San Francisco, USA.

## References

1. Box G E and Jenkins G M. *Time Series Analysis: Forecasting and Control.* Holden-Day, San Francisco, (1971).
2. Hammacher K. In *Gynaekologie und Geburtshilfe,* Thieme, Stuttgart, 793-803, II (1967).
3. Hammacher K et al. *Gynaekologische Rundschau 14,* Suppl.1, 61-63 (1974).
4. Somville T, Abels T, Bender K and Morgenstern J. Eine Methode zur Berechnung der fetalen Herzfrequenz-Oszillationen. In *Perinatale Medizin,* edited by E Schmidt, J W Dudenhausen and E Saling, Vol X, S.198. Stuttgart, Thieme (1983).
5. Streitberg B. *Vector Correlations of Time Series and the Box-Jenkins Approach to ARMA Identification.* Institute of Applied Statistics, 4/83, Free University of Berlin, Berlin.

Chapter 38

# A digital system for rapid transmission and distant computer-processing of antepartum fetal heart rate recordings

**N A J Gough, A J Dawson**

## Introduction

Regular antepartum fetal heart rate recording has become an important method of fetal surveillance. A technique for telemetry of fetal heart rate from patients' homes was recently reported (2). In carefully selected cases, distant telemetry could be applied safely and economically with patient-acceptability. The reported system operated in real time, with transmission of the analogue audio signal using the public telephone network. We now report a system which employs digital data transmission for distant telemetry of fetal heart rate with a short transmission and processing time. There is an independent portable unit at the patient's (peripheral) end which collects and retains a recording for up to several hours. The system is suited to the rapid transmission of data by telephone or radio using acoustic couplers. A microcomputer in the obstetric department displays the trace on a visual display unit (VDU) and makes a permanent record on 5 and a quarter inch disc, and on paper.

## Method

The system can be considered in three parts; the scheme is shown in Figure 1.

### Data collection

The data collection apparatus comprises a Huntleigh D500 Fetal Heart Detector, an audio signal processor enclosed with a digital storage telemeter, and a K&N 800 Series Acoustic Coupler. It operates by mains or battery power.

The envelope waveform from the 2 MHz ultrasound fetal heart detector is filtered and amplified by an audio signal processor (3) to produce trigger pulses which in turn drive the interval timing circuitry of the digital storage telemeter. Once a trigger pulse has been generated the trigger pulse circuit is disabled for 250 ms, causing any secondary heart signals to be ignored.

The interval timing circuitry, referenced to a 1 KHz crystal oscillator, measures the intervals between pulses in milliseconds. There are 2 twelve-bit counters, A and B, each having a capacity of 4095 ms. The 1 kHz clock pulses are channelled alternately to each counter by a bistable. The bistable itself is switched by the trigger

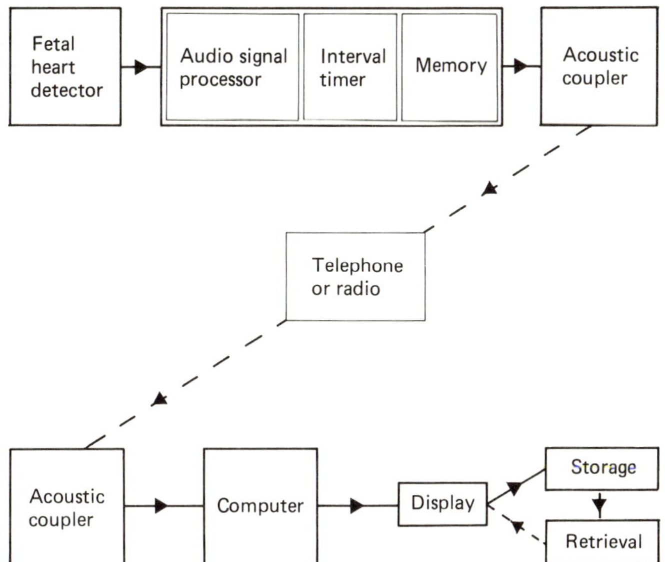


*Figure 1.* Flow diagram showing the components of the system. The interval timer and memory, together with their control circuits, comprise the digital storage telemeter

pulse, or by the current twelve-bit counter should this reach its capacity. When the bistable is switched, counter A is stopped and counter B started. The value in counter A is passed to a location in static random access memory (RAM), and counter A is then reset to zero, ready for the next trigger pulse.

The memory array of 16k by 12 bits is sufficient for a normal recording of more than 2 hours. Twelve-bit binary values have been used to accommodate rates down to 60 beats per minute. This also has the advantage of minimal memory use during periods of signal loss.

Once a recording is completed, the input and timing circuitry is disabled, and the instrument is set to a standby condition, ready for transmission.

## Data transmission

The telephone link to the hospital can be established at any time after the recording has been completed, providing the instrument remains powered and in the standby

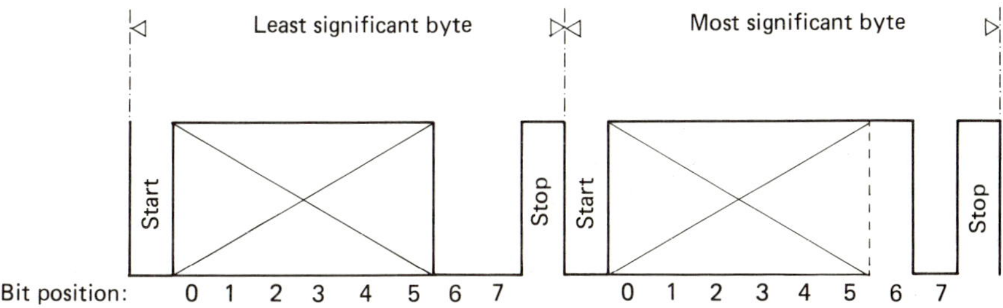


*Figure 2.* Representation of the two eight-bit words which carry the two halves of one twelve-bit value during transmission. Bits 6 and 7 are identity bits. Bit 6 is set to identify the most significant byte

condition. Once the link has been established, a prompt from the acoustic coupler in the hospital signals that sequential data transfer from the memory may commence, set at 300 baud.

Because of hardware limitations each twelve-bit value is transmitted as two six-bit values, each contained within an eight-bit word. The word format is shown in Figure 2.

The acoustic coupler at the hospital detects the incoming data, passing it to the RS 423 serial input port of the BBC Micro model B computer. The computer will indicate when all the data have been received. The hospital acoustic coupler can be used to signal that voice communication may be re-established.

### Data processing

In the hospital, data processing, display and storage are carried out using the BBC microcomputer, VDU, disc operating system (DOS) and dot matrix printer. Because of the limit of computer memory, software is divided into three consecutive programs, automatically chained.

The twelve-bit values are reconstituted by a machine code routine and stored in an array before the main processing program, written in BBC BASIC, is continued. Intervals are processed through an error algorithm for validation (3). An average value is calculated from validated intervals for each epoch of 3750 ms (4). The recording is stored permanently, with identity, as a series of epoch values by the DOS. A fetal heart rate trace constructed from the epoch values is displayed on the VDU for immediate assessment and a hardcopy printed out for inclusion in the patient's records.

The controls of the recording device have been carefully planned for simplicity of operation. There are just three colour-coded press-button controls and an on-off switch. Light-emitting diodes have been used to indicate which mode the instrument is in (recording, standby, or transmitting), and also to indicate the recognition of fetal pulses whilst recording.

## Results

The operation of the system has so far been tested with 30 supervised recordings, in 18 women between 26 weeks gestation and term. Recordings usually lasted for 21 minutes. Transmission took about 3.5 minutes per recording, and processing to the point of display, a further minute. All but five recordings were interpretable, and the cause of signal loss was sub-optimal fetal heart detection in each case.

Failure times averaged 73% (s.d. ± 16%) crude, and 42% (s.d. ± 22%), corrected for averaging over epochs.

The system has been tested from a patient's home, and also using the 2 m amateur radio band for transmission. Its output has been compared with that of a Hewlett-Packard 8030A Cardiotocograph in a number of simultaneous recordings. All features on the cardiotocographs were clearly visible in the transmitted form on the computer screen. Repeated transmissions of one recording were made to check reproducibility and the effect of noise on the telephone line. Occasionally minor durational differences of a few seconds between transmissions of the same recording could be detected, but no obvious change to the visual trace occurred.

## Discussion

Routine, regular antepartum fetal heart rate monitoring has become an established practice in the management of some high-risk pregnancies. A recent report (2) has shown the feasibility of monitoring fetal heart rate from long distances using the telephone network. Our system for distant screening of fetal heart rate tracings shares the important features of that previously reported. Additionally, it is independent of a telephone until the time of transmission, and indeed, the pregnant woman does not have to be a telephone subscriber. The system is light and portable; it could be kept at the woman's home, the surgery, or health centre; it could be carried by the general practitioner or midwife in their car.

Controls have been kept simple and bright, allowing for confident use by attendants or the patient herself, after supervised instruction.

The use of computer, telephone, and staff time is efficient and economical, and the system has a low capital cost. One computer would be able to service quickly a number of peripheral units. The system is still computationally relatively slow, partly limited by the size of the computer's memory, and partly because of the use of unreduced transmitted data. The use of radio would allow for faster transmission; the telephone system has a limitation of 300 baud. The present system functions as expected, but it still depends on being supplied with a carefully maintained fetal heart signal. A modification of the audio signal processor described elsewhere (3) has been retained because of its known properties determined in extensive use.

The future application of such a system will particularly be in large geographical areas served by central obstetric units, at home or abroad. It has potential for increasing the involvement of community staff in the management of selected high-risk pregnancies. Further, one recent controlled trial (5) has suggested that the main benefit of antepartum cardiotocography may be in avoiding, or reducing the duration of, hospital admissions. Other reports (1, 6) also lead to the observation that weekly recordings may be too infrequent to provide measurable clinical benefit. A distant telemetry system could help to reduce further hospital admissions and possibly enable more frequent recordings to be made economically and conveniently, apart from providing reassurances to mothers.

Such telemetric techniques still await definition of their clinical application; full evaluation of their clinical and social benefit must follow.

## Acknowledgements

We thank Professor Hibbard for his support, Tim Tomkins of University College Cardiff for his advice, and Huntleigh Medical Ltd for their donation of the D500 Fetal Heart Detector. Our thanks are also due to Paul Fulgoni and Tony Royston, licensed amateur radio operators. AJD was supported by the Heart Research Fund for Wales.

## References

1. Brown V A, Sawers R S, Parsons R J and Duncan S L B. The value of antenatal cardiotocography in the management of high-risk pregnancy: a randomized controlled trial. *British Journal of Obstetrics and Gynaecology*, 89, 716-722 (1982).

2. Dalton K J, Dawson A J and Gough N A J. Long distance telemetry of fetal heart rate from patients' homes using the public telephone network. *British Medical Journal,* 286, 1545 (1983).

3. Dalton K J, Hemp J, Dawson A J and Gough N A J. TELEPLOT: a computerised system for objective analysis of fetal heart rate recordings. *International Journal of Biomedical Computing,* 15,23-24 (1984).

4. Dawes G S, Visser G H A, Goodman J D S and Redman C W G. Numerical analysis of the human fetal heart rate: the qualtity of ultrasound records. *American Journal of Obstetrics and Gynecology,* 141, 43-52 (1981).

5. Flynn A M, Kelly J, Mansfield H, Needham P, O'Conor M and Viegas O. A randomized controlled trial of non-stress antepartum cardiotocography. *British Journal of Obstetrics and Gynaecology,* 89, 427-433 (1982).

6. Lumley J, Lester A, Anderson I, Renou P and Wood C. A randomized controlled trial of weekly cardiotocography in high-risk obstetric patients. *British Journal of Obstetrics and Gynaecology,* 90, 1018-1026 (1983).

Chapter 39

# The use of a purpose-built microcomputer for the automatic diagnosis of fetal distress

**Christopher J Chandler, R John Parsons and Alan Palmer**

## Introduction

Continuous fetal heart rate monitoring is aimed at the early detection of fetal hypoxia. The extent to which it reliably achieves this continues to be a matter of vigorous discussion (3). It has recently been suggested (2) that there is a need for the application of microcomputers to produce a 'new generation of more intelligent fetal heart rate monitors'.

Professor K Maeda of Tottori University in Japan has designed an algorithm for the interpretation of cardiotocographic traces (1). This has been used to programme a small, dedicated on-line microcomputer which can rest on top of the fetal monitor. The algorithm evaluates baseline fetal heart rate, variability, accelerations and decelerations in association with the strength, duration and frequency of uterine contractions. An 'evaluation score' is given to each of these parameters and the sum of evaluation scores after five minutes provides a 'fetal heart rate score'.

Other abnormalities, including loss of variability, prolonged tachycardia, prolonged bradycardia and typical late deceleration patterns, are also recognised and used in conjunction with the fetal heart rate score to produce a fetal distress index when adverse features appear.

The fetal heart rate score and a summary of the parameters from which it is derived are printed out every five minutes. The total fetal distress index generated over a 15 minute period activates an audible and visible alarm, when appropriate. There are three levels of alarm:

Fetal distress index 1 = warning of possible distress requiring further careful monitoring

Fetal distress index 2 = suspected fetal distress

Fetal distress index 3 = established fetal distress.

## Patients and methods

The aim of our study was to assess the validity of the microcomputer interpretation of cardiotocographs by comparing the fetal distress index (if present) with outcome in terms of Apgar score and umbilical cord blood pH. Patients were assigned to conventional or computerised monitoring at random, although as the study progressed an increasing number of high risk pregnancies and those with abnormal fetal heart rate tracings were monitored with the computer. At delivery the umbilical cord was clamped in two places approximately 10 centimetres apart and blood was withdrawn from the umbilical vein (and artery in later cases) into a previously heparinised syringe. The blood samples were immediately analysed using an Instrumentation Laboratory System 1302 pH/blood gas analyser.

## Results

Complete data are available from 71 patients. In 28 the computer found no evidence of fetal distress and in this group there were no babies with one minute Apgar scores less than 7 and no operative deliveries for fetal distress. The mean pH was 7.29 0.071.

There were 19 cases in which the fetal distress index was 1 (warning of possible fetal distress). There were no Apgar scores less than 7 and no operative deliveries for fetal distress in this group and the mean pH was identical to that of the normal group (7.29 0.071).

In 11 cases the fetal distress index was 2 (suspected fetal distress) and in this group there was one baby with a one minute Apgar score of 6 (cord venous pH 7.11). Another baby in this group was delivered using the Kielland's forceps for a persistent occipito-posterior position associated with fetal distress. The pH of this baby at birth was 7.17 with an Apgar score of 8 at one minute. The mean of pH in this group was 7.29 with a standard deviation of 0.094.

In the established fetal distress group (fetal distress index greater than 3) there were 13 patients, four of whom had babies with Apgar scores of less than 7 (pH 7.10, 7.20, 7.20, 7.26). Only one of these four had an operative delivery for fetal distress. There were, however, five other operative deliveries for fetal distress in this group but in only one was the cord pH less than 7.2. The difference between the mean pH of the normal and the established fetal distress group is highly significant (p less than 0.005).

The sensitivity and selectivity of the system have been calculated by comparing the number of babies with a cord blood pH of greater or less than 7.25 in the normal and established fetal distress group.

## Discussion

Cardiotocographic tracings alone have been shown to be unreliable in the prediction of significant fetal distress. Recently, Sykes *et al* (3) published a series in which only 14% of patients having operative deliveries for fetal distress had a low pH and, even more worrying, 8% of babies delivered normally had a low pH but fetal distress had not been suspected in spite of continuous electronic monitoring of the fetal heart. Although this paper has been heavily criticised, the fundamental conclusion that cardiotocography alone is an unsatisfactory way of monitoring the fetus, is unavoidable. The addition of fetal blood sampling for pH estimation in all cases where the cardiotocograph is abnormal will improve the false positive rate (selectivity) but can do nothing to prevent the birth of acidotic fetuses when either the cardiotocograph is normal or has not been recognised as being abnormal.

In this series the umbilical cord vein pH has been measured in all cases. Although arterial values should, in theory, give a more accurate assessment of fetal condition, the correlation between arterial and venous pH in the 20 cases in which both were measured was so good ($r = 0.8, p$ less than 0.001) that we feel justified in publishing our preliminary results using venous levels. The study is, however, still in progress and we now measure both cord blood arterial and venous pH as well as $pCO_2$, $pO_2$ and base deficit. From the regression line a venous pH of 7.25 (which we have taken as the lower limit of normal) corresponds with an arterial value of 7.14. (Sykes *et al* took an arterial value of 7.12 as their lower limit of normal on the basis that, for their population, this represents one standard deviation below the mean).

Although the mean pH in the established fetal distress group (index greater than or equal to 3) is significantly lower than that of the normal group there were a considerable number of false positive and false negative results. In four cases the computer diagnosed fetal distress but the babies were born with a normal pH (false positive). Three of these four babies had operative deliveries for fetal distress (one Caesarean section and two forceps deliveries). We would agree with Selwyn-Crawford (3) that the normal pH in these babies is probably accounted for by the resuscitative efforts (stopping oxytocin, change in maternal position, inhalation of oxygen) made between the time that fetal distress was recognised and delivery.

It is also of interest to note that only three of the nine babies with a low pH and predicted as having established fetal distress were, in fact, delivered operatively. In other words the obstetrician preferred his own interpretation of the trace to that of the computer.

Of the six cases with a low pH in the 'normal' group, only two had a pH less than 7.2 and in both of these the cardiotocograph trace in the second stage was very poor and probably difficult to interpret by the computer. The last reliable computer prediction was, therefore, some 30-50 minutes before delivery.

It is tempting to speculate from our small series that the application of continuous computer analysis of the CTG may provide a reliable and non-invasive means of improving the value of fetal heart rate monitoring. Further evaluation is required and we are currently enlarging our series and measuring umbilical arterial pH and base deficit, since this should give a more accurate reflection of the state of the baby at birth.

The presence of the microcomputer with its various alarm signals does not appear to increase significantly patient anxiety, however, the noise of the printer every five minutes is unduly intrusive. We would hope to modify the system so that the microcomputer only prints out information when a fetal distress index is generated. In addition, the quality of recording in the second stage is sometimes poor and little reliance can be placed on the computer interpretation in such cases. Hopefully, it will be possible to alter the sensitivity of the fetal heart rate monitor during the second stage to overcome this problem.

We believe that, with minor modifications, the Toitu Fetal Heart Rate Monitor and microcomputer represent a significant advance in fetal monitoring technique.

## Acknowledgements

The authors would like to thank Mrs C Turner and the staff of the Labour Ward at the Maternity Hospital Hull for their co-operation in carrying out this study. This work would not have been possible without the generosity of Professor K Maeda and the Toitu Co Ltd who provided the monitor and computer and also much useful advice.

## References

1. Maeda K. Computerised fetal heart rate analysis and automatic fetal distress diagnosis utilising external monitoring techniques with on-line and real-time processing. *International Congress Series No. 512, Gynaecology and Obstetrics, Proceedings of the 9th World Congress of Gynaecology and Obstetrics*, Tokyo 1979.

2. Sawers R S. Fetal monitoring during labour. *British Medical Journal*, 287, 1649-1650 (1983).

3. Sykes G S, Molloy P M, Johnson P, Stirratt G M and Turnbull A C. Fetal distress and the condition of newborn infants. *British Medical Journal*, 288, 567-569 (1984).

Part 6

# Developing Countries

Chapter 40

# Perinatal technology transfer and impact of neonatal intensive care on neonatal mortality in a developing country - Saudi Arabia

**Y K Abu-Osba, A A Thalji, A T Doyle, M S AhmadA M Al-Habbal**

## Introduction

Perinatal mortality and morbidity are indicators of health care in the community at large. Facilities for adequate maternal and neonatal care are lacking in developing countries, and maternal, fetal and neonatal mortality rates are high (11, 33). Despite improvements in health services during the last decade, perinatal mortality is still high in the various provinces of Saudi Arabia (33).

The development of neonatal intensive care and regionalization of these services has lowered neonatal mortality and morbidity in various developed countries (21, 27). Neonates with respiratory failure who were declined admission to a regional neonatal intensive care unit (NICU) and remained in their maternity unit of birth had double the mortality rate compared to infants transferred to a regional NICU (22).

The impact of neonatal intensive care on neonatal and perinatal mortality in a developing country (Saudi Arabia) is described in this paper.

## Newborn medicine in ARAMCO Medical Organization

ARAMCO Medical Organization provides health care to Arabian- American Oil Company (ARAMCO) employees (about 50 000) and their dependents (about 150 000). The facilities consist of a 360-bed hospital in Dhahran and six major outlying district clinics (DC). Dhahran Health Center (DHC) serves as a referral centre for consultation and hospitalization. In 1981 approximately 5000 newborn infants were delivered at ARAMCO health facilities.

## Phases of newborn care

Antenatal care is provided through mother and child health (MCH) clinics and the Obstetric/Gynaecology Department. Normal pregnancies are followed and delivered in the outlying MCH clinics by a physician or a midwife. Infants born by normal delivery are observed for 6 hours, and, if well, are discharged to be seen in 3 and 7 days postpartum. High-risk pregnancies are referred to the high-risk clinic and delivered at DHC by an obstetrician. Complications of the mother or infant arising during parturition result in referral to DHC.

Care for the newborn infants in ARAMCO developed in three phases:

Phase I: the period prior to the development of a neonatal intensive care unit (up to December 1979). During this period the majority (63%) of ARAMCO hospital deliveries took place in local private hospitals (LPH) with minimal NICU facilities.
Phase II: the period of 9 months in which a NICU was established in DHC (December 1979) staffed by general paediatricians, and only 9% of all ARAMCO uncomplicated deliveries took place in the same local private hospitals.
Phase III: the period starting September 1980 when two trained neonatologists joined the DHC paediatric staff and neonatal intensive care.

## Problems faced in the development of neonatal intensive care

In the process of establishing the newborn intensive care service, several problems were solved through the cooperation of various departments concerned with the care of the newborns. Neonatal intensive care is costly and sophisticated, and requires teamwork beginning with a sensitive and sympathetic hospital administration (2, 34). Supportive services, including respiratory therapy, laboratory, radiology, biomedical engineering and blood banking, which are able to meet the demands of the service are of the utmost importance. Well educated, specially trained nurses are rare, even in advanced countries. It was necessary to develop our neonatal intensive care nursing education programme which consisted of three parts: a basic education programme, continuous on-the-job practical training, and a didactic course of 36 lectures explaining the pathophysiology of the newborn.

Some of the sick newborns and high-risk mothers are referred from distant places. A maternal-neonatal transport team, well experienced and well equipped, is essential for the transfer of such patients. Another important problem was the shortage of neonatal beds resulting from an ever-increasing numb[illegible] infants. As the neonatal mortality decreased, more premature infants were saved and stayed longer in the hospital. The neonatal unit - which is a combined intensive and intermediate unit - began with eight neonatal beds in December 1980 and was enlarged to 30 beds in 1983.

## Methods

Perinatal-neonatal data were extracted from the medical records for equivalent time periods from each phase to evaluate the impact of the main changes in each phase on neonatal mortality.

To calculate neonatal mortality in the outlying clinics, all infants born in the districts and who died within 28 days of age were considered as neonatal deaths from the districts. Neonatal mortality at DHC and LPH included deaths of all infants delivered in these hospitals. All ARAMCO deliveries and neonatal deaths included the sum of the deliveries and the neonatal deaths of the districts, DHC and LPH. The American Academy of Pediatrics' definitions were used for the calculation of perinatal mortality rates (2). The chi square test was used when appropriate.

## Result

### Comparison of phase I and phase III

Medical records for the year 1979 (the last year before full establishment of neonatal intensive care) and 1981 (the first year after full establishment of the neonatal intensive care) were considered as representative of phase I and phase III respectively. Stillbirth rates are shown in Table 1. In phase I, the stillbirth rate in the local district clinics was significantly lower than that of the local hospitals - 11.8 and 22.4 respectively (p less than 0.05) - but similar to DHC. Most of the high-risk pregnancies (23% of all district pregnancies) were referred and delivered at LPH. Similarly, in phase III the stillbirth rate in the DC was significantly lower than at DHC (p less than 0.01) where all high-risk pregnancies (27% of all district pregnancies) were referred and delivered. The percentage of cases referred from the districts to deliver in the hospitals was similar in phase III and in phase I. The stillbirth rate showed a trend to increase, rising from 13.9 to 21.2 per 1000 births in phases I and III respectively, but this was not statistically significant. The stillbirth rate for all ARAMCO was virtually unchanged in phase III as compared to phase I, being 13.9 and 14.3 per 1000 births.

The neonatal mortality rates are shown in Table 1. In 1979 (phase I) it was similar in the districts, local private hospitals and Dhahran Health Center: 25.7, 26.5 and 26.8 per 1000 live births respectively.

The district neonatal mortality in phase III was significantly lower than that in phase I: 14 and 25.7 per 1000 live births respectively (p less than 0.02). These figures include infants born in the districts and those transferred to the referral hospitals, thus reflecting the changes in medical care in both the districts and the referral hospitals. DHC neonatal mortality decreased significantly in phase III as compared to phase I: 6.7 and 26.8 per 1000 live births respectively (p less than 0.001). DHC neonatal mortality in phase I was similar to LPH and DC: 26.8, 26.5 and 25.7/1000 live births respectively.

All ARAMCO neonatal mortality decreased significantly, from 23.2 to 9.4 per 1000 live births in phases I and III respectively (p less than 0.001). Similarly, perinatal mortality dropped from 36.8 to 21.1 per 1000 births in phases I and III respectively (p less than 0.001).

### Comparison of phase II and phase III

Data were summarized for equal time periods from phase II and phase III for comparison. Statistical analysis was performed to evaluate the impact of trained neonatologists joining a modern neonatal service. Neonatal mortality for the infants delivered at Dhahran Health Center dropped significantly to 4.2 per 1000 live births in phase III from 15.9 per 1000 live births for an equal period in phase II (p less than 0.001) (Table 2). This represents a decrease of almost 75% in the neonatal mortality. The stillbirth rates were very similar: 16.9 and 16.7 per 1000 deliveries in phases II and III respectively. This apparently high stillbirth rate at DHC probably resulted from all high-risk pregnancies having been transferred to DHC for delivery.

Neonatal mortality for all infants admitted to NICU decreased significantly in phase III compared to phase II (4.1% vs 16.7%, p less than 0.001). Similarly, the mortality rate of the infants transferred from the districts to the NICU in phase III was lower than that in phase II (4.3% vs 15.9%, p less than 0.05).

**TABLE 1. Perinatal mortality statistics for ARAMCO in 1979 (phase 1) and 1981 (phase III).**

| | *Live Births* (≥500 g) | | *Stillbirths* (≥500 g) | | *Neonatal death* (<28 days) | | *Stillbirth rate* | | *Neonatal mortality rate* | | *Perinatal mortality rate* | |
|---|---|---|---|---|---|---|---|---|---|---|---|---|
| | *Phase I* | *Phase III* | *Phase I* | *Phase III* | *Phase I* | *Phase III* | *Phase I* | *Phase III* | *Phase I* | *Phase III* | *Phase I* | *Phase III* |
| District clinics | 1671 | 2141 | 20 | 20 | 43 | 30 | 11.8 | 9.3* | 25.7 | 14.00** | 37.3 | 23.1** |
| Local hospital | 1134 | 177 | 26 | 2 | 30 | 0 | 22.4 | 11.2* | 26.5 | 0.0† | 48.3 | 11.2† |
| Dhahran Health Center | 710 | 2396 | 10 | 52 | 19 | 16 | 13.9 | 21.3* | 26.8 | 6.7‡ | 40.3 | 27.8* |
| All Aramco*** | 3972 | 5115 | 56 | 74 | 92 | 46 | 13.9 | 14.3* | 23.2 | 9.4‡ | 36.8 | 21.1‡ |

* Differences not significant.
** $p < 0.02$.
*** Figures include deliveries en route to hospital and in emergency room.
† $p < 0.05$ (a very small number of infants were delivered in phase III).
‡ $p < 0.001$.

**TABLE 2. Comparison of perinatal mortality statistics in phases II and III at Dhahran Health Center.**

| | *Phase II* | | *Phase III* | | *Percent Change Phase III/II* | *p* |
|---|---|---|---|---|---|---|
| | *Number* | *Per 1000* | *Number* | *Per 1000* | | |
| DHC live births | 1570 | | 2116 | | +34.8% | |
| DHC NICU admissions | 148 | 94.3 | 222 | 105 | +50% | NS |
| Total NICU admissions | 192 | | 291 | | +51% | |
| NICU neonatal deaths | 32 | 166.7* | 12 | 41.2* | −75.3% | <0.001 |
| DHC neonatal deaths | 25 | 15.9* | 9 | 4.3 | −73% | <0.001 |
| DHC stillbirths | 27 | 16.9 | 36 | 16.7 | − 1.2% | NS |
| DHC perinatal deaths | 52 | 32.6 | 45 | 10.9 | −35.9% | <0.05 |

*Deaths during the first 28 days of life/1000.

### Phase III perinatal statistics for Dhahran Health Center

Total deliveries inside the hospital during the first 2 years (1981 and 1982) post-NICU establishment were 6056. There were 102 stillborns and 53 infants less than 28 days who died. This gives a stillbirth rate of 16.6 per 1000 deliveries, a neonatal mortality for infants delivered in hospital of 8.7 per 1000 live births; and a perinatal mortality of 25.6 per 1000 births. Early neonatal mortality for all infants born at DHC was 6.7 per 1000 live births.

Corrected neonatal mortality for infants below 1000 g was 4.7 per 1000 live births. Neonatal mortality corrected for major congenital anomalies and infants weighing less than 1000 g was 2.9 per 1000 live births.

Very-low-birthweight infants (751-1500 g) constituted 1.1% of all live newborns delivered at DHC and the survival rate was 78.3%. Low-birthweight infants (below 2500 g) constituted 8.3% of all live newborns delivered at DHC and had a survival rate of 94%. Infants with a birthweight over 2500 g (92% of all infants delivered) had a survival rate of 99.6%.

## Discussion

Several reports from the advanced countries have shown the importance of neonatal intensive care management in decreasing neonatal mortality and morbidity. However, some authors still debate the impact of neonatal intensive care units on neonatal mortality and morbidity and their impact under actual field conditions in total populations (4, 7, 8, 12, 24, 25). This is the first report, to our knowledge, which demonstrates the impact of intensive care management on neonatal mortality in a developing country. Our figures compare favourably with the results obtained in centres in more advanced countries following the establishment of neonatal intensive care units (Tables 3 and 4). Survival rate figures for very-low-birthweight infants at Dhahran Health Center are comparable with the recent reports from centres with long experience in neonatal intensive care (3, 9, 13, 18-20, 31). These figures are affected by the fact that, since the establishment of the NICU, all high-risk pregnancies in ARAMCO are transferred to deliver at DHC.

During the study period stillbirth rates were unchanged and the obstetric practices and antenatal care policies did not change significantly. Also the population served

**TABLE 3. Comparison of neonatal mortality before and after neonatal intensive care institution in various centres.**

| Centre (reference) | | Neonatal mortality per/1000 live births | | | | |
|---|---|---|---|---|---|---|
| | | Before NICU | | After NICU | | |
| | | *Year* | *Mortality* | *Year* | *Mortality* | *Percent Change* |
| Johns Hopkins Hospital, Baltimore, Md, USA | (21) | 1961 – 1962 | 21.6 | 1963 – 1968 | 13.6 | −37% |
| University Women's Hospital and Children's Hospital, Helsinki, Finland | (16) | 1963 – 1964 | 14.9 | 1966 – 1967 | 12.4 | −17% |
| University of Mississipi Jackson, Miss., USA | ( 1) | 1968 | 26.0 | 1972 | 10.8 | −58% |
| Metropolitan Toronto, Canada | (28) | 1961 | 15.4 | 1972 | 10.1 | −34% |
| Dhahran Health Center Dhahran, Saudi Arabia | | 1979 | 26.8 | 1981 | 6.7 | −74% |

during the study period did not change significantly as judged by the employment figures and nationalities. Minimal social and cultural changes would occur over a 1-year period to account for the significant change in the neonatal mortality. We believe that the rapid decline in neonatal mortality demonstrated in this study was mainly due to the establishment of a modern, well-staffed and well-equipped neonatal intensive care centre. This study demonstrates that the establishment of neonatal intensive care units in a developing country is both feasible and successful.

A neonatal follow-up clinic was established simultaneously with the beginning of phase III, and all NICU survivors are followed up through the clinic by one of the neonatologists. It will be interesting to see the effect of this experience on the quality of life of these survivors.

Infant mortality is very high in most developing countries (10, 33). Ghosh reported a perinatal mortality rate of 75.6 per 1000 deliveries, and early neonatal mortality of 40 per 1000 births in Safdarjang hospital, New Delhi, India (6). Neonatal mortality in developing countries accounted for 38-45% of the total infant mortality early in this century and in the seventies (15, 32). This trend probably changed only slightly, if at all. Neonatal mortality is a major health and development problem for countries such as Saudi Arabia, Iraq and Libya which have a relatively high annual income, a low population density and ambitious development plans.

Neonatal intensive care implies costly and sophisticated management which depends on the transfer of medical technology. Some rich developing countries have ambitious health care plans and the required resources to implement them. Eradication of endemic and infectious diseases, immunization programmes and the battle against malnutrition remain high priorities in most of the developing countries. Mother and child health care centres with their well established functions can play a major role in decreasing maternal and perinatal mortality. Improving antenatal and obstetric care and better maternal nutrition will further decrease mortality. These measures

**TABLE 4. (Comparison of neonatal survival rates in relation to birthweight after neonatal intensive care institution (per/1000 live births).**

| Centre (Reference) | | Years | Birthweight (g) and survival rate (%) | | | | | |
|---|---|---|---|---|---|---|---|---|
| | | | 1001 | 1001 – 1500 | 1001 – 2500 | 1501 – 2000 | 2001 – 2500 | 2501 |
| Johns Hopkins Hospital, Baltimore, MD, USA | (21) | 1967–68 | 15 | 81.8 | — | 92.4 | 98 | — |
| University Women's Hospital and Children's Hospital, Helsinki, Finland | (16) | 1966–67 | 14 | 60 | — | 85 | 94.7 | — |
| Medical Center Hospital, Columbus, GA, USA | (29) | 1971–72 | — | 65.9 | — | 89.3 | 97.3 | — |
| Province of Quebec (First Week Mortality), Canada | (30) | 1972 | — | 59 | 92.8 | — | — | — |
| New Jersey, USA | ( 5) | 1969–71 | — | — | — | — | — | 89 |
| Vanderbilt University Hospital, Nashville, Tenn., USA | (25) | 1963–68 | — | — | 93.5 | — | — | 87.9 |
| Capital Regional Perinatal Center, New York, USA | ( 8) | 1975–79 | 20 | 71 | — | — | — | — |
| Hamilton-Wentworth Region, Hamilton, Ontario, Canada | (20) | 1973–78 | 31.9 | 82.6 | — | — | — | — |
| Dhahran Health Center, Dhahran, Saudi Arabia | | 1981–82 | 42.8 | 83 | 95.8 | 94 | 98 | 93.6 |

are long-term solutions and require considerable time before their effect can be appreciated. In addition, their institution and success are affected by many social, cultural, educational and economic factors.

## Conclusion

From the newborn medicine experience in the ARAMCO Medical Organization we conclude that, in a developing country, the establishment and regionalization of neonatal intensive care medicine is an efficient way to decrease perinatal mortality. This requires well co-ordinated efforts of administrators, physicians, nurses and supportive services.


## Acknowledgements

We thank Drs M A Zaru, J J Aboud and Ms R Quast for their help in obtaining the statistics, and Mr S Rafiuddin, EDP programmer. We also thank the Neonatal Intensive Care Unit staff for their very valuable help.

This paper was presented in part at the 7th Saudi Medical Meeting, Dammam, Saudi Arrabia (1982), and at the Second Kuwait International Medical Sciences Conference, Kuwait (1984).

## References and further reading

1. Brann A W Jr. Perinatal health care in Mississipi 1973. In *Regionalization of Perinatal Care*, Report of the Sixty-Sixth Ross Conference in Pediatric Research, edited by P Sunshine, Columbus, Ohio, Ross Laboratories (1974).
2. Brann A W Jr and Cafalo R C (Ed). *Guidelines for Perinatal Care*, Evanston-Washington, DC, American Academy of Pediatrics and American College of Obstetricians and Gynecologists (1983).
3. Britton S B, Fitzhardinge P M and Ashby S. Is intensive care justified for infants weighing less than 801 g at birth? *Journal of Pediatrics*, 99, 937 (1981).
4. David R J and Siegel E. Decline in neonatal mortality, 1968 to 1977: better babies or better care? *Pediatrics*, 71, 531 (1983).
5. Ellis W C, Bharara J and Snyder R. The regional newborn center: effect on neonatal mortality of referring hospital (abstract). *Pediatric Research*, 6, 409 (1972).
6. Ghosh S, Bhargava S K, Sazena H M K and Sagreiya K. Perinatal mortality-report of a hospital based study. *Annals of Tropical Pediatrics*, 3, 115 (1983).
7. Hughes-Davies T H. Conservative care of the newborn baby. *Archives of Disease in Childhood*, 54, 59 (1979).
8. Knobloch H, Malone A, Ellison P H, Stevens F and Zdeb M. Considerations in evaluating changes in outcome for infants weighing less than 1501 grams. *Pediatrics*, 69, 285 (1982).
9. Koops B L, Morgan L J and Battaglia F C. Neonatal mortality risk in relation to birth weight and gestational age: update. *Journal of Pediatrics*, 101, 969 (1982).
10. Nortman D L and Fisher J. *Population and Family Planning programs: a compendium of date through 1981*, New York, Population Council (1982).
11. Ohlsson A and Serenius F. Perinatal mortality at King Faisal Specialist Hospital and research center 1976-1981. Abstract presented at the Eighth Saudi Medical Conference, Riyadh, Saudi Arabia, (30 October-3 November 1983).
12. Paneth N, Kiely J L and Wallenstein S. Newborn intensive care and neonatal mortality in low-birth-weight infants. A population study. *New England Journal of Medicine*, 307, 149 (1982).
13. Philip A G S, Little G A, Polivy D R and Lucey J F. Neonatal mortality risk for the eighties: the importance of birth weight/gestational age groups. *Pediatrics*, 68, 122 (1981).
14. Pomerance J J. Cost of living for infants weighing 1000 grams or less at birth. *Pediatrics*, 61, 908 (1978).
15. Puffer R R and Serrano C V. *Patterns of Mortality in Childhood*, Scientific Publication No. 262, Washington DC, Pan American Health Organization (1973).
16. Raiha N. Experiences with neonatal intensive care in Finland. In *Problems of Neonatal Intensive Care Units*, Report of the Fifty-ninth Ross Conference on Pediatric Research, edited by J F Lucey, Columbus, Ohio, Ross Laboratories (1969).
17. Rawlings G, Reynolds E O R, Stewart A and Strang L B. Changing prognosis for infants of very low birth weight. *Lancet*, 1, 516 (1971).
18. Robertson N R C. Intensive care and the very low birth weight infant. *Lancet*, 1, 362 (1979).
19. Rothberg A D, Maisels M J, Baganto S *et al.* Outcome for survivors of mechnical ventilation weighing less than 1250 g at birth. *Journal of Pediatrics*, 98, 106 (1981).
20. Saigal S, Rosenbaum P, Stoskopf B V and Milner R. Follow up of infants 501-1500 g birth weight delivered to residents of a geographically defined region with perinatal intensive care facilities. *Journal of Pediatrics*, 100, 606 (1982).
21. Schaffer A J and Avery M E. *Diseases of the Newborn*, Philadelphia and London, Saunders (1966).
22. Shannon D C. Survival, cost of hospitalization, and prognosis in infants critically ill with respiratory distress syndrome requiring mechanical ventilation. *Critical Care Medicine*, 9, 94 (1981).
23. Sims D G, Wynn J and Chiswick M L. Outcome for newborn babies declined admission to a regional neonatal intensive care unit. *Archives of Disease in Childhood*, 57, 334 (1982).
24. Sinclair J C, Torrance G W, Boyle M H, Horwood S P, Saigal S and Sackett D L. Evaluation of neonatal-intensive-care programs. *New England Journal of Medicine*, 305, 489 (1981).
25. Stahlman M T. What evidence exists that intensive care has changed the incidence of intact survival. In *Problems of Neonatal Intensive Care*, Report of the Fifty-ninth Ross Conference on Pediatric Research, edited by J F Lucey, Columbus, Ohio, Ross Laboratories (1969).
26. Steiner E S, Sanders E M, Phillips E C K and Maddock C R. Very low birth weight children at school age: comparison of neonatal management methods. *British Medical Journal*, 281, 1237 (1980).
27. Stewart A L and Reynolds E O R. Improved prognosis for infants of very low birthweight. *Pediatrics*, 54, 724 (1974).

28. Swyer P R and Hardiem J. Reproductive medicine in Toronto with particular reference to neonatal care in the Hospital for Sick Children. In *Neonatal Intensive Care,* edited by J B Stetson and P R Swyer, St Louis, Mo, Warren H Green (1976).
29. Thompson R E, Souma M L, Cassady G and Sumners J. Impact of intensive care on neonatal mortality in a community hospital. *Southern Medical Journal,* 69, 688 (1976).
30. Usher R H. The special problems of the premature infant. In *Neonatology, Pathophysiology and Management of the Newborn,* edited by G B Avery, Philadelphia and Toronto. J B Lippincott (1975).
31. Walker G J A and Simpson H. Mortality rates and neonatal intensive care for very small babies. *Archives of Disease in Childhood,* 57, 112 (1982).
32. Woodbury R M. The relation between breast and artificial feeding and infant mortality. *American Journal of Hygiene,* 2, 668 (1922).
33. *World Health Statistics Annual,* 2, 1980.
34. Wynn M and Wynn A. Prevention of handicap of perinatal origin. London, Foundation for Education and Research in Childbearing (1976).

Chapter 41

# A suggested regional newborn screening programme for the Arabian Gulf States, and ARAMCO newborn screening programme experience in Saudi Arabia

**Y K Abu-Osba, A A Thalji, A R Sa'di, M S Ahmad, A M Al-Habbal**

## Introduction

Screening programmes for congenital diseases of newborn infants have been in effect for many years in the advanced countries. Such programmes include hypothyroidism (4, 5, 23, 29), cystic fibrosis (12), galactosaemia (3), phenylketonuria (27), abnormal haemoglobins (7, 28, 31, 40), glucose-6-phosphate dehydrogenase deficiency (G6PD) (17, 18) and many aminoacidopathies (10, 34, 38). The list of diseases which can be screened for in the neonatal period exceeds 25, and this list is constantly growing (10, 11, 13, 35). Developing countries lack newborn screening programmes due to several factors. Control of infectious diseases, gastroenteritis and malnutrition are top priorities in most of these countries. Some of the developing nations have changed their priorities following their great success in implementing immunization programmes against childhood communicable diseases such as measles, poliomyelitis and diphtheria. Several of these countries have the economic resources to enable them to concentrate more on the quality of life of their population and to pay more attention to the less urgent problems. Control of genetic diseases and detection of treatable congenital disease or prevention of its complications became a priority alongside other public health problems. During the past decade several reports have been published describing various screening programmes for a variety of diseases. Which one of these diseases should we screen for in these countries? And which has the priority? One of the major obstacles is lack of knowledge of the accurate incidence of these diseases in most of the developing countries, and of whether the natural history of the disease and its complications are similar to that which was published in Western countries.

The populations of various Arab countries have a closely related genetic background, and various regional health organizations are in operation. The Arabian Gulf States have a cooperation council, 'The Gulf Cooperation Council' (19), through which are implemented several projects of common interest. Planning for health services in the region is one of the major targets for these joint efforts. Healthcare has improved a great deal in the past decade, and programmes for compulsory immunization against childhood communicable diseases, such as measles, diphtheria, pertussis, tetanus and poliomyelitis, are in operation in the region. Although continuity of such programmes is undoubtedly a priority, it is now time to put some effort into the battle to control or prevent other potentially disastrous diseases for these young societies with very high crude birth rates ranging from 39.8 per 1000 in Bahrain to 52.3 per 1000 in

Kuwait (39). Improving antenatal and neonatal care is one of the major areas of concern, and perinatal screening programmes are one of its essential aspects. Such programmes are lacking on national and regional levels. Major medical centres and modern sophisticated medical laboratories are very few. The technical experience and the human resources required to organize separate programmes in every individual country are lacking.

The cost/benefit for a comprehensive neonatal screening programme as described later is shown in this example. Saudi Arabia has a population of 9 229 000 and crude birth rate of 46.9 per 1000 (39). The cost to screen all the infants born in 1 year (based on the cost of tests in the commercial laboratories) is about 14 million dollars (32 dollars per infant), and the cost for taking care of all hypothyroid infants born every year for an estimated life span of 10 years is about 71 million dollars (660 000 dollars per child). The projected saving in 1 year is 57 million dollars, putting aside the incalculable amount of human suffering for the individuals and the detrimental social impact on the families with a mentally- or physically-handicapped child. Added to that is the loss of projected economic production which could have been achieved by these future citizens. The implication is tremendous for future national planning. It should be noted that these savings in money were considered for one disease only based on private commercial cost. The actual cost for a national screening programme run by the government would be much less, due to mass screening and development of cheaper methods. In a mass screening laboratory handling 50 000 - 100 000 specimens per year, the cost for neonatal thyroid screening approximates 1 dollar (20), and for haemoglobinopathies 3 cents (16). Regionalization and automated testing of a single specimen simultaneously for several defects would further decrease the cost for a comprehensive genetic screening programme.

## Problems and obstacles

Several problems and obstacles will face establishment of a newborn screening programme for the whole region. Similar problems were encountered during the development of the ARAMCO programme, and solutions were found. These can be summarized by the following.

### Manpower

Who will collect the blood samples and identify them properly? Transporting the blood samples fit for analysis to the appropriate laboratory, performing the tests, reporting the results and keeping records of these results require a good deal of manpower. Results should be readily available in the medical records for the practising physician. A precise mechanism should be defined for recalling all patients with abnormal results, and the person responsible for that should be identified. Experienced physicians should be available for consultation. A group of experts should be responsible for the planning, organization, analysis of the results and overall administration of the programme.

### Technical difficulties

These can be summarized as: (1) proper collection, identification and transportation of the samples; (2) appropriate equipment, test procedures and technical expertise; (3) quality control programmes.

### When to collect the blood samples

The appropriate time to collect the blood samples is of major importance and has to be defined for the various groups of babies born in the hospital, at home, en route to hospital and those discharged early from hospital.

### Confirmation, treatment and follow up

A precise mechanism has to be defined for the immediate notification to the primary physician of the abnormal results, for performing the appropriate confirmatory tests, for starting the treatment if indicated and for providing family counselling. A specialty consulting service should be available for the practising physician.

### Appropriate funds

Sufficient funds should be available for the preparatory stage, laboratory facilities, operational cost and follow up.

## How to start a newborn screening programme

The following options are available to establish a mass screening programme for the newborn:

1. Affiliate with an established programme and a laboratory abroad. Advantages include: a quick start and a relatively short period for preparation; it is economic for small-scale screening and a short-term plan; and there are no worries about technical problems and quality control. Disadvantages include: problems with transportation and communication; delay in receiving some results that are needed for immediate care; and the fact that this programme is very costly for mass screening and not suitable for long-term plans.
2. Establish or designate a central laboratory provided with the necessary staff and equipment, and develop a local programme with all its requirements. Advantages of such a programme include: fewer problems with transportation and communication; and it is suitable for long-term plans and economic for mass screening. A central laboratory can be used as a nucleus for a research laboratory affiliated to one of the universities to perform sophisticated highly technical tests for the whole region. The disadvantages of such a programme are few; it will require more time to establish and it may face several problems, including technology transfer, professional expertise and quality control. These, however, are solvable problems with good planning and appropriate funding. Cooperation with an established programme or laboratory for quality control and technical assistance will help to overcome several of these problems.

## ARAMCO perinatal screening programme

ARAMCO Medical Organization provides health services for all Arabian American Oil Company (ARAMCO) employees (about 50 000) and their dependents (about

150 000). In 1983 about 6500 newborn infants were delivered in ARAMCO health care facilities.

Various aspects of preventive medicine are emphasized in the practices of health care in ARAMCO Medical Organization. Antenatal screening is performed for all pregnant mothers attending the maternal and child health clinics or the obstetric clincs, or at the time of delivery for those who have not received antenatal care. All mothers are screened for blood type and Rh, syphilis, hepatitis B, abnormal haemoglobins, G6PD deficiency, anaemia and rubella.

A newborn screening programme is performed for all ARAMCO newborn infants. The tests carried out are dictated by several factors. Previous reports indicated a high incidence of G6PD deficiency (17, 18) and sickle cell anaemia in the Eastern Province and other parts of Saudi Arabia (6, 28, 32); the natural history of these problems is not yet well studied. The severity of these diseases and the complications do not seem as benign as was first thought (2, 6, 24, 25, 30). Blood group identification and incompatibility are required for clinical reasons, especially with the presence of the above-mentioned risk factors for the management of neonatal jaundice. Congenital hypothyroidism, phenylketonuria and galactosaemia are dangerous but treatable diseases and their incidence in this area is not known. The cost-effectiveness and the successful applications of the screening programmes for these diseases have been documented from various countries (20).

A comprehensive newborn screening programme (NBSP) was implemented in November 1980 to screen for blood group and incompatibility, G6PD deficiency, abnormal haemoglobins, congenital hypothyroidism, phenylketonuria and galactosaemia. Tests to identify these problems are performed in our medical laboratory at Dhahran Health Center (DHC). Neural tube defects and trisomies seem to have high incidence in this area (37). Several infants with aminoacidopathies were diagnosed in the past 2 years and it seems not very rare in our institution. Ambiguous genitalia and adrenogenital syndrome seem to have a high incidence compared to other countries (26). Cystic fibrosis seems very rare in this area; only one case has been documented in the past 10 years in ARAMCO (33). For various reasons we do not screen routinely for these problems although it is very important so to do. Chromosomal studies and good genetic and metabolic laboratories are required to deal with these diseases. Most of the laboratory tests required to establish a definite diagnosis are not available in our laboratory and have to be performed abroad, with the various problems associated with this practice.

The following paragraphs will describe ARAMCO NBSP as designed and operated and the preliminary results of this programme. We will conclude with a suggested programme for the Arabian Gulf States.

## Collecting the blood samples

Midwives and physicians attending the deliveries collect the blood samples from the cord, and the laboratory technicians and nurses collect the venous or capillary blood samples according to standard procedures for the following:

1. Blood group and incompatibility, abnormal haemoglobins, G6PD and hypothyroidism: (a) cord blood is collected from every delivery at ARAMCO health facilities; (b) for infants born at home, other non-ARAMCO facilities or en route to it, venous or capillary blood is collected on admission to hospital or on first visit to the clinic.
2. Phenylketonuria and galactosaemia: (a) heel prick sample on filter paper after 48

hours of milk feeding for all in-hospital newborns; (b) early newborn discharges before 48 hours of milk feeding - a blood sample on filter paper is drawn at the time of discharge and at the first clinic visit after one week; (c) for infants born in a non-ARAMCO facility - a blood sample on filter paper is drawn in the first clinic visit.

## Processing the blood samples

All blood samples are labelled properly and transported to Dhahran Medical Laboratory (DML) where all the tests required are performed according to DML procedures. Quality control for all tests is carried out according to DML policies. A copy of the results is distributed to each of medical records, outpatient file, the screening physician and the co-ordinator of the screening programme.

## Laboratory methods

Glucose-6-phosphate dehydrogenase deficiency in red blood cells is detected by the visual quantitative detemination described by Berger (9). Total serum thyroxine is determined by radioimmunoassay using a commercially available kit Tetra-Tab RIA (36). Thyroid-stimulating hormone is measured by radioimmunoassay for all infants with a cord blood thyroxine value of 2 s.d. below the mean for all the group. Abnormal haemoglobins are tested for by screening haemoglobin electrophoresis. Confirmatory tests such as citrate agar electrophoresis are utilized to verify haemoglobins migrating in the same area S,C,H and Bart's (15). Blood typing is done by slide and tube procedures. Phenylketonuria is tested for by the Guthrie method (20).

## Responsibilities and follow up

1. Newborn screening programme physician: every ARAMCO medical district has a designated paediatrician responsible for the following: (a) recall and follow up all infants with abnormal results and perform the appropriate confirmatory tests; (b) contact with appropriate consultants for any problem as necessary; (c) refer to the NBSP manual for specific problems.
2. Co-ordinator of newborn screening programme: the co-ordinator of the programme has the following responsibilities: (a) review the NBSP policies, procedures and revise them as necessary; (b) perform statistical analysis of the results. (c) provide guidance to the physicians and nurses with regard to the programme; (d) initiate a quality assurance programme; (e) maintan, review and update the NBSP manual.

## Resources for consultation

The following resources are available for procedural and clinical consultations: (a) the newborn screening programme manual, which explains in detail the purposes, procedures, interpretation of the results, confirmatory tests for the diagnosis, and treatment and follow up of the confirmed cases; (b) paediatric endocrinologist for consultation on phenylketonuria galactosaemia and hypothyroidism; (c) paediatric haematologist for consultation on blood incompatibilities, G6PD deficiency and abnormal haemoglobins; (d) developmental paediatrician for growth and development; (e) coordinator of the NBSP for any procedural and administration problem.

## Quality assurance programme

A programme for quality assurance is implemented. Frequent audits are conducted to evaluate the operation of the programme and corrective action is instituted if a deficiency found.

## Preliminary results of the ARAMCO NBSP

More than 20 000 newborn infants have been screened in our programme. Results are reported and distributed as already described for clinical management. A computer program was designed to provide a cumulative record of all the results to facilitate the analysis. One weekly report for all the normal results and another for all the abnormal results from the various medical districts will be distributed to the various screening physicians to serve as a quick reference. About 12 000 infants' results have been entered in the program so far. Our aim is to report and enter the results directly and to have direct print-out to the various medical districts. Computer terminals located in the various MCH clinics are planned for the future, and these wll be connected to the laboratory in order to give direct access by the practising physician to the screening results.

Preliminary analysis of our results for the various problems showed the following.

### *Blood groups and incompatibility*

Infants' blood groups for the Saudi Arabs and all other nationalities are shown in Table 1. The most common blood group in the Saudi Arab infants is group O, which

**TABLE 1. Newborns blood groups (ARAMCO).**

| *Country* | *Blood group (%)* | | | |
|---|---|---|---|---|
| | A | B | AB | O |
| Saudi Arabs | 23.5 | 22.7 | 3.7 | 50.0 |
| Other nationalities | 30.0 | 18.6 | 6.4 | 45.0 |
| USA (white) | 45.0 | 8 | 4 | 43.0 |
| USA (black) | 29.0 | 17 | 4 | 50.0 |

is similar in incidence to the black Americans and slightly higher than the white Americans. Blood group B is much more common than in white and black Americans, and group A is less common than in both. Blood groups varied significantly between infants from various villages.

Mother and infant blood group incompatibilities in Saudi Arabs are different from those in other countries. Mothers with blood group O and infant with blood group A or B (ABO set up) were found in 14% of the cases. ABO set up and direct Coombs test were positive in 4% of the infants. Mothers with Rh negative and infant with Rh positive were 5.1% and those with positive direct Coombs test were 4.3 per 1000.

### *G6PD deficiency*

Erythrocyte deficiency of glucose-6-phosphate dehydrogenase was found in 17.7% of all Saudi Arab infants (Table 2). Several infants from other nationalities (including

**TABLE 2. G6PD deficiency screening programme (ARAMCO).**

| *Country* | *Total no.* | *Normal no.* | *Deficient no.* | *%* |
|---|---|---|---|---|
| Saudi Arabia | 9643 | 7935 | 1708 | 17.7 |
| Bahrain | 3 | 2 | 1 | 33.3 |
| Jordan | 80 | 79 | 1 | 1.3 |
| Lebanon | 28 | 25 | 3 | 10.7 |
| Pakistan | 171 | 168 | 3 | 1.8 |
| Sudan | 68 | 67 | 1 | 1.5 |
| USA | 372 | 360 | 12 | 3.2 |
| Total* | 10505 | 8776 | 1729 | 16.5 |

* Including 140 newborns from Britain, India, Egypt, Canada, Philippines and Sri Lanka all were normal.

Jordan, Bahrain, Lebanon, Pakistan, Sudan and the USA) were also found to be G6PD deficient. The incidence of G6PD deficiency among the Saudi Arab varied from one village to another.

### *Cord blood abnormal haemoglobins*

Screening haemoglobin electrophoresis of the cord blood of the Saudi Arab newborns showed that 27% of the Saudi Arab newborns had one or more abnormal haemoglobin (Table 3). Bart's haemoglobin was present in 16.4% and sickle cell haemoglobin in 16.6% of the Saudi Arabs screened. Thirty infants from Jordan, Egypt, India, Pakistan, the USA, Yemen, Sudan and Britain were found to have Bart's or sickle cell haemoglobin.

**TABLE 3. Saudi Arabs cord blood screening haemoglobin electrophoresis.**

| | *Number of newborns* | *% from all newborns screened* |
|---|---|---|
| F | 486 | 4.838 |
| FA | 6312 | 62.837 |
| FAB | 1229 | 12.235 |
| FAS | 909 | 9.049 |
| FASB | 284 | 2.827 |
| FB | 103 | 1.025 |
| FBS | 32 | 0.319 |
| FS | 144 | 1.434 |

### *Congenital hypothyroidism*

Cord blood total serum thyroxine is show in Table 4. The mean value for thyroxine was 10.25 and s.d. 2.19 μg/dl (132 and s.d. 28.25 mmol/l). Three infants had confirmed congenital hypothyroidism. Twenty infants had transient hyperthyrotropinaemia. Details of the analysis for congenital hypothyroidism are in preparation.

**TABLE 4. Cord blood thyroxine values ARAMCO newborns.**

| *Country of origin* | *No.* | *Mean (μg/dl)* | *s.d.* | *s.e.* |
|---|---|---|---|---|
| Saudi Arabia | 7321 | 10.25 | 2.19 | 0.03 |
| Canada | 23 | 9.83 | 1.94 | 0.04 |
| USA | 285 | 10.81 | 2.09 | 0.12 |
| Jordan | 64 | 9.98 | 2.29 | 0.29 |
| Lebanon | 19 | 10.6 | 2.17 | 0.29 |
| Egypt | 12 | 10.8 | 1.77 | 0.51 |
| India | 39 | 10.17 | 2.00 | 0.32 |
| Pakistan | 136 | 10.15 | 2.14 | 0.18 |
| Sudan | 57 | 10.85 | 2.43 | 0.32 |
| Philippines | 8 | 9.78 | 2.51 | 0.89 |

### *Galactosaemia and phenylketonuria*

All infants tested for phenylketonuria had normal levels. About 3000 infants were screened for galactosaemia, with a positive/confirmed result in only one. The programme was stopped because of some technical problems.

### Conclusions from ARAMCO NBSP

About 20 000 newborn infants have been screened since the programme was started 3 years ago. Several problems were encountered during the operation which required modifications to the programme. From this experience we conclude that a comprehensive NBSP modified to the needs and resources available can be achieved. Valuable epidemiological data have been gathered and important information for direct clinical use obtained.

## A regional NBSP for the Arabian Gulf States

The justification for a similar or modified programme for all the Arabian Gulf States is similar to that of ARAMCO. Published data regarding the incidence and presence of the various metabolic and genetic diseases other than in Saudi Arabia and Kuwait are very scarce, and this emphasizes the need for pilot screening programmes in certain areas. On the other hand, several reports have indicated the high incidence or the presence of certain genetic diseases (1, 8, 14, 21, 22).

These States have a 'cooperation council' which encourages various aspects of cooperation including health services, and several projects have already been put into operation. Health service plans are ambitious. Programmes for the prevention of communicable diseases are in practice and much progress has been achieved in this field. The theme for the WHO week in 1984 was 'Children's health is future wealth': this is a great challenge. One of the aims of NBSP is the promotion of children's mental and physical health, and the prevention of complications.

Several limitations face the establishment of a NBSP in this respect. Among these are *the limited number of experts in the field and the problems related to technology transfer* . Human and economic resources for the successful operation of such a programme are available but are limited. A joint plan can be adopted by the various States and modified according to the circumstances of each. Such a plan should take into consideration the above limitations. An *ad hoc* committee should be set up to define the programme's objectives, procedures, operational plans, quality assurance, statistical analysis and evaluation. A central laboratory affiliated to one of the universities to perform the sophisticated tests for all the region can serve as a reference laboratory. This laboratory may be supported by the local laboratories which will perform the simple tests for follow up. Such a plan should make use of the limited number of experts in the region and maximize their expertise by joint planning and operation. A unified training programme in the deficient areas should be dealt with. Cost for the whole joint programme will be much less than if every country plans its own programme.

## Acknowledgements

We thank Drs N Al-Masri, B Bascom, Cherian Mathew, A Mallouh, P M Mathew, Salwa Abdul Hadi and J J Shamma for their valuable help in the follow up; Mr S Rafiuddin, EDP programmer, for his help in designing the screening computer program; and Dr D J Goodwin and Ms C Tidwell for their valuable help in the analysis. We also thank Mr M Naseer for the secretarial help.

This paper was presented in part at the Second Kuwait International Medical Sciences Conference, Kuwait (1984).

## References

1. Al-Awadi S A, Teebi A S, Farag T I, Naguib K and El-Khalifa M Y. Scope of inherited metabolic disease in Kuwait. An overview from Medical Genetics Centre. Paper presented at the Second Kuwait International Sciences Conference, Kuwait (4 - 8 March 1984).

2. Al-Away B, Pearson H A, Wilson W A and Naeem M. Function of the spleen in Saudi Arabian patients with sickle cell anaemia. Abstract presented at the Seventh Saudi Medical Meeting, Dammam, Saudi Arabia (3 - 6 May 1982).

3. Alm J and Larsson A. Evaluation of a nationwide neonatal metabolic screening program in Sweden 1965 - 1979. *Acta Paediatrica Scandinavica,* 70, 601-607 (1981).

4. Alm J, Larsson A and Zetterstrom R. Congenital hypothyroidism in Sweden. Psychomotor development in patients detected by clinical signs and symptoms. *Acta Paediatrica Scandinavica,* 70, 907-912 (1981).

5. American Academy of Pediatrics Committee on Genetics. Screening for congenital metabolic disorders in the newborn infant: congenital deficiency of thyroid hormone and hyperphenylalaninemi a. *Pediatrics,* 60, 389 (1977).

6. Babiker M A and Taha S A. Two different patterns of sickle cell disease in children in Saudi Arabia. *Annals of Tropical Paediatrics,* 2, 179-181 (1982).

7. Barnes M G, Komarmy L and Novack A H. A comprehensive screening program for hemoglobinopathies. *Journal of the American Medical Association,* 219, 701-705 (1982).

8. Basalamah A H, Serebour F and Al-Amoudi S. Maternal serum alphafetoprotein (AFP) screening in pregnancy in Jeddah - social problems. Abstract presented at the Eighth Saudi Medical Conference (30 October-3 November 1983).

9. Berger L.*Glucose-6-Phosphate Dehydrogenase Deficiency in Red Cells.* St Louis, Mo, Sigma Chemical Company (1980).

10. Burton B K and Nadler H L. Clinical diagnosis of the inborn errors of metabolism in the neonatal period. *Pediatrics,* 61, 398 (1978).
11. Cacciari E, Balsamo A, Cassio A *et al.* Neonatal screening for congenital adrenal hyperplasia *Archives of Disease in Childhood,* 58, 803-806 (1983).
12. Committee Report. Neonatal screening for cystic fibrosis. Position paper. *Pediatrics,* 72, 741-745 (1983).
13. Dahlquist G, Gustavsson K H, Holmgren G *et al.* The incidence of diabetes mellitus in Swedish children 0-14 years of age. *Acta Paediatrica Scandinavica,* 71, 7-14 (1982).
14. El-Hazmi M A F, Jabbar F A and Al-Faleh F Z. The frequency of red cell glucose-6-phosphate dehydrogenase pyruvate kinase and hexokinase deficiency in Riyadh, Hafoof and Khaiber - comparative studies. Abstract presented at the Eighth Saudi Medical Conference (30 October-3 November 1983).
15. Evans D I K. Haemoglobin electrophoresis on cellulose acetate using whole blood samples. *Journal of Clinical Pathology,* 24, 877-878 (1971).
16. Garrick M D, Dembure P and Guthrie R. Sickle-cell anemia and other hemoglobinopathies: procedures and strategy for screening employing spots of blood on filter paper as specimens. *New England Journal of Medicine,*288, 1265-1268 (1973).
17. Gelpi A P. Glucose-6-phosphate dehydrogenase deficiency, the sickling trait and malaria in Saudi Arab children. *Tropical Pediatrics,* 71, 138-146 (1967).
18. Gelpi A P. Glucose-6-phosphate dehydrogenase deficiency in Saudi Arabia: a survey. *Blood,* 25, 486-493 (1965).
19. Gulf Cooperation Council consists of Saudi Arabia, Kuwait, Qatar, Bahrain, United Arab Emirates and Oman.
20. Guthrie R. Organization of a regional newborn screening laboratory. In *Neonatal Screening for Inborn Errors of Metabolism,* edited by H Bicket, R Guthrie and G Hammersen, pp 259-270. Berlin, Heidelberg and New York, Springer Verlag (1980).
21. Killander J and Gumaa K. Diagnostic facilities for metabolic diseases in Kuwait - present and planned procedures with some results. Paper presented at the Second Kuwait International Medical Sciences Conference, Kuwait (4-8 March 1984).
22. Kollberg H. Cystic fibrosis in Kuwait. Paper presented at the Second Kuwait International Medical Sciences Conference,Kuwait (4-8 March 1984).
23. Larson A, Ljunggren J G and Lundberg K. TSH and thyroxine in stored neonatal filter-paper blood samples from patients with congenital hypothyroidism. *Acta Paediatrica Scandinavica,* 71, 39-41 (1982).
24. Mallouh A, Burke L, Ahmad M S, Salamah M M and Habbal A. The TC99 scan in Saudi patients with sickle cell anemia. Abstract presented at the Seventh Saudi Medical Meeting, Dammam, Saudi Arabia, (3-6 May 1982).
25. Mallouh A and Salamah M. Pneumococcal meningitis in patients with sickle cell anemia. Abstract presented at the Eighth Saudi Medical Conference (30 October-3 November 1983).
26. Mathew P M, Abu-Osba Y K, Thalji A A, Hann R W and Hamdan J A. Ambiguous genitalia and adrenogenital syndrome in Saudi infants. Abstract presented at the Eighth Saudi Medical Conference (30 October-3 November 1983).
27. McCabe E R B, McCabe L, Mosher G A, Allen R J and Berman J L. Newborn screening for phenylketonuria. Predictive validity as a function of age. *Pediatrics,* 72, 390-398 (1983).
28. Perrine R P, John P, Pembrey M and Perrine S. Sickle cell disease in Saudi Arabs in early childhood *Archives of Disease in Childhood,* 56, 187-192 (1981).
29. Report of the Newborn Committee of the European Thyroid Association. Neonatal screening for congenital hypothyroidism in europe. *Acta Endocrinologica,* Suppl. 223, 4-14 (1979).
30. Salamah M, Thalji A, Mallouh A and Hamdan J A. Acute splenic sequestration crisis in homozygous sickle cell disease in children in Saudi Arabia 'ASSC'. Abstract presented at the Eighth Saudi Medical Conference (30 October-3 November 1983).
31. Schneider R G, Hightower B, Hosty T S *et al.* Abnormal hemoglobins in a quarter million people. *Blood,* 48, 629-637 (1976).
32. Selchouk S, Acquaye J, Ganeshaguru K *et al.* The incidence of Hb variants and thalassaemia in south western Saudi Arabia. A study on hospital population. Abstract presented at the Eighth Saudi Medical Conference (30 October-3 November 1983).
33. Smith, R. Personal communication.
34. Talbot H W, Sumlin A B, Naylor E W and Guthrie R. A neonatal screening test for argininosuccinic acid lyase deficiency and other urea cycle disorders. *Pediatrics,* 70, 526-531 (1982).
35. Task Force on Genetic Screening. The pediatrician and genetic screening (every pediatrician a geneticist). *Pediatrics,* 58, 757 (1976).
36. Tetra-Tab RIA. $T_4$ diagnostic kit for the quantitative determination of total serum thyroxine by radioimmunoassay. Dallas, Tx, Nuclear-Medical Laboratories Inc. (1980).

37. Thalji A A, Abu-Osba Y K and Ahmad M S. Congenital malformations: a major cause of neonatal mortality at Dhahran Health Center; pattern and incidence. Abstract presented at the Seventh Saudi Medical Meeting, Dammam, Saudi Arabia (3-6 May 1982).
38. Thomas G H and Scott C L. Laboratory diagnosis of genetic disorders, *Pediatric Clinics of North America,* 20, 105 (1973).
39. United Nations Economic Commission for Western Asia, Population Division. *Demographic and related socio-economic indicators for countries of the ECWA region, 1980.* Beirut, Lebanon (1981).
40. World Health Organization Working Group. Hereditary anaemias. Genetic basis, clinical features, diagnosis and treatment. *Bulletin of the World Health Organization,* 60, 643-660 (1982).

Chapter 42

# Perinatal technology in a developed country - Japan

**R John Parsons**

## Introduction

International comparisons of perinatal mortality rates are frequently used by the media and commentators, often ignoring the underlying problems of definitions and epidemiological considerations. One of the countries which is repeatedly used in such comparisons is Japan. Figure 1 shows the fall in perinatal mortality rate (PNMR) in Japan, England and Wales, and Sweden over the last three decades. In 1951 the Japanese PNMR was greater than the England and Wales figure by some 20% (4) but this difference disappeared by the late 1960s.

The trend has since continued and the Japanese PNMR now ranks amongst the lowest in the world. The positional improvement is demonstrated in Table 1 in a rank order table amongst selected countries over the period 1955-1975. Japan climbed from twelfth to eighth position compared with the England and Wales overall decline from eleventh to thirteenth. It is well known that the reasons for changes in PNMR are multifactorial but the increasing use of technology has been quoted as a major factor contributing to observed PNMR reductions (5). Over this same period there was certainly a large growth in the Japanese electronics industry but from the literature it was not clear whether this had been accompanied by an increasing use of such technology in their obstetrics. Therefore how much, if any, of the PNMR decline was due to technology was not obvious. A Winston Churchill Travelling Fellowship to Japan enabled the author to gain some experience of the utilization of technology and its impact on Japanese obstetrics and its possible influence on PNMR.

## Background

There are many striking similarities and differences between the UK and Japan. Both are island groups positioned off large continental masses. Both rely on trade to sustain a large population but the UK can rely on many more raw material sources than the volcanic mass of the Japanese archipelago. The peoples could not be more different, though. The British are a very mixed population having experienced much immigration over the centuries, whereas Japan over the last 300 years at least has been very much a closed community.

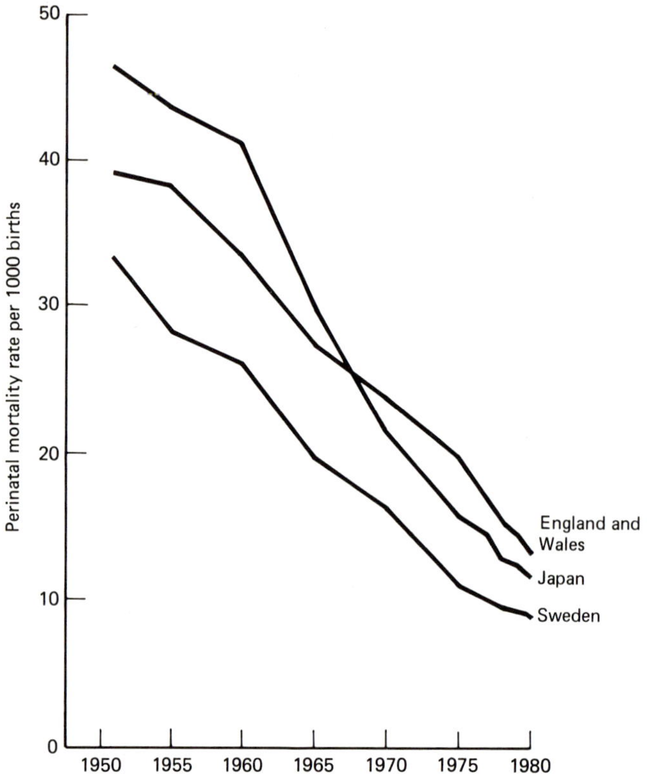


*Figure 1.* Perinatal mortality rate — selected countries 1950–1980

**TABLE 1. Perinatal mortality rates (per 1000 births)—rank order 1955/1975.**

| *Rank* | | *1955* | *1975* | | *Rank* |
|---|---|---|---|---|---|
| 1 | 26.0 | Norway | Sweden | 11.3 | 1 |
| 2 | 28.2 | New Zealand | Finland | 12.5 | 2 |
| 3 | 28.4 | Sweden | Denmark | 13.4 | 3 |
| 4 | 29.3 | Netherlands | Switzerland | 13.5 | 4 |
| 5 | 30.4 | USA | Netherlands | 14.0 | 5 |
| 6 | 30.9 | Switzerland | Norway | 14.2 | 6 |
| 7 | 31.5 | Canada | Canada | 15.4 | 7 |
| 8 | 33.9 | Denmark | Japan | 16.0 | 8 |
| 9 | 34.0 | France | New Zealand | 16.5 | 9 |
| 10 | 34.1 | Finland | France | 18.3 | 10 |
| 11 | 38.3 | England and Wales | USA | 18.3 | 11 |
| 12 | 43.9 | Japan | West Germany | 19.4 | 12 |
| 13 | 44.0 | West Germany | England and Wales | 19.9 | 13 |
| 14 | 46.2 | Italy | Italy | 24.2 | 14 |

The intention of the Fellowship was to visit many hospitals and universities across Japan to give a sampled view of obstetric practice. Although it cannot be claimed that a random sample was visited, it was reasonably representative because efforts were made to visit a wide range of centres. Contacts were arranged at many rural hospitals, less well-provided-for hospitals and many grades of private clinics which provide about one-half of the obstetric services in Japan. During the Fellowship some 23 institutions were visited in the south and west of Japan on two of the major islands, Honshu and Shikoku. Table 2 lists the main centres visited and a few details about the type of work seen.

**TABLE 2. Centres visited.**

| *Centre* | *Type* | *Comments* |
|---|---|---|
| Tokyo | 2 University clinics | Established contacts<br>Ultrasound/monitoring |
| | 4 Private clinics | Introduction to private clinics |
| | National Medical Center Hospital | 'Overview' and epidemiological discussions |
| | Japan Red Cross Medical Center | Highest delivery rate seen |
| Kyoto | University | Monitoring/research |
| | National Hospital | Monitoring |
| | City Hospital | Monitoring |
| | 2 Private clinics | Including one using traditional Japanese style beds |
| Osaka | University | Research centre |
| | Osaka Prefecture Perinatal Center | New high-risk centre |
| | National Cardiovascular Hospital | New high-risk centre |
| | 1 Private clinic | General discussions |
| | 1 municipal hospital | General discussions |
| Okayama and | 3 University clinics | General discussions |
| Inland Sea | 1 municipal hospital | Island community |
| Tottori | University | Medical electronics discussions |

## Impressions

Like the UK, Japan has seen an increasing tendency towards hospital confinements, changing from 4.6% in 1950 to 99.3% in 1973 (6). England and Wales has only changed from about 62% to 98% hospital confinement rate over the same period (1). However, about 45% of all their deliveries occur in small private clinics with less than 20 beds (4), and even in the larger hospitals the number of deliveries is very low, averaging between 700 and 1000 a year in most units. As with facilities in the UK disparities still occur. Labour wards in the affluent areas of the large cities are very well equipped, showing the international influence of technological progress. However, in some of the less affluent suburbs and the rural areas, hospitals carrying an equal workload, measured by the number of deliveries, managed with many fewer monitors and doctors. Most units utilized Western beds but one clinic still retained traditional Japanese tatami floors and beds in first stage rooms.

The extent of penetration of technology into obstetrics, as in the UK, other parts of Europe and the USA, varied enormously from centre to centre. Very few units were aiming for total monitoring. Only one purpose built high-risk unit was setting out to achieve this. Others adopted a mean level of about 20-30% monitoring. One monitor per 600 deliveries per annum was a very rough approximation in the hospitals seen - a figure somewhat higher than that recommended in the UK (2). As expected, the American influence is very strong and most monitors are of American origin. That is now changing as Japanese companies develop their own types. Only one UK-manufactured machine was seen although undoubtedly there are more distributed within the system. The latest Japanese machines utilize microcomputers and modern miniaturzation techniques to make what is in many cases a very functional and non-obtrusive unit.

Several workers in Japan have been considering the automatic diagnosis of fetal distress using microcomputers. A Tocoputer was developed some years ago and involved the operator in the choice of a large number of variable limits, but the latest Toitu microcomputer development requires very little interference from the clinician. It accepts either ultrasound or ECG signals from a monitor and produces an automatic diagnosis of fetal condition every five minutes. This machine is based on an analysis produced by Maeda (3) which utilizes many of the concepts accepted by most as important for fetal heart analysis (i.e. basal heart rate, lag time, beat-to-beat etc). Preliminary results of clinical trials held in the UK have now been reported (Chandler *et al*, see p.279).

Automatic oxytocin infusion systems were also seen but seemed very rarely used. Induction rates are generally very low indeed and the use of oxytocin is by no means common. In contrast with these observations on labour ward technology, *every* unit visited was seen to possess a real-time ultrasound machine. Yet again this ranged from just one machine in the very small private clinics to perhaps an overprovision in some of the large university hospitals. It was very striking to note the use of ultrasound and the reliance placed upon the results. Clinicians (i.e. obstetricians) ran this service exclusively.

## Discussion

The main conclusion to be drawn from these observations is that technology has played a part in the fall in perinatal mortality rates in a rather indirect way. Socioeconomic improvements and changes in epidemiological factors are probably more important.

First, the rates of congenital abnormalities between our two countries are very different. Spina bifida is the prime example. The difference in rates is approximately eight times between Japan and England, borne out by the observations of many Japanese clinicians that they could not remember when they had delivered such an infant. Secondly, low birthweight rates are well known as an indicator of overall perinatal mortality rate. Japanese women are well educated and very concerned about their health and welfare, hence they attend antenatal clinics early and are very conscious of their pregnancy. They tend to marry after the age of 20 and have fewer children which, together with a liberal abortion policy, leads to very few teenage or elderly pregnancies going to term. All this affects their low birthweight rate and, hence, the perinatal mortality rate. These low rates are also due in no small way to the growth of the socioeconomic status of the Japanese people, to which they are inversely proportional. The mothers who delivered in the 1950s had been brought up in times of great deprivation following the end of the war and perhaps it is only in the past 20 years that we have seen the true reproductive potential of the Japanese. Therefore technology, by raising the economic status of the Japanese nation, has in fact played an indirect but very important part in the fall in PNMR, but in the labour ward it has perhaps contributed very little to these figures.

In contrast to the great improvement in PNMR in Japan maternal mortality figures have not improved so dramatically. By our standards they are still high; about 2.0

per 10 000 in 1980, for example. It seems that the facilities available in the small clinics, similar to those described, are not sufficient to deal with emergencies arising during labour and the puerperium. There is very little co-ordination between hospitals, leading to the transfer of patients or doctors to deal with such emergencies. The Japanese are envious of our flying squads and also of our confidential enquiry system. It will be interesting to see if they can make as much progress towards reducing their maternal mortality rate over the next few years as they have in reducing their perinatal mortality figures since the last war.

## Conclusions

From this very brief examination of the Japanese obstetric scene it would seem that developing nations would be better advised to concentrate on improvements in socioeconomic status rather than on the use of complex high technology. Both ultrasound and fetal heart rate monitoring have a role to play in the detection of acute obstetric situations but other problems are much more likely to be keeping perinatal mortality rates high. Like the UK, Japan has an economy geared to the use of technology, but in many developing countries this is lacking. They may be able to purchase expensive pieces of equipment but unless these can be repaired and maintained locally then their usefulness soon evaporates. Most companies fail to provide such repair services, particularly in developing countries; until these are made available from within a nation's own resources then the value of monitors and ultrasound equipment is very doubtful. Developing countries should examine their own local conditions carefully before committing themselves to large expense.

## Acknowledgement

The author thanks the Winston Churchill Memorial Trust for making the visit possible and all his Japanese colleagues who gave so freely of their own time and energy to make the visit worthwhile.

## References

1. Department of Health and Social Security. *Annual Reports,* London, HMSO.
2. Editorial, Intrapartum fetal monitoring for all? *British Medical Journal,* 2, 1466 (1976).
3. Maeda K. Computerised FHR analysis and automatic fetal distress diagnosis utilizing external monitoring techniques with on-line and real-time processing. International Congress Series No 512 Gynaecology and Obstetrics. *Proceedings of the IX World Congress of Gynaecology and Obstetrics, Tokyo 1979* .
4. Ministry of Health and Welfare. *Statistics relating to Maternal and Child Health in Japan,* Tokyo (1981).
5. Parer J T. Fetal heart-rate monitoring. *Lancet,* 2, 632 (1979).
6. Wagatsuma T. Achievements in maternal and neonatal health survival in Japan. *First International Congress on Maternal and Neonatal Health,* Manila, Philippines (1981).

Chapter 43

# Predictive value of cervimetric progress indicated by the inductopartogram

**H M Maarof and A L Fazary**

## Introduction

Parturition has been referred to as the most perilous journey in an individual's life. A thorough understanding of the physiology and pathophysiology of the process involved is essential if this journey is to be completed safely by both mother and fetus. Though basically a physiological process, abnormalities can and do occur. Early recognition and prompt and appropriate management can do much in furthering the goal of modern obstetrics - optimizing maternal and neonatal outcome.

Modern obstetrics has reached a point where clinical assessment of a patient's progress in labour can be best appreciated on graphic records. These records aid the recognition of abnormal labour by allowing the events in labour to be seen at a glance, and make an early decision possible whenever necessary.

Since his original work on the graphic analysis of labour in 1955, Friedman (3) has transformed the subjective evaluation and management of labour into a predictive science. In 1971, in an article entitled *The Functional Divisions of Labour,* (4) Friedman divided labour into three functional phases: preparatory (latent), dilatatory (active) and pelvic. Cervical dilatation and descent of a fetal presenting part were illustrated on a cervicograph. Philpott and Castle (7,8) added two new concepts to the cervicograph, 'alert' and 'action' lines.

Pauls (5) evaluated the partograph at the Mama Yemo Hospital, Kinshasa, Zaire, where 42 000 - 44 000 mothers are delivered annually. He analysed 10 000 cases and found an increase of maternal and perinatal mortality and morbidity when the labour course crossed the 'alert and action' lines.

The partogram was introduced into Riyadh Maternity Hospital a few years ago, but no 'alert' or 'action' lines were used. The purpose of this limited study was to evaluate the suitability of such indicator lines for our women, although originally they were constructed and used in an inductopartogram for Malayasian women. These lines included only 'plot' and 'alert' lines but no 'action' line as it was felt by the preliminary investigator that these lines were more than adequate in the evaluation of the progress of labour (H M Maarof, unpublished observations).

## Materials and methods

Riyadh Maternity and Children's Hospital is the only public maternity hospital in the capital of Saudi Arabia.

It is also one of the teaching hospitals for the King Saud University as well as for postgraduate students for the Diploma in Obstetrics and Gynaecology, conducted jointly by the Ministry of Health for Saudi Arabia and the Institute of Obstetrics and Gynaecology, London. The hospital has nine consultant obstetricians and gynaecologists and conducts 20 000-24 000 deliveries per year.

The study reported here was a prospective one in which the course of labour of 30 patients of different parities and nationalities was charted on the above mentioned inductopartogram. There are two sections of this inductopartogram, the inductogram which is used to plot the dilatation, descent and a modified Bishop score in early labour, and the partogram which has the 'plot' and 'alert' lines.

The patients in active and established labour were immediately plotted on the partogram. In view of the difficulty of determining the exact time of onset of labour, particularly in those patients admitted to the labour ward after the onset of their labour at home, the time of admission to the labour ward was taken as the starting point for plotting. The cervicogram is only applicable after the cervix has dilated to at least 3 cm. All patients were examined on admission, at two hourly intervals thereafter, when the membranes were ruptured or when patients were found bearing down, indicating the onset of the second stage.

Established labour was defined as the presence of one contraction every 5 minutes, or more frequent, and cervical dilatation 3 cm or more. This would represent patients described by Friedman (4) as in the dilatatory (functional) stage of labour. Patients who were started on the inductogram were transferred to the partogram once they were in established labour.

The plot and alert lines were drawn with a slope of 1 cm/h which is the lower limit of the cervical dilatation rate in the active phase of labour, in the three ethnic groups of Malaysian patients. They were then classified into two groups based on whether they were in established labour or not, and the progress of patients was classified into three groups:-

1 Those who reached full dilatation left of the plot line.
2 Those whose dilatation fell between the plot and alert lines.
3 Those who crossed to the right of the alert line.

**TABLE 1. Distribution of patients according to nationality and parity.**

| | *Primigravid* | | | *Multigravid* | | | *Total* | | |
|---|---|---|---|---|---|---|---|---|---|
| | *Saudi* | *Non-Saudi* | *Total* | *Saudi* | *Non-Saudi* | *Total* | *Saudi* | *Non-Saudi* | *Total* |
| Group 1 | 5 | 3 | 8 | 12 | 4 | 16 | 17 | 7 | 24 |
| Group 2 | 2 | 0 | 2 | 0 | 0 | 0 | 2 | 0 | 2 |
| Group 3 | 1 | 0 | 1 | 2 | 0 | 2 | 3 | 0 | 3 |
| Total | 8 | 3 | 11 | 14 | 4 | 18 | 22 | 7 | 29 |

The distribution of patients according to nationality, parity and labpour performance groups were as follows.

Of the thirty patients initially selected, one was not included in the study as she was found not to be in labour. The rest have been shown in Table 1. The Saudi patients who formed the bulk of the patients, were composed of eight primigravidae and 14 multigravidae.

The distribution of the patients according to the progress of labour into groups as mentioned before were eight primigravida and multigravida in group 1, two primigravida only in group 2, and one primigravida and two multigravida in group 3.

## Results

The delivery performance of the 29 patients is shown in Table 2 below.

**TABLE 2. The delivery performance of the 29 patients.**

| | *Group 1* | *Group 2* | *Group 3* |
|---|---|---|---|
| *Vaginal delivery* | | | |
| Primigravid | 8 | 2 | 1 |
| Multigravid | 16 | 0 | 0 |
| *Caesarian section* | | | |
| Primigravid | 0 | 0 | 0 |
| Multigravid | 0 | 0 | 2 |

The 11 primigravidae in the three groups and the 16 multigravidae patients in group 1 and 2 delivered spontaneously, while the two multigravidae in group 3 needed Caesarian section. A closer analysis of these patients revealed that both had overdistended uterus the gravida 6 with hydramnios and a persistently high head and the other a gravida 8 had a twin pregnancy indicating the possibility of abnormal uterine activity leading to a poor progress despite efforts at augmentation.

## Discussion

Due to the shortage of doctors and specialists in developing countries, inadequate care in labour is still a major problem in most of the maternity units of these countries. A simple and reliable means of detecting problems which require immediate and adequate intervention is therefore an urgent need. The partogram appears to meet the above requirements.

The use of the alert (attention) and action (interference) lines provided an accurate and reliable guideline for these delivery units.

In this study deliveries with surgical interference occurred in Group 3 patients when the labour curve crossed the alert line.

The term 'alert line' was used here rather than 'action line' to indicate the need for alertness to the relatively inefficient progress of labour so that simple causative factors, such as uterine hypotonia, could be looked for and corrected (e.g. by using oxytocics) and checking to see whether or not the progress regains its 'slope'. Although it has not been calculated in detail, it seems that our regional parameters for the functional divisions of labour (i.e. latent, active and pelvic phases and the dilatation of the cervix during active phase) fit well with those calculated for Malaysian women. Furthermore, the lowest limit of the rate of cervical dilatation in the active phase of 1 cm/h seems to fit both our nulliparous and multiparous patients. In Rhodesia, Philpott and Castle (7) established a similar rate of 1 cm/h. However, according to Friedman, the rate in the United States is 1.2 cm/h and 1.5 cm/h for primigravidae and multigravidae respectively.

In the 29 labours assessed in this study, there was no maternal or fetal morbidity or mortality.

Although the study was limited in size, it seemed to highlight the usefulness and appropriateness of partographic recording in reducing the risks of inadequate care in labour, especially in crowded labour wards such as ours. The results obtained were encouraging and a plan to widen the aims of the study is in preparation in order to establish an optimum partogram for Saudi patients.

## Conclusion

Considering the fact that physicians are scarce in most developing countries, it is important that Obstetric services develop effective but simple methodologies for the recognition of abnormalities in labour.

This study emphasizes the value of prognostic indicator lines in prompting the early recognition of abnormal progress of labour and helping to make appropriate intervention. The partogram has demonstrated its value in many settings. We would like to reiterate together with Friedman, Cardozo et al (1) and others (2,6,9) that the partogram should have universal application in the management of labour.

## References

1. Cardozo et al. Predictive value of cervimetric labour pattern in primigravida. *British Journal of Obstetrics and Gynaecology,* 89, 33 (1982).
2. Drouin et al. The value of the partogramme in the management of labour. *Obstetrics and Gynecology,* 53, 741 (1979).
3. Friedman E A. Primigravida labour, graphico-statistical analysis. *American Journal of Obstetrics and Gynecology,* 6, 567 (1955).
4. Friedman E A. The functional divisions of labour. *American Journal of Obstetrics and Gynecology,* 109, 274 (1971).
5. Pauls F. Une analyse de 10,000 cas de femmes en travail suivies par le partogramme modifie de Friedman. *Federation des Societes de Gynecologie et Obstetrie de Langue Francaise,* pp.435-437 (1972).
6. Peng W W and Aun L M. Pattern of normal labour in Malaysian women. *Medical Journal of Malaysia.* 30, 261 (1976).
7. Philpott R H and Castle W M. Cervicographs in the management of labour primigravidae: 1. The alert line for detecting abnormal labour. *Journal of Obstetrics and Gynaecology of the British Commonwealth,* 79, 592 (1972).
8. Philpott R H and Castle W M. Cervicographs in the management of labour primigravidae: 2. The action line and treatment of abnormal labour. *Journal of Obstetrics and Gynaecology of the British Commonwealth,* 79, 599 (1972).
9. The Iowa perinatal letter; conduct of labor. September/October (1981).

Chapter 44

# Organization of neonatal intensive care and perinatal mortality in Libya

**N A Mir, Z Albin, A Faquih, A Soni, J Kishan, A Elzouki**

## Introduction

Perinatal and neonatal mortality are high in developing countries (4). One of the major concerns of perinatal paediatric care in the developing countries is the high costs, particularly for services which depend upon sophisticated technology, as the units for intensive care are costly to equip and run. Special care nurseries require trained and experienced personnel, both medical, nursing and technological. The conflict between the high costs and the limitations of resources make it imperative to examine the effectiveness of these services.

## Methods

As part of a comprehensive neonatal health care programme, two neonatal intensive care units were established in Benghazi, the second largest city in Libya, in January 1981. Over 95% of the deliveries in the city (about 16 500 per annum) take place at the Jamahiria Maternity Hospital and the special care baby unit (SCBU) was established here. The neonatal intensive care unit (NICU) was organized at the Benghazi Children's Hospital which serves as a referral centre for the eastern part of Libya.

A period of 5 months (August to December 1980) was spent in planning and organization, and hence serves as a control.

The results of 3.5 years of experience with the intensive care units are presented.

## Results and discussion

Prior to the commencement of the neonatal programme in Benghazi, perinatal mortality rate (PNMR) was over 34/1000 births and the mortality rate, in one of the neonatal units, over 43% (2). About 21% of the pregnancies are high risk (2) and perinatal asphyxia has been the leading cause of PNM in Libya (1).

The impact of intensive care on the survival rate of neonates is shown in Figure 1 and Table 1. Over a period of 3 years, PNMR was reduced from 34.16 to 26.7. With

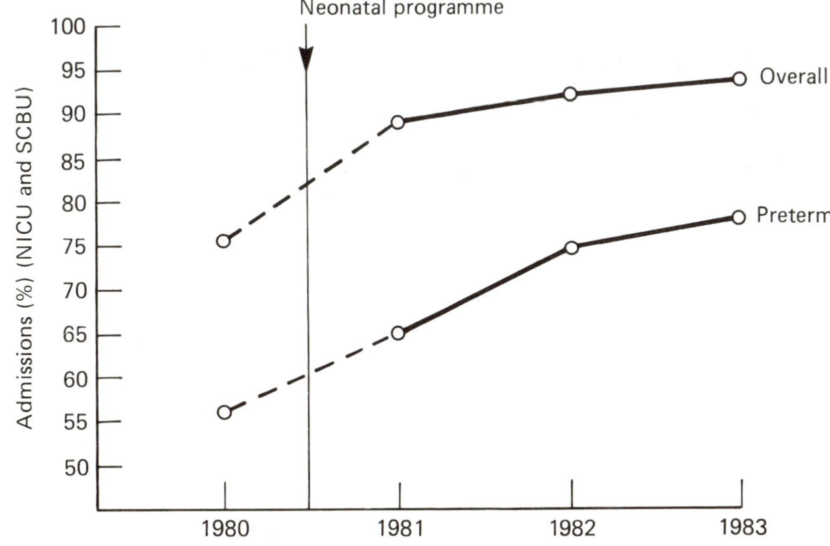


*Figure 1.* Survival rate

**TABLE 1. Perinatal mortality in Libya.**

| | *Before the neonatal programme July–December 1980* | *After the neonatal programme 1981* | *1982* | *1983* |
|---|---|---|---|---|
| Total births | 7580 | 16465 | 16946 | 16884 |
| Still births | | | | |
| n | 122 | 242 | 211 | 204 |
| per 1000 births | 16.0 | 14.0 | 12.4 | 12.0 |
| 1st week deaths | 137 | 263 | 259 | 247 |
| per 1000 births | 18.0 | 15.9 | 15.0 | 14.6 |
| Perinatal mortality | 259 | 505 | 470 | 451 |
| per 1000 births | 34.16 | 30.6 | 27.7 | 26.7 |
| Neonatal deaths (% of admissions to NICU and SCBU) | 13.1 | 10.6 | 8.3 | 7.2 |

the perinatal paediatric service, a significant achievement was a steady decline in the neonatal mortality from birth asphyxia (Figure 2).

During 1982, of 3639 babies admitted to the SCBU, 1185 (32.5%) required level three intensive care. Because of the large number of babies requiring intensive care, mechanical ventilation was offered only to infants of birthweight greater than 2500 g (1981), 1500 g (1982) and 750 g (1983). In infants over 1500 g birthweight, the main indications for intermittent positive pressure ventilation (IPPV) were: respiratory distress syndrome (40.4%), pneumonia (32.4%), sepsis (18.9%) and asphyxia (4.2%).

The incidence of low birthweight (less than 2650 g) babies was 8.94%, prematurity (less than 37 weeks) 4.2% and intrauterine growth retardation 4.7% (3). Overall survival rate of preterm infants increased steadily from 56.2% (1980) to 77.4% (1983).

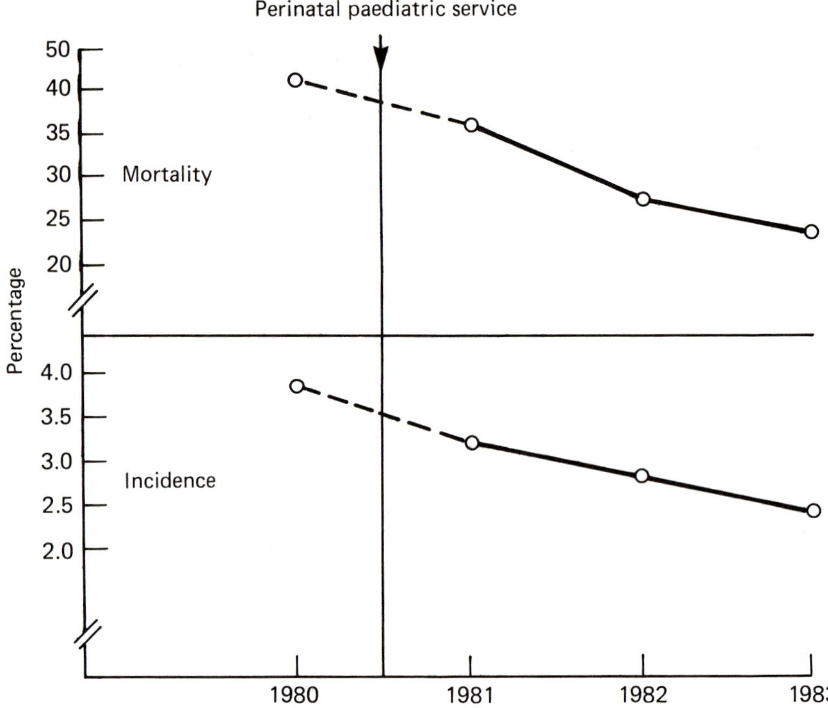


*Figure 2.* Incidence of and mortality from birth asphyxia

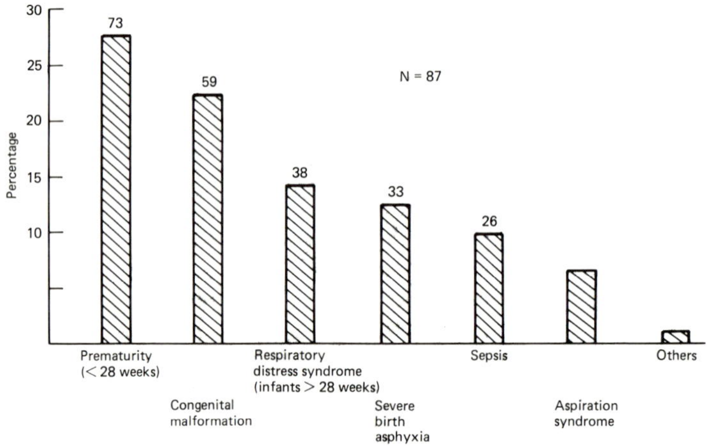


*Figure 3.* Perinatal mortality: causes of 1st week deaths

As shown in Figure 3, extreme prematurity (less than 28 weeks) was the major cause of first week deaths in 1982. With an increasing number of babies of 750-1500 g birthweight being ventilated in 1983, congenital malformations rank as the principal cause of first week deaths in 1983.

## Conclusion

With improvements in the perinatal paediatric service and use of advanced technology in the neonatal care units, the survival rate of sick neonates can be significantly improved in the developing countries. A multiphase introduction of level three intensive care and organization of perinatal paediatric services, with emphasis on the regional priorities, is of paramount importance to achieve the best possible results.

## Acknowledgements

We thank Dr Murad Lenghi, former Dean of Faculty of Medicine, Dr M Legnain, Chairman Department of Obstetrics and Gynaecology and all the medical, nursing and technical staff involved in the care of neonates in NICU and SCBU.

## References

1. Abudejaja A, Gupta R S, Khan A U et al. Perinatal mortality in Benghazi in 1977. *Garyounis Medical Journal,* 4, 15-25 (1981).
2. Mir N A and Mowla R. Comments on neonatal care in Benghazi. *Garyounis Medical Journal,* 4, 103-106 (1981).
3. Mir N A, Albin Z et al. Pattern of neonatal diseases in Libya (in preparation).
4. WHO. *Annual vital statistics and causes of death.* Table 5, 16-20, Geneva (1979).

Part 7

# Appendix

Chapter 45

# Positron emission tomography in the newborn: regional CBF in the preterm infant with intraventricular haemorrhage and haemorrhagic intracerebral involvement and in the asphyxiated term infant

**Joseph J Volpe**

## Introduction

The two major causes of neurological morbidity and mortality related to definable events in the neonatal period are intraventricular haemorrhage (IVH) with haemorrhagic intracerebral involvement in the preterm infant and hypoxic-ischaemic encephalopathy in the asphyxiated term infant. In this presentation studies of regional cerebral blood flow (CBF) by positron emission tomography (PET) in these two important groups of infants are reviewed.

### Intraventricular haemorrhage with haemorrhagic intracerebral involvement in the preterm infant

Periventricular-intraventricular haemorrhage (PVH-IVH) is the most common serious neurological lesion encountered in the preterm infant (28). The incidence of PVH-IVH is high, approximately 35-45% (25). In our institution, a recent prospective study of 460 infants of less that 2000 g birthweight by serial real-time ultrasonography revealed an incidence of PVH-IVH of 39% (16). Of all patients with PVH-IVH, those with haemorrhagic intracerebral involvement exhibit the highest rates of mortality and neurological morbidity and, indeed, account for the vast majority of all neurologically impaired infants with PVH-IVH. To prevent this lesion, an understanding of its pathogenesis and basic nature will be necessary.

Two possibilities concerning the pathogenesis and basic nature of the haemorrhagic intracerebral involvement with severe PVH-IVH seem most worthy of consideration. First, the intracerebral blood could represent localized extension of blood from the germinal matrix or lateral ventricle into previously normal white matter, or second, the intracerebral blood could represent a component of a larger, primary parenchymal lesion. We reasoned that assessment of regional CBF could provide highly valuable information for the resolution of these possibilities. However, until now, elucidation of regional CBF in the newborn has not been possible. PET has been shown recently to be highly effective in the study of regional CBF in older patients (20).

In this study, we utilized PET to measure regional CBF in six preterm infants with severe IVH and haemorrhagic intracerebral involvement to obtain insight into the basic nature of the parenchymal involvement. The findings demonstrate the value and feasibility of PET for the determination of regional CBF in the newborn with severe IVH and haemorrhagic intracerebral involvement and clarifies the basic nature of the parenchymal involvment.

### Hypoxic-ischaemic encephalopathy in the asphyxiated term infant

Hypoxic-ischaemic encephalopathy in the term newborn is the most frequently recognized cause of the subsequent non-progressive motor deficits often grouped under the rubric, 'cerebral palsy' (28). These deficits consist most commonly of spastic weakness of extremities, usually symmetrical. The magnitude of the problem of hypoxic-ischaemic encephalopathy relates not only to the essential gravity of the lesions, but also to the relatively high and unchanging prevalence of the encephalopathy (4). Indeed, unlike the decline in neurological sequelae attributable to hypoxic-ischaemic encephalopathy in the preterm infant with the advent of neonatal intensive care, there has been little or no decrease in such sequelae in the term infant (11).

Further insight into the basic nature and pathogenesis of the major brain injury assoicated with neonatal hypoxic-ischaemic encephalopathy is needed to devise interventions to decrease the seriously high prevalence of the neurological sequelae. Obtaining such insight from neuropathological observations has been difficult because relatively few infants die in the neonatal period, i.e. approximately 10 to 15%, and these, as expected, represent the most severely affected infants. Diffuse cerebral changes, confirmed by CT (9), are common and obscure critical elemental lesions. We reasoned that insight into the basic nature and pathogenesis of the brain injury in *surviving* infants could be provided by measurements of regional CBF in the acute period of illness. Recently, we have demonstrated the feasibility and value of PET in the study of regional CBF in the newborn (29). Thus, we undertook the present study to measure regional CBF during the acute period of illness in term infants with hypoxic-ischaemic encephalopathy and to attempt to provide insight into the basic nature and pathogenesis of the associated brain injury.

## Methods

### Measurement of regional cerebral blood flow by positron emission tomography

Positron emission tomography was performed with the PETT VI tomograph. The design and performance characteristics of this system have been described elsewhere (26,30). Data are recorded simultaneously from seven slices with a centre-to-centre separation of 14.4 mm. The in-plane resolution is 11.7 mm. Each PET slice is performed in the horizontal plane parallel to the orbitomeatal line. Head positioning is accomplished with the aid of a vertical laser line, which indicates the level of the lowest PET slice.

For the measurement of regional CBF, an emission scan, 40 seconds in duration, is obtained following an intravenous bolus injection of $^{15}O$-labelled water, 0.7 mCi/kg, in 0.5 ml of saline. In those studies in which an arterial catheter had been placed for the infant's intensive care, collection of arterial samples was carried out approximately every 5 seconds. These samples were weighed and counted and the radioactivity corrected for the physical decay of $^{15}O$, as previously described (29). Calibration of the tomograph to obtain the regional isotope concentration in brain from the reconstructed image was carried out as described elsewhere (29).

The scan data and blood curve were analysed according to the general principles of inert gas exchange, developed by Kety (12) and later embodied in a tissue autoradiographic technique for the measurement of local CBF in laboratory animals (13,23). We have described the details of this analysis (29) and have established the validity of this technique in the adult baboon (21). The correlation between CBF determined by PET, and CBF determined with $^{15}O$-labelled water and standard tracer principles, was excellent. Because of the near linear relationship between local tissue counts and CBF that is obtained with the PET autoradiographic approach, it is possible to measure accurately relative differences in local blood flows in different brain regions. This is particularly important because the majority of the infants studied herein did not have arterial lines in place and, thus, absolute blood flow quantitation could not be performed.

The total absorbed radiation dose, in a representative 1 kg subject receiving an intravenous bolus injection of 0.7 mCi of $^{15}0$-labelled water, is 63 mrem for the whole body. The critical organs, i.e. those receiving the largest radiation exposure, are the brain, heart, kidney, liver and gastrointestinal tract. These high-flow organs receive 76 mrem.

### Other measurments

Continuous measurements of arterial blood pressure were made from an indwelling umbilical artery catheter. Intracranial pressure was determined at the anterior fontanelle with the Ladd monitor. Cranial ultrasonography was performed with an ATL sector scanner. Computerized tomography and technetium radionuclide brain scanning were performed by standard techniques.

## Results

### Intraventricular haemorrhage with haemorrhagic intracerebral involvement in the preterm infant

*Clinical features*

The birthweights of the six infants studied ranged from 920 to 1200 g. Four of the six infants sustained varying degrees of perinatal asphyxia, since their 1 minute Apgar scores were 3, or below, and their 5 minute scores, below 6. Each of these four infants experienced probable intrauterine insults, e.g. fetal bradycardia, worsening maternal hypotension, precipitous delivery, and second born of twins. Two infants had large patent ductus arteriosus at the time of the PET study, and all six had severe respiratory distress syndrome. The PET scans were performed on the fifth day of life in two of the infants, the sixth day in one, the tenth day in two, and the seventeenth day in one. The latter infant had a second PET study on the ninetieth day. Four infants expired in the neonatal period, and the two survivors are only four and five months of age.

In a typical case, the cranial ultrasound scan shows bilateral subependymal haemorrhage and IVH, much more marked on the left, and marked haemorrhagic intracerebral involvement on the left. The left sagittal scan demonstrates that the haemorrhagic intracerebral involvement was confined to frontal white matter.

*PET determinations of regional cerebral blood flow*

Each patient exhibited the essential PET findings which include: (i) on the side opposite to the intraparenchymal lesion, highest blood flows laterally in the region adjacent and overlapping frontal-temporal-cortex, i.e. Sylvian cortex, and in some slices, basal ganglia; (ii) anteriorly and posteriorly, in the midline, highest blood flows in adjacent, right and left medial frontal and occipital cortex; and, most significantly, (iii) in the hemisphere containing the intraparenchymal blood, decreases in regional blood flow that are much more extensive in distribution than can be accounted for by the locus of the intracerebral blood. Indeed, in the involved left hemispheres, marked diminutions of regional CBF are apparent, not only anteriorly in frontal white matter, the site of the haemorrhagic intracerebral involvement, but also in posterior cerebral white matter and, to a lesser extent, in frontal-temporal-parietal cortex (especially Sylvian cortex).

*Structural correlate of the extensive impairment of cerebral blood flow in the involved hemisphere*

Neuropathological study of three of the cases defined the structural correlate of the extensive impairment of CBF in the hemisphere containing the intraparenchymal haemorrhagic involvement. Thus, the blood clot in the left frontal white matter was found to be continuous with extensive non-haemorrhagic softening of the posterior frontal, parietal and occipital white matter.

**Hypoxic-ischaemic encephalopathy in the asphyxiated term infant**

*Clinical features*

The essential clinical features of the 14 infants were characteristic of neonatal hypoxic-ischaemic encephalopathy (28). The severity of the asphyxial insults is emphasized by Apgar scores of less than 4 at 5 minutes in 11. The likelihood that the Apgar scores reflected depression secondary to intrauterine asphyxia is supported by the findings of fetal distress in 10 of the 12 infants for whom adequate intrauterine data were recorded. One infant sustained a primarily *postnatal* hypoxic-ischaemic event, i.e. cardiorespiratory arrest at 4 hours, aetiology unknown.

The neurological features were similar and conformed to the neurological syndrome previously described (28). Eight of the infants experienced neonatal seizures, with onset consistently on the first postnatal day. All infants were treated with phenobarbital, as previously described (28).

Twelve of the infants exhibited proximal limb weakness. Affection of upper more than lower extremities was consistent, as we have previously described (28). The two infants who did not exhibit definite proximal limb weakness also did not exhibit seizures and, on the basis of clinical course, appeared to be the least affected patients in the group.

The PET studies were performed on postnatal days 3-5 in 12 infants, on day 7 in one, and on day 20 in one. At the time of the PET studies, all infants had normal blood gases, haematocrit, intracranial pressure and systemic blood pressure.

*PET determinations of regional cerebral blood flow*

The normal, or near normal pattern of regional CBF in the term newborn is apparent in the PET scan obtained from the infant least affected on the basis of clinical findings.

(For ethical considerations, no clinically normal infants have been studied thus far.) The major PET findings include an external ribbon of relatively higher flows in regions of cerebral cortex. CBF to frontal and parietal cortical regions are approximately 50% higher than to corresponding cerebral white matter. Of the cortical regions, relatively higher flows are especially apparent anteriorly and posteriorly in the midline, in adjacent right and left medial frontal and occipital cortex. Laterally, CBF to adjacent and overlapping frontal-temporal-parietal cortex, i.e. Sylvian cortex, is approximately 10% higher than CBF to adjacent frontal or parietal cortex. In addition to cerebral cortical regions, relatively higher flows are observed also centrally, in the region of thalamus and basal ganglia.

The abnormalities of regional CBF in the infants constitute a continuum of deviation from the normal or near normal pattern just described. The consistent and apparently unifying abnormality was a relative decrease in CBF to parasagittal regions, generally symmetrical and more marked posteriorly than anteriorly.

In the least affected patients, CBF to posterior parasagittal regions is approximately 25% lower than CBF to Sylvian cortex, and in the most affected infants, parasagittal CBF values are approximately 40% lower than those to Sylvian cortex. The relative decreases in parasagittal CBF are slightly less marked in the anterior parasagittal regions. A consistent feature in the affected parasagittal areas is a loss or even reversal of the cortical grey matter versus white matter gradient of regional CBF.

The number of infants who were studied with arterial lines in place and for whom, therefore, absolute values for CBF are available is too small to permit generalizations about the severity of the deviation of parasagittal CBF from normal. In three such infants, the absolute values in the posterior parasagittal regions ranged from 30 to 50 ml/100 g per minute, and in the corresponding Sylvian regions, from 60 to 80 ml/100 g per minute.

### *Correlates of the parasagittal abnormality in regional cerebral blood flow*

To determine the structural correlates, if any, of the decrease in CBF in parasagittal regions, initially we turned to the CT scan. However, clear topographic correlation of the CT findings with the PET findings was not possible. Thus, CT scans obtained within several days of the PET scans showed more diffuse abnormalities, usually diffuse hypodensity of cerebral white matter, as described in previous studies of asphyxiated term infants (9).

We next evaluated correlation with the radionuclide brain scan. Thus far, the two infants evaluated by technetium brain scan have exhibited nearly identical findings. A striking pattern of increased uptake of the radionuclide in the parasagittal regions, bilaterally, posteriorly more than anteriorly, was observed. The close correlation of this abnormality with the abnormality of regional CBF is apparent.

Neuropathological correlation of the parasagittal abnormality in CBF was obtained in the one infant who died. At postmortem examination, softening was apparent in parasagittal parietal cortex bilaterally. Coronal sections of the fixed brain revealed regions of softening in the parasagittal cerebral cortex and subcortical white matter, especially posteriorly. The involvement extended into periventricular white matter. Microscopic sections of the affected areas showed occasional cortical neurons with faintly eosinophilic cytoplasm and/or pyknotic nuclei and pyknotic nuclei in cerebral white matter; there was no definite tissue reaction, the latter not unexpected in view of the short duration of survival. (Similar cellular changes were observed also in caudate nucleus, ventral pons and Purkinje cell layer of cerebellum.)

## Discussion

### Intraventricular haemorrhage with haemorrhagic intracerebral involvement in the premature infant

The current observations indicate that the haemorrhagic intracerebral involvement in the infants with severe PVH-IVH is a component of a larger, primary *ischaemic* lesion. This conclusion is based on consideration of the topography of the abnormality of CBF, shown by PET, and on the nature of the anatomical abnormality, shown by neuropathological study. Concerning the topography - the lesion involves periventricular white matter and, apparently, frontal, temporal and parietal cortex, although because of the limits of resolution of PET, it remains possible that the lesion involves only white matter. Periventricular white matter is a region vulnerable to ischaemic injury in the preterm newborn (28). Thus, DeReuck and co-workers have demonstrated the presence of periventricular arterial border zones and end zones, i.e. 'watershed' regions, at the sites of occurrence of ischaemic neonatal periventricular white matter injury (8). Within the periventricular region, two sites, one anterior and one posterior, are especially likely to be affected by periventricular leukomalacia (24), and, in this regard, it is of particular interest that in the infant with the least severe parenchymal involvement, separate anterior and posterior lesions appeared to be present. Our conclusion that the haemorrhagic intracerebral lesion observed in these patients is a component of a primary ischaemic lesion is compatible with our own neuropathological observations and those reported by Flodmark *et al* (9), who concluded that virtually all of the haemorrhagic parenchymal lesions in their series of preterm infants with severe PVH-IVH were haemorrhagic infarcts. In keeping with this formulation is our demonstration, in the single patient who had a second PET scan, that the relative extent and severity of the decreased CBF in the left hemisphere persisted (data not shown); thus, the ischaemia was not a transient acute event, but rather a reflection of a fixed structural lesion.

The aetiology and timing of the ischaemic injury in our infants remain unclear. The ill preterm infant is considered to be especially susceptible to ischaemic cerebral injury, often secondary to systemic hypotension, because of the occurrence of a pressure-passive cerebral circulation (15). In this regard, it is noteworthy that four of our six infants experienced perinatal asphyxia, as judged by depressed Apgar scores, and two had a large patent ductus arteriosus, which we have shown to be associated with decreased cerebral blood flow velocity (19). It also remains possible that the ischaemic lesion present in our patients was not caused by prior systemic hypotension, but rather by the secondary effects of blood in the lateral ventricle, the cerebral parenchyma or subarachnoid space. Thus, the topography of the lesion is compatible with ischaemia in the distribution of the middle cerebral artery. Such a formulation raises the possibility of spasm of the middle cerebral artery, secondary to subarachnoid or intraventricular blood, the former a well-documented event in older patients, or of compression of branches of the middle cerebral artery by local brain swelling.

Why does the intracerebral haemorrhage occur principally anteriorly in a primary parenchymal lesion that also extends far posteriorly? The consistent relation between the laterality of the intraparenchymal blood and the laterality of the more extensive degree of IVH may provide a clue. Thus, as observed in this study of six cases and in our previous ultrasonographic study of 33 cases (16), the haemorrhagic intracerebral component almost invariably occurs on the side of most marked IVH. This relation raises at least three potential explanations for the anterior placement of the haemorrhage. First, as noted above, the large amount of intraventricular blood could impair venous drainage in the affected hemisphere, and the resulting increased venous pressure, with a propensity for haemorrhage into an infarcted area, would be greatest at the anterior site because of the previously described anatomical peculiarities of the deep venous drainage anteriorly (14). Second, the intracerebral blood may emanate from the anteriorly-placed germinal matrix and may extend into the periventricular white matter because the latter is infarcted. Third, the intracerebral blood may emanate from the blood-laden lateral ventricle and extend into the infarcted white matter through the external angle of the lateral ventricle because of a combination of pressure effects, related to the large volume of intraventricular blood, and a relative weakness of the ependymal barrier, related to the presence of the anteriorly-placed germinal matrix.

### Hypoxic-ischaemic encephalopathy in the asphyxiated term infant

These observations, the first measurements of regional CBF in the term newborn, are of particular importance with regard to the basic nature and probable pathogenesis of the major brain injury in the asphyxiated infant. In addition, the data provide important new information concerning normal regional CBF in the newborn.

Regarding normal regional CBF in the newborn, the data define approximately 50% higher flows to cerebral cortex than to subcortical white matter. It is likely that the true difference between CBF to cerebral cortex and to subcortical white matter is greater than this because of the 'partial volume averaging' effect of the PET technique. Thus, because of the current spatial resolution of PET, 11.7 mm in the image plane, it is not possible to sample pure grey or white matter, and measurements of local tissue radioactivity will receive contributions from both grey and white matter. As a consequence, blood flow is slightly underestimated in cerebral cortex and slightly overestimated in subcortical white matter. In addition to the cortical grey matter-white matter differences, our data indicate that CBF in basal ganglia and thalamus is at least as high as to cerebral cortex. These observations are compatible with regional differences in CBF measured in neonatal animals by tissue autoradiographic techniques (5).

Regarding the major brain injury in the asphyxiated infant, a consistent abnormality has been identified, i.e. a relative decrease in CBF to parasagittal regions, posterior regions affected more than anterior. A continuum of this abnormality was observed. The absolute severity of the defects in parasagittal CBF is difficult to quantitate precisely because of our lack of 'normal' values for CBF and the relatively small number of the asphyxiated infants in whom absolute values of CBF could be obtained. However, we consider the parasagittal deficits in CBF to be indicative of tissue injury. In support of this conclusion are, first, the findings on the delayed radionuclide brain scans in the two patients so studied. Thus, increased uptake of the radionuclide in the parasigittal regions, posteriorly more than anteriorly, correlated closely with the findings on the PET scans. Second, in the single patient studied at post-mortem examination, injury to parasagittal cerebral cortex and subcortical white matter, especially posteriorly, could be identified. It is similarly noteworthy that the few available neuropathological studies of long-term survivors with 'cerebral palsy' emphasize and illustrate the parasagittal distribution of cerebral cortical and subcortical white matter injury (6,10).

Our CBF findings suggest that parasagittal cerebral injury is an extremely common feature of neonatal hypoxic-ischaemic encephalopathy, at least in patients who survive the perinatal insult. Previous studies of asphyxiated term infants by radionuclide brain scans, by ourselves (27) and others (18), showed that this distribution of injury, although the most common single type, nevertheless is demonstrable in only the minority of asphyxiated infants. It is reasonable to speculate that the less marked degrees of disturbance of parasagittal CBF, defined by PET, reflect degrees of tissue injury that would not be detected by radionuclide brain scan. Whether such injury is associated with neurological deficts will require long-term follow-up for resolution.

The pathogenesis of the parasagittal brain injury in these asphyxiated infants is not established by our measurements, but the characteristic parasagittal topography is indicative of ischaemia as the principal pathogenetic factor. Thus, the parasagittal cerebral injury occurs in the border zones between the end fields of the major cerebral arteries, i.e. the anterior, middle and posterior cerebral arteries. This characteristic topography was defined initially by Meyer in a series of primarily adult patients (one of the series was an infant who had experienced birth asphyxia) and was related by Meyer to systemic hypotension (17). Experimental support for this 'watershed' concept was provided in the monkey by Brierley and co-workers who reproduced similar parasagittal lesions by producing rapid, profound systemic hypotension while preventing hypoxaemia (3). As we observed in our asphyxiated infants, more marked injury was demonstrable in the monkeys in the posterior cerebrum, an observation also made by Brierley and co-workers in affected adult human patients (1).

Our observations emphasize the critical importance of ischaemia in the pathogenesis of the brain injury with neonatal hypoxic-ischaemic encephalopathy, but do not establish the timing or precise cause of the ischaemia. At least one major component of the ischaemia may occur with systemic hypotension in association with the intrauterine asphyxia. Thus, evidence for fetal distress was common in our patients, and the occurrence of systemic hypotension (7), impaired CBF (22), and parasagittal cerebral injury (2) in asphyxiated fetal animals is well documented. However, the additive role of *postnatal* hypotension, perhaps in association with difficulties with resuscitation, as evidenced by the depressed Apgar scores, could be considerable. In addition, the possibilities that postnatal hypoxaemia, hypercarbia, acidaemia or brain oedema could play additive roles in impairing cerebral perfusion and/or energy metabolism must be considered. Further studies of regional CBF, coupled with the determinations of regional oxygen metabolism, could provide considerable insight into several of these issues. Clearly, PET should be of great value in such subsequent studies.

## References

1. Adams J H, Brierley J B, Connor R C R and Treip C S. The effects of systemic hypotension upon the human brain: clinical and neuropathological observations in 11 cases. *Brain,* 89, 235 (1966).

2. Brann A W Jr and Myers R E. Central nervous system findings in the newborn monkey following severe *in utero* partial asphyxia. *Neurology,* 25, 327 (1975).

3. Brierley J B and Excell B J. The effects of profound systemic hypotension upon the brain of M Rhesus: physiological and pathological observations. *Brain,* 88, 269 (1966).

4. Brown J K. Infants damaged during birth. In *Recent Advances in Paediatrics,* edited by D Hull, p.234, London, Churchill Livingstone (1976).

5. Cavazzuti M and Duffy T E. Regulation of local cerebral blood flow in normal and hypoxic newborn dogs. *Annals of Neurology,* 2, 247 (1982).

6. Courville C B. *Birth and Brain damage* . Pasadena, Courville (1971).

7. Dawes G S. *Foetal and Neonatal Physiology* . Chicago, *Year Book* (1968).

8. DeReuck J, Chattha A S and Richardson E B Jr. Pathogenesis and evolution of periventricular leukomalacia in infancy. *Archives of Neurology,* 27, 229 (1972).
9. Flodmark O, Becker L E, Harwood-Nash D C, Fitzhardinge P M, Fitz C R and Chuang S H. Correlation between computed tomography and autopsy in premature and full-term neonates that have suffered perinatal asphyxia. *Radiology,* 137, 93 (1980).
10. Friede R S. *Developmental Neuropathology.* New York, Springer-Verlag (1975).
11. Hagberg B, Hagberg G and Olow I. The changing panorama of cerebral palsy in Sweden in 1970 to 1974. II Analysis of the various syndromes. *Acta Paediatrica Scandinavica,* 64, 193 (1975).
12. Kety S S. The theory and applications of the exchange of inert gas at the lungs and tissues. *Pharmacology Review,* 2, 1 (1951).
13. Landau W M, Freygang W H Jr, Rowland L W and Sokoloff L. The local circulation of the living brain: values in the unanesthetized and anesthetized cat. *Transactions of the American Neurological Association,* 80, 125 (1955).
14. Larroche J C. *Developmental Pathology of the Neonate.* New York, Excerpta Medica (1977).
15. Lou H C, Lassen N A and Friis-Hansen B. Impaired autoregulation of cerebral blood flow in the distressed neewborn. *Journal of Paediatrics,* 94, 118 (1979).
16. McMenamin J B, Shackelford G D and Volpe J J. Outcome of periventricular-intraventricular haemorrhage with apparent intraparenchymal haemorrhage. *Annals of Neurology,* (in press).
17. Meyer J E. Uber die lokalisation fruhkindlicher hirschadenin arteriellen grenzebieten. *Archive für Psychiatrie und Nervenkrankheiten,* 190, 328 (1953).
18. O'Brien M J, Ash M J and Gilday D L. Radionuclide brain scanning in perinatal hypoxia-ischaemia. *Developmental Medicine and Child Neurology,* 21, 161 (1979).
19. Perlman J M, Hill A and Volpe J J. The effect of patent ductus arteriosus on flow velocity in the anterior cerebral arteries: ductal steal in the premature newborn infant. *Journal of Pediatrics,* 99, 767 (1981).
20. Raichle M E. Quantitative *in vivo* autoradiography with positron emission tomography. *Brain Research,* 1, 47 (1979).
21. Raichle M E, Martin W R W, Herscovitch P, Mintun M and Markham J. Brain blood flow measured with intravenous $H_2{}^{15}O$. II. Implementation and validation. *Journal of Nuclear Medicine,* 24, 790 (1983).
22. Reivich M, Brann A W Jr, Shapiro H M and Myers R E. Regional cerebral blood flow during prolonged partial asphyxia. In *Research on the Cerebral Circulation,* edited by J S Meyer, M Reivich, H Lechner and O Eichorn, pp. 216-227. Springfield, Thomas (1972).
23. Sakurada O, Kennedy C, Jehle J, Brown J D, Carbin G L and Sokoloff L. Measurement of local cerebral blood flow with iodo[$^{14}$C]lantipyrine. *American Journal of Physiology,* 234, H59 (1978).
24. Shuman R M and Selednik L J. Periventricular leukomalacia. A one-year autopsy study. *Archives of Neurology,* 37, 231 (1980).
25. Tarby T J and Volpe J J. Intraventricular haemorrhage in the premature infant. *Pediatric Clinics of North America,* 29, 1077 (1982).
26. Ter-Pogossian M M, Ficke D C, Hood J T, Yamamoto M and Mullani N A. PETT VI: a positron emission tomograph utilizing cesium fluoride scintillation detectors. *Journal of Computed Assisted Tomography,* 6, 125 (1982).
27. Volpe J J and Pasternak J. Parasagittal cerebral injury in neonatal hypoxic-ischemic encephalopathy: clinical and neuroradiologic features. *Journal of Pediatrics,* 91, 472 (1977).
28. Volpe J J. *Neurology of the Newborn,* Philadelphia, W B Saunders (1981).
29. Volpe J J, Herscovitch P, Perlman J M and Raichle M E. Positron emission tomography in the newborn: extensive impairment of regional cerebral blood flow with intraventricular hemorrhage and hemorrhagic intracerebral involvement. *Pediatrics,* 72, 589 (1983).
30. Yamamoto M, Ficke D C and Ter-Pogossian M M. Performance study of PETT VI, a positron computed tomography with 288 cesium fluoride detectors. *IEEE Transactions on Nuclear Science,* NSO29, 529 (1982).

## Contributors


**T Abels** Biomedical Technique Unit, Department of Obstetrics and Gynaecology University of Dusseldorf, Dusseldorf, West Germany

**Y K Abu-Osba** Neonatal Intensive Care Unit, Pediatric Services, Dhahran Health Center, Saudi Arabia

**M S Ahmad** Neonatal Intensive Care Unit, Pediatric Services, Dhahran Health Center, Saudi Arabia

**A M Al-Habbal** Neonatal Intensive Care Unit, Pediatric Services, Dhahran Health Center, Saudi Arabia

**N A Albin** Department of Pediatrics, University of Caryounis, Benghazi, Libya

**D P Alexander** Department of Pediatrics and Physiology, St Mary's Hospital Medical School, London, UK

**S Alexander** Department of Obstetrics and Gynaecology, Hopital Erasme, Universite Libre de Bruxelles, Brussels, Belgium

**D C Alverson** University of New Mexico School of Medicine, Department of Pediatrics, Albuquerque, New Mexico, USA

**D C Andrews** Nuffield Department of Obstetrics and Gynaecology, John Radcliffe Hospital, Oxford, UK

**K J Antila** Cardiorespiratory Research Unit, University of Turku, Turku, Finland

**J M Arnold** Department of Obstetrics and Gynaecology Maternity Hospital, Bristol

**D J Bekedam** Department of Obstetrics and Gynaecology, University Hospital of Groningen, Groningen, The Netherlands

**M Benthin** Teltec Ltd, Lund, Sweden

**A Berec** University of Zurich, Zurich, Switzerland

**W Berman** University of New Mexico School of Medicine, Department of Pediatrics, Albuquerque, New Mexico, USA

**N Bernard** Service de Gynecologie-Obstetrique, Centre Medico-Chirurgical, Paris-Suresnes, France

**T Blomquist** University of New Mexico School of Medicine, Department of Pediatrics, Albuquerque, New Mexico, USA

**H G Britton** Department of Pediatrics and Physiology, St Mary's Hospital Medical, School London, UK

**P N Burns** Department of Obstetrics and Gynaecology, Maternity Hospital, Bristol, UK

**F Cantraine** Department of Scientific Calculation, Faculty of Medicine, University Libre de Bruxelles, Brussels, Belgium

**M C Carter** Perinatal Equipment Evaluation Unit, Department of Obstetrics and Gynaecology, St Mary's Hospital Medical School, London, UK

**B Castle** Nuffield Department of Obstetrics and Gynaecology, John Radcliffe Hospital, Oxford, UK

**M Cooper** Department of Pediatrics and Physiology, St Mary's Hospital Medical School, London, UK

**P Dahl** Teltec Ltd, Lund, Sweden

**G S Dawes** Nuffield Institute for Medical Research, University of Oxford, Oxford, UK

**A J Dawson** Department of Obstetrics and Gynaecology, Welsh National School of Medicine, Heath Park, Cardiff, UK

**O De Bakker** Department of Obstetrics and Gynaecology, Academic Hospital, Free University, Amsterdam, The Netherlands

**G De Toffoli Konishi** Institute of Human Physiology. University of Padova, Padua, Italy

**T Dillon** University of New Mexico School of Medicine, Department of Pediatrics, Albuquerque, New Mexico, USA

**M S Dodgson** Department of Anaesthesia, Ulleval Sykehus, Oslo 4, Norway

**A T Doyle** Neonatal Intensive Care Unit, Pediatric Services, Dhahran Health Center, Saudi Arabia

**P M Dunn** Department of Child Health (Perinatal Medicine), University of Bristol, Southmead Hospital, Bristol UK

**M Eldridge** University of New Mexico School of Medicine, Department of Pediatrics, Albuquerque, New Mexico, USA

**A Elzouki** Department of Pediatrics, University of Caryounis, Benghazi, Libya

**P S Eriksen** Department of Obstetrics and Gynaecology, Malmo Allmanna Sjukhus, Malmo, Sweden

**J M Evans** Department of Obstetrics and Gynaecology, Maternity Hospital, Bristol, UK

**F Fallenstein** University of Zurich, Zurich, Switzerland

**A Faquih** Department of Pediatrics, University of Caryounis, Benghazi, Libya

**A L Fazary** Maternity and Children's Hospital, Jeddah, Saudi Arabia

**G Gennser** Department of Obstetrics and Gynaecology, Malmo Allmanna Sjukhus, Malmo, Sweden

**R W Gill** Ultrasonics Institute, 5 Hickson Road, Millers Point, New South Wales, Australia

**N A J Gough** Department of Obstetrics and Gynaecology, Welsh National School of Medicine, Heath Park, Cardiff, UK

**P Grella** Department of Obstetrics and Gynaecology, University of Padova, Padua, Italy

**V Martino** Department of Physiology, Stanford University, USA

**H J Hoogland** Department of Obstetrics and Gynaecology, Ziekenhuis St Annadal State University, Maastricht, The Netherlands

**A Huch** University of Zurich, Zurich, Switzerland

**R Huch** University of Zurich, Zurich, Switzerland

**T C Jansen** Department of Pediatrics, Erasmus University Medical School, Rotterdam, The Netherlands

**O Jensen** Department of Biomedical Engineering, Rikshospitalet, Oslo 1, Norway

**P Johnson** Nuffield Department of Obstetrics and Gynaecology, John Radcliffe Hospital, Oxford, UK

**N-P Jorgensen** Department of Obstetrics and Gynaecology, University Hospital, Trondheim, Norway

**V Kariniemi** Department of Obstetrics and Gynaecology, Helsinki University Central Hospital, Helsinki, Finland

**J Kishan** Department of Pediatrics, University of Caryounis, Benghazi, Libya

**J Kuzniar** Department of Obstetrics and Gynecology and Internal Medicine, District Hospital, Rzeszow, Poland

**R Leblanc** Biomedical Technique Unit, Department of Obstetrics and Gynaecology, University of Dusseldorf, Dusseldorf, West Germany

**K Lindstrom** Department of Biomedical Engineering, Malmo Allmanna Sjukhus, Malmo, Sweden

**G Lingman** Department of Obstetrics and Gynaecology, University Hospital, Malmo, Sweden

**D W Lubbers** Max Planck Institut fur Systemphysiologie, Dortmund, West Germany

**H M Maarof** Maternity and Children's Hospital, Jeddah, Saudi Arabia

**I Z Mackenzie** Nuffield Department of Obstetrics and Gynaecology, John Radcliffe Hospital, Oxford, UK

**P H Magne** Service de Gynecologie-Obstetrique, Centre Medico-Chirurgical, Paaris-Suresnes, France

**K Marsal** Department of Obstetrics and Gynaecology, University Hospital Malmo, Sweden

**R Martino** Institute of Human Physiology, University of Padova, Padua, Italy

**J Melchior** Service de Gynecologie-Obstetrique, Centre Medico-Chirurgical, Paris-Suresnes, France

**N A Mir** Department of Pediatrics, University of Caryounis, Benghazi, Libya

**J Morgenstern** Biomedical Technique Unit, Department of Obstetrics and Gynaecology, University of Dusseldorf, Dusseldorf, West Germany

**A J Murrills** Wessex Regional Department of Medical Physics, Southampton General Hospital, Southampton, UK

**J H Nagel** Zentralinstitut fur Biomedizinische Technik, Universitat Erlangen-Nurnberg, Erlangen, West Germany

**U Naumann** Biomedical Technique Unit, Department of Obstetrics and Gynaecology, University of Dusseldorf, Dusseldorf, West Germany

**C Nickelsen** Department of Obstetrics and Gynaecology, Rigshospitalet, University of Copenhagen, Denmark

**M F Niermeijer** Department of Clinical Genetics, Erasmus University, Rotterdam, The Netherlands

**R T Oja** Cardiorespiratory Research Unit, University of Turku, Turku, Finland

**R J Parsons** Department of Medical Physics, The Princess Royal Hospital, Hull, UK

**A Piela** Department of Obstetrics, Gynaecology and Internal Medicine, District Hospital, Rzeszow, Poland

**C W G Redman,** Nuffield Deparment of Obstetrics and Gynaecology, John Radcliffe Hospital, Oxford, UK

**D Redstone** Department of Pediatrics and Physiology, St Mary's Hospital Medical School, London, UK

**P Rolfe** Bio-Engineering Unit, University of Oxford, John Radcliffe Hospital, Oxford, UK

**G D Ryan** Department of Pediatrics and Physiology, St Mary's Hospital Medical School, London, UK
**A R Sa'di** Neonatal Intensive Care Unit, Pediatric Services, Dhahran Health Center, Saudi Arabia
**H Schettler** Biomedical Technique Unit, Department of Obstetrics and Gynaecology, University of Dusseldorf, Dusseldorf, West Germany
**S Schmidt** Arbeitsgruppe Perinatale Medizin, The Free University of Berlin, Berlin, West Germany
**J Schwers** Department of Obstetrics and Gynaecology, Hopital Erasme, University Libre de Bruxelles, Brussels, Belgium
**F Sharp** University Department of Midwifery, Queen Mother's Hospital, Glasgow, UK
**J Sheddon** Department of Obstetrics and Gynaecology, Maternity Hospital, Bristol, UK
**A S I Siimes** Cardiorespiratory Research Unit, University of Turku, Turku, Finland
**A Skret** Department of Obstetrics and Gynecology and Internal Medicine, District Hospital, Rzeszow, Poland
**N C Smith** University Department of Midwifery, Queen Mother's Hospital, Glasgow, UK
**T Somville** Biomedical Technique Unit, Deparment of Obstetrics and Gynaecology, University of Dusseldorf, Dusseldorf, West Germany
**A Soni** Department of Pediatrics, University of Caryounis, Benghazi, Libya
**D P Southall** Institute of Obstetrics and Gynaecology, Queen Charlotte's Hospital, London, UK
**W P Soutter** University Department of Midwifery, Queen Mother's Hospital, Glasgow, UK
**J A D Spencer** Nuffield Department of Obstetrics and Gynaecology, John Radcliffe Hospital, Oxford, UK
**P A Stewart** Department of Obstetrics and Gynaecology, Erasmus University. Rotterdam, The Netherlands
**L Svenningsen** Department of Obstetrics and Gynaecology, Ulleval Sykehus Oslo, Norway
**Z Szmigiel** Department of Obstetrics and Gynaecology and Internal Medicine, District Hospital, Rzeszow, Poland
**D G Talbert** Institute of Obstetrics and Gynaecology, Queen Charlotte's Hospital, London, UK
**A A Thalji** Neonatal Intensive Care Unit, Pediatric Services, Dhahran Health Center, Saudi Arabia
**S G Thomsen** Department of Obstetrics and Gynaecology, Rigshospitalet, University of Copenhagen, Copenhagen, Denmark
**H M Tonge** Department of Obstetrics and Gynaecology, Erasmus University, Rotterdam, The Netherlands
**O Th Uttendorfsky** Department of Obstetrics and Gynaecology, St Lambertus Teaching Hospital, Helmond, The Netherlands
**I A Valimaki** Cardiorespiratory Research Unit, University of Turku, Turku, Finland
**A R Van der Wiel** Department of Pediatrics, Erasmus University Medical School, Rotterdam, The Netherlands
**D Veersema** Department of Obstetrics and Gynaecology, St Lambertus Teaching Hospital, Helmond, The Netherlands

**C Velussi** Institute of Human Physiology, University of Padova, Padua, Italy

**A Verhoeff** Department of Obstetrics and Gynaecology, Erasmus University Medical School, Rotterdam, The Netherlands

**K Vetter** University of Zurich, Zurich, Switzerland

**G H A Visser** Department of Obstetrics and Gynaecology, University Hospital of Groningen, Groningen, The Netherlands

**M Vossen** Department of Obstetrics and Gynaecology, St Lambertus Teaching Hospital, Helmond, The Netherlands

**H C S Wallenburg** Department of Obstetrics and Gynaecology, Erasmus University Medical School, Rotterdam, The Netherlands

**T Weber** Department of Obstetrics and Gynaecology, Rigshospitalet, University of Copenhagen, Copenhagen, Denmark

**T Wheeler** Department of Human Reproduction, Princess Anne Hospital, Southampton, UK

**T H Wilmshurst** Department of Electronics, University of Southampton, Southampton, UK

**J W Wladmiroff** Department of Obstetrics and Gynaecology, Erasmus University, Rotterdam, The Netherlands

**P Wolf** Biomedical Technique Unit, Department of Obstetrics and Gynaecology, University of Dusseldorf, Dusseldorf, West Germany

**J C Wollner** Nuffield Institute for Medical Research, University of Oxford, Oxford, UK

**R S Wolton** Bio-Engineering Unit, University of Oxford, John Radcliffe Hospital, Oxford, UK

**T Zaczek** Department of Obstetrics, Gynecology and Internal Medicine, District Hospital, Rzeszow, Poland

# Index

0 411 980 00 D4